# Handbook of Experimental Pharmacology

Continuation of Handbuch der experimentellen Pharmakologie

## Vol. 65

# Teratogenesis and Reproductive Toxicology

Contributors

S. T. Chao · K. P. Chepenik · M. S. Christian · B. E. G. Gabel
J. H. Greenberg · R. M. Greene · H. E. Holden · D. E. Hutchings
R. P. Jensh · E. M. Johnson · M. R. Juchau · N. W. Klein
D. M. Kochhar · D. W. Nebert · L. M. Newman · L. J. Pierro
L. W. Rampy · K. S. Rao · D. S. Salomon · C. A. Schreiner
B. A. Schwetz · J. L. Sever · S. A. Waldmann · J. F. Young

Editors

E. M. Johnson and D. M. Kochhar

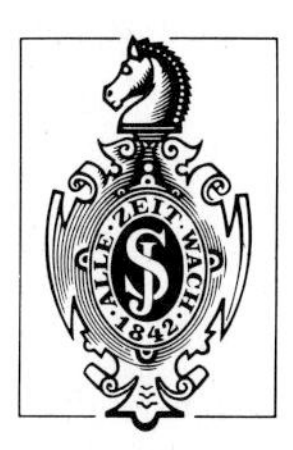


Springer-Verlag Berlin Heidelberg New York 1983

Professor E. MARSHALL JOHNSON, Ph.D.
Chairman of Department of Anatomy, Director of Daniel Baugh Institute,
Jefferson Medical College, 1020 Locust Street, Philadelphia, PA 19107/USA

Professor DEVENDRA M. KOCHHAR, Ph.D.
Department of Anatomy, Daniel Baugh Institute, Thomas Jefferson University,
1020 Locust Street, Philadelphia, PA 19107/USA

With 69 Figures

ISBN 3-540-11906-X Springer-Verlag Berlin Heidelberg New York
ISBN 0-387-11906-X Springer-Verlag New York Heidelberg Berlin

Library of Congress Cataloging in Publication Data. Main entry under title: Teratogenesis and reproductive toxicology. (Handbook of experimental pharmacology; v. 65) Includes bibliographies and index. 1. Fetus–Effect of drugs on. 2. Teratogenesis. 3. Behavioral toxicology. 4. Behavioral assessment. I. Johnson, E. M. (Elmer Marshall), 1930–. II. Kochhar, D. M. (Devendra M.), 1938–. III. Chao, S. T. IV. Series. [DNLM: 1. Abnormalities, Drug-induced. 2. Prenatal exposure delayed effects. W1 HA51L v. 65/QS 679 T313] QP905.H3 vol. 65 [QM691] 615'.ls [616'.043] 82-19581. ISBN 0-387-11906-X (U.S.)



Typesetting, printing, and bookbinding: Brühlsche Universitätsdruckerei Giessen.
2122/3130-543210

# List of Contributors

Dr. S. T. CHAO, Ph.D., Department of Pharmacology, SJ-30 School of Medicine, University of Washington, Seattle, WA 98195/USA

Dr. K. P. CHEPENIK, Ph.D., Associate Professor, Department of Anatomy, Daniel Baugh Institute of Anatomy, Jefferson Medical College, Thomas Jefferson University, 1020 Locust Street, Philadelphia, PA 19107/USA

Dr. M. S. CHRISTIAN, Ph.D., Director of Research, Argus Research Laboratories, 935 Horsham Road, Horsham, PA 19044/USA

Mr. B. E. G. GABEL, Department of Anatomy, Daniel Baugh Institute, Jefferson Medical College, 1020 Locust Street, Philadelphia, PA 19107/USA

Dr. J. H. GREENBERG, Ph.D., National Institute of General Medical Sciences, Medical Institutes Westbard, National Institutes of Health, Westwood Building, Room 920, 5333 Westbard Avenue, Bethesda, MD 20205/USA

Dr. R. M. GREENE, Ph.D., Assistant Professor, Department of Anatomy, The Jefferson Medical College, 1020 Locust Street, Philadelphia, PA 19107/USA

Dr. H. E. HOLDEN JR., Ph.D., Safety Evaluation Department, Pfizer Central Research, Groton, CT 06340/USA

Dr. D. E. HUTCHINGS, Ph.D., New York State Psychiatric Institute, 722 West 168th Street, New York, NY 10032/USA

Dr. R. P. JENSH, Ph.D., Associate Professor, Anatomy and Radiology, Department of Anatomy, 561 Jefferson Alumni Hall, Thomas Jefferson University, 1020 Locust Street, Philadelphia, PA 19107/USA

Dr. E. M. JOHNSON, Ph.D., Professor and Chairman of Department of Anatomy, Director of Daniel Baugh Institute, Jefferson Medical College, 1020 Locust Street, Philadelphia, PA 19107/USA

Dr. M. R. JUCHAU, Ph.D., Department of Pharmacology, SJ-30, School of Medicine, University of Washington, Seattle, WA 98195/USA

Dr. N. W. KLEIN, Ph.D., Department of Animal Genetics, University of Connecticut, Storrs, CT 06268/USA

Dr. D. M. KOCHHAR, Ph.D., Department of Anatomy, Daniel Baugh Institute, Thomas Jefferson University, 1020 Locust Street, Philadelphia, PA 19107/USA

Dr. D. W. NEBERT, Ph.D., Developmental Pharmacology Branch, Building 10, Room 8C-420, National Institute of Child Health and Human Development, National Institutes of Health, Bethesda, MD 20205/USA

Dr. L. M. NEWMAN, Ph.D., Daniel Baugh Institute, Department of Anatomy, Jefferson Medical College, 1020 Locust Street, Philadelphia, PA 19107/USA

Dr. L. J. PIERRO, Ph.D., Department of Animal Genetics, University of Connecticut, Storrs, CT 06268/USA

Dr. L. W. RAMPY, Ph.D., Health and Environmental Sciences, Building 1803, Dow Chemical Co., Midland, MI 48640/USA

Dr. K. S. RAO, Ph.D., Health and Environmental Sciences, Building 1803, Dow Chemical Co., Midland, MI 48640/USA

Dr. D. S. SALOMON, Ph.D., Laboratory of Tumor Immunology and Biology, National Cancer Institute, National Institute of Health, Bethesda, MD 20205/USA

Dr. C. A. SCHREINER, Ph.D., Supervisor Genetic Toxicology, Toxicology Division, Mobil Oil Corporation, P.O. Box 1026, Princeton, NJ 08540/USA

Dr. B. A. SCHWETZ, D.V.M., Ph.D., Director, Toxicology Research Laboratory, Health and Environmental Sciences, Building 1803, Dow Chemical Co., Midland, MI 48640/USA

Dr. J. L. SEVER, M.D., Ph.D., Chief, Infectious Disease Branch, IRP, National Institute of Neurological and Communicative Disorders and Stroke, National Institutes of Health, Building 36, Room 5D06, Bethesda, MD 20205/USA

Dr. S. A. WALDMANN, Ph.D., Department of Anatomy, Daniel Baugh Institute of Anatomy, Jefferson Medical College, Thomas Jefferson University, 1020 Locust Street, Philadelphia, PA 19107/USA

Dr. J. F. YOUNG, Ph.D., Division of Teratogenesis Research, National Center for Toxicological Research, DHHS/FDA/EPA, Jefferson, AR 72079/USA

# Preface

The resolution of links between exposure to components of our complex environmental and causation of reproductive effects in the population constitutes an important problem in the field of toxicology. The focus of this volume is developmental toxicology, which represents one aspect of reproductive toxicology dealing with the study of adverse effects on the developing conceptus.

Developmental toxicology, which includes teratogenesis as one of its manifestations, provides a fertile field for research in several basic and clinical disciplines; this field also receives input from several disciplines such as developmental and molecular biology, pathology, pharmacology and toxicology, pediatrics and neonatology, and epidemiology. More recently we have seen an emergence of interest in other fields such as perinatal physiology and postnatal behavior which have now become incorporated into the mainstream of research in this discipline. The present volume is an effort to provide a sampling of concepts currently under active investigation in several of the above fields. The authors have endeavored to provide up-to-date information on the following topics: detection and analysis of potential hazards to the conceptus in the workplace, pharmacokinetic aspects of the maternal/placental/fetal complex and its relationship to human birth defects, and probable mechanisms of teratogenesis as uncovered in certain well-defined situations. Also included are summaries of newer investigations on the emerging field of postnatal functional evaluations, i.e., adverse effects on adult activities resultant from in utero exposure to toxic substances. Explanation of some experimental methods in use for the detection of hazards to in utero development under well-controlled laboratory investigations are a further area of some uniqueness and immediate practical interest.

This text is organized into four general segments. The first part provides a brief yet pointed awareness of human in utero exposure in one context. The second segment deals with several aspects of mechanisms thought to underlie abnormal development. An important third part concentrates upon on the subtle postnatal manifestations of prenatal exposure to toxic concentrations of specific substances. This section is a pioneering effort to provide an awareness of the diverse nature and extent to which in utero exposure can influence function of several organ systems in later life. Last but not least is a section on methods presently available for the more rapid detection of environmental hazards to the cenceptus. These systems may prove to be germane to assessing the degree to which specific industrial and other exposures pose a hazard to development of the next generation.

This volume will be of interest to investigators in the fields of developmental biology and toxicology – those interested in basic mechanisms underlying abnormal development, to individuals in industry who bear responsibility for workplace safety, to persons who face the myriad and complex considerations necessary for regulatory decisions regarding potential hazards to the conceptus, and to informed physicians who wish to remain conversant with advances in the field of environmental toxicology.

THE EDITORS

# Contents

## Epidemiology and Bioavailability

## Mechanisms of Teratogenesis

CHAPTER 6

**Hormonal Involvement in Palatal Differentiation**
R. M. GREENE. With 8 Figures



CHAPTER 7

**Membrane Lipids and Differentiation.** K. P. CHEPENIK and S. A. WALDMANN
With 2 Figures



CHAPTER 8

**Hormone Receptors and Malformations.** D. S. SALOMON. With 1 Figure

CHAPTER 13

**Postnatal Alterations of Gastrointestinal Physiology, Hematology, Clinical Chemistry, and Other Non-CNS Parameters.** M. S. CHRISTIAN. With 8 Figures



## In Vitro Screens of Teratogenic Potential

CHAPTER 14

**Detection of Teratogens Using Cells in Culture**
J. H. GREENBERG. With 1 Figure



CHAPTER 15

**Embryonic Organs in Culture.** D. M. KOCHHAR. With 3 Figures

# Epidemiology and Bioavailability

CHAPTER 1

# Assessment of Potential Hazards to the Unborn in the Workplace

B. A. Schwetz, K. S. Rao, and L. W. Rampy

## A. Introduction

A controversial occupational health issue being faced today by scientists, administrators, managers, lawyers, employers, and employees is how to protect the unborn in the workplace. This issue is complex because it involves not only scientific judgment, but also legal and social considerations. A sense of urgency has arisen primarily because of an increase in the number of women entering the workplace and an increase in the number of agents being identified as potential teratogens or fetotoxins.

Women in the workplace are subject to essentially the same potential occupational hazards as men. One major difference from men, however, is women's ability to bear children. It is actually the fetus that is the focal point of concern associated with the placement of women in the workplace. In consideration of how to protect the unborn, the policies and restrictions, when necessary, have been directed necessarily toward the mother. A rational goal must be to provide a safe work environment for the adults of both sexes as well as the unborn individual who might unknowingly be present in the work environment. Practices which unnecessarily limit the placement of women in certain jobs or, on the other hand, unnecessarily present a hazard to the unborn are unacceptable and unnecessary.

## B. Management of the Hazard

Approaches to managing the potential problem of hazard to the unborn range from one extreme to another. One approach is to eliminate the potential problem by refusing to allow women into jobs which involve any exposure to agents which may have an adverse effect on the unborn. This approach would theoretically eliminate women from all jobs, since any chemical or other form of stress has the potential, under some conditions, to affect the outcome of pregnancy adversely. However, the need for such a policy is not supported by scientific facts of toxicology. A similarly unreasonable posture, but in the opposite direction, is that no special precautions are needed to protect the unborn in the workplace. This posture is not supported by scientific facts and could jeopardize the well-being of the developing embryo and fetus.

Another approach between these two extreme positions is reasonable and defendable, one permitting women to work in almost all work environments without unreasonable risk to the unborn. There can be no blanket policy covering all agents; instead, each agent must be considered on an individual case-by-case basis for potential adverse effects on the unborn, just as it is for other toxic manifestations, including such effects as potential toxicity to the liver, kidney, heart or other organs, central nervous system depression, or any other adverse effect. All data, from humans as well as laboratory animals, must be considered in selecting a level of exposure at which the risk to the unborn is acceptable.

## C. Environmental Agents

There are numerous examples of environmental agents which either cause or are suspected to cause adverse effects on the developing embryo and fetus of humans. These agents are not widespread and they are very heterogeneous. Agents which are considered potentially to alter the development of the unborn include iodine deficiency (causing endemic cretinism), carbon monoxide, X-rays, toxoplasmosis, rubella, and organic mercury. Other agents known to be teratogenic in humans are cytomegalic inclusion disease, aminopterin, virilizing progesterones, thalidomide, chronic alcoholism, certain anticonvulsants, and warfarin.

The level of concern by the public regarding possible adverse effects of environmental agents on the unborn has increased in recent years. An increasing number of reports in the news media has been devoted to the spread of information regarding alleged health hazard of polluted air, water, and soil. As a result, there is significant public belief that many human malformations are caused by exposure to toxic agents in the environment. In contrast to this misconception, scientific surveys and case reports in the medical literature suggest that no more than 4%–5% of the malformations in humans are causally related to drugs or chemicals (WILSON 1977).

In a recent report released by the *Center* for *Disease Control* (1978), Atlanta, Georgia, on congenital malformation surveillance, data are presented on the incidence of 16 selected malformations reported through the Birth Defects Monitoring Program for the period 1970–1978. The report concludes that there is no evidence for an overall increase or decrease in malformation rates since 1970. In fact, the frequencies of critical marker malformations such as anencephaly and spina bifida were notably decreased in this survey. These data suggest that there is no increase of birth defects in the United States as a result of increased production and use of chemicals during the last decade.

## D. Protective Measures

Protection of the unborn from unreasonable risks from agents encountered in the workplace is obviously achieved by preventing exposure of women to unacceptable levels of agents in the workplace. Agents which might be encountered in the workplace to which the unborn is uniquely sensitive compared with adults are rare, but must be identified; thorough examination of all available data has generally indicated that exposure levels which are sufficiently low to protect one sex also protect the opposite sex. There are certain cases, however, where the developing embryo or fetus is more sensitive to certain chemicals than are the adult male or female. Protection of the unborn from overexposure to such agents may necessitate a downward adjustment of the permitted exposure level. A reasonable approach limits exposure to levels which are not hazardous to adults or the unborn, but does not unnecessarily exclude women from the workplace. The upper limit of the exposure level should be selected to provide some margin of safety from exposure levels which are known to cause adverse effects in humans or in laboratory animals.

To protect the women of childbearing capability and the fetus, existing standards for acceptable exposure levels must be examined carefully. Epidemiologic and toxicologic research has been conducted on certain agents to provide sufficient data to make judgments regarding the relative hazard of agents to women and the unborn. Such data must be used where applicable to make rational decisions.

## E. Safety Standards

How does one select standards for exposure levels which provide safety to both the unborn and adult? All available data must be evaluated, not just the results of teratology, reproduction, or epidemiologic studies. The most relevant determination is whether or not parameters involving embryonal and fetal development are more sensitive than other manifestations of toxicity. It is in these cases where the standard for permissible exposure is determined by the sensitivity of the developing conceptus. For other chemicals where the conceptus is not the most sensitive organ, levels of exposure which protect against other manifestations of toxicity should logically be sufficient to protect against adverse effects on the unborn. In those cases where the unborn is uniquely sensitive to an agent, the choice is either to: (a) set the standard at a level which protects the unborn; or (b) exclude women from working in an environment including that agent. There is considerable evidence to indicate the existence of a threshold for teratogenic agents. Thus, a general policy that prohibits women of childbearing potential from working in any area with known animal or human teratogens, regardless of the level of exposure, is scientifically unsound since it ignores the principles of threshold and dose-response. Furthermore, such a policy would be inconsistent with the approach to other manifestations of toxicity.

Women of childbearing capacity should not work in areas where one cannot be reasonably assured that exposure to toxic levels of certain chemicals will not occur. When actual exposure of women of childbearing capacity is likely to exceed the standard for an agent to which the unborn is uniquely sensitive, temporary exclusion of women should be considered until corrective actions to reduce exposure can be taken. Such exclusion should be only temporary, until the necessary engineering changes or protective equipment can be put into place to prevent exposure above the selected standard.

There is another circumstance in which women of childbearing capacity should perhaps be at least temporarily excluded from a work environment. In the case where new data have just been collected which indicate through animal studies or epidemiologic data that an agent is a teratogen and a no-observed-effect level has not been established, precautions should be taken to avoid exposure of women until a level of exposure can be defined which does not represent an unreasonable risk to the unborn. Until such data can be collected to permit definition of an appropriate standard, women should not be permitted to work in such an environment because of the unknown risk to a positive agent of unknown potency.

This does not mean that women should be automatically excluded from work areas that involve any risk of a chemical spill or other type of exposure. Such an approach would be unnecessarily restrictive. However, women capable of childbirth should be excluded or given special protection in certain situations (e. g., a spill or runaway process) where there is unreasonable risk of exposure to toxic levels of certain chemicals, those to which the unborn is uniquely sensitive. These situations are seen as temporary and must be handled individually as they arise in isolated situations.

This means in practical terms that women capable of childbearing will be excluded from certain work areas only when an acceptable level of exposure has not been defined for an agent which is known to be teratogenic, or when the exposure level of an agent exceeds the permitted exposure standards. For a plant supervisor to prohibit women from working in a certain area, he or she must declare that the potential for exposure to a toxic amount of a known teratogen is great and that there is no reasonable assurance that such an overexposure can be prevented. In such a situation, action should be taken, as feasible, to reduce the exposure to a level in compliance with the recommended standard. In the case of an agent which has been identified as a teratogen but no safe level of exposure has been identified, the necessary information should be acquired by research or analogy from existing data to define a health standard which would pose no unreasonable risk to the unborn.

## F. Summary

In summary, the goal is to maintain a healthy work environment for all employees: men, women, and the unborn. Intelligent use of all available data from studies in humans and laboratory animals should generally allow one to set standards which would allow men and women to work safely in the presence of agents, even those which may at some high level of exposure represent a hazard to the unborn. Through the wise use of sound toxicologic and engineering principles, health standards can be defined which do not unreasonably exclude employees from the workplace and which also provide protection from unreasonable health hazard. Through such an approach there is no need to compromise either the protection of the unborn or the right of women to work.

## References

Center for Disease Control (1978) Congenital malformations surveillance report, April 1977–March 1978. Center for Disease Control, Washington DC

Wilson JG (1977) Current status of teratology – general principles and mechanisms derived from animal studies. Embryotoxicity of drugs in man. In: Wilson JG, Fraser FC (eds) Handbook of teratology, vol 1. Springer, Berlin Heidelberg New York, pp 47–74

CHAPTER 2

# Pharmacokinetic Modeling and the Teratologist

J. F. YOUNG

## A. Introduction

Pharmacokinetics has proven to be an exceptional tool in pharmaceutical and pharmacologic research. Its development has enhanced the capabilities of providing optimum dosing schedules and formulations for delivery of ethical drugs by relating blood levels of a particular drug to its therapeutic efficacy. Likewise, perturbations in the pharmacokinetic parameters of a compound produced by interactions with a second chemical or with liver or kidney insufficiency, for example, have provided a more logical basis for the study of drug–drug or drug–chemical interactions, as well as effects of disease states in clinical pharmacology.

Pharmacokinetic concepts have direct application in the broad area of toxicology. Utilization of pharmacokinetic approaches early in the development of a new drug or chemical in preclinical and clinical evaluations, as well as in basic mechanistic studies and interspecies comparisons, offers on approach to the quantification of data, which can provide a better basis for safety evaluations. This area has been recognized by the pharmaceutical scientists; however, the research toxicologist is only now becoming aware of the potential of pharmacokinetics. In general, many, if not most, toxicologists do not fully understand the concepts and advantages, nor the pitfalls, in the applications of pharmacokinetics.

The objective of this chapter is to stimulate toxicologists to use and apply pharmacokinetic principles in their research. Concepts of modeling and simulation are presented as the basis for an introduction to the area. Although the experienced pharmacokineticist may find this review oversimplified and the equations too detailed, the needs of the toxicologist as presented herein will hopefully stimulate these researchers to broaden their mathematical thinking and develop and incorporate these concepts into their research.

## B. Pharmacokinetic Modeling and Simulation

Pharmacokinetics is the study of the time course of absorption, distribution, metabolism, and elimination of a chemical in an intact organism (GARRETT 1970). To aid in the evaluation of this time course, a mathematical model is proposed to imitate the real biologic system. The model is kept as simple as possible, but at the same time must be consistent with physiologic reality (BERLIN et al. 1968; GARRETT 1969; HIMMELSTEIN and LUTZ 1979). The internal parts of the mathematical model are known as compartments (CUTLER 1978). The compartments represent theoretical areas of the system in which the chemical acts homogeneously in transport and transformation. The extent of the compartment is described by its volume of distribution, and may or may not be consistent with physiologic reality; i.e., several organ systems may be lumped together for simplification of the mathematical model that describes the biologic system. In pharmacokinetic modeling, the term most often used to describe the time interval required for physiologic action upon a compound is the half-life. The half-life of a chemical is the amount of time elapsed while the chemical goes from one concentration to half that concentration.

When the proper model has been created which "imitates" the biologic system, one can then simulate experimental data and obtain a set of rate constants as pharmacokinetic parameters. These rate constants may then be used to predict the time course at a dose that has not been experimentally determined. Modeling also allows one to predict the concentration–time curve of tissues or compartments that have not been sampled or may not be convenient to sample. The keyword is "predict"; the analysis allows one to describe the biologic system mathematically and assign a set of numbers to that system. This mathematical description allows for quantitative comparison between individuals either within or between species. The investigator is no longer limited by the biologic quantitation of "+++ versus ++" or "larger versus largest"; but is able to describe the system in a more exacting manner with a set of differential equations having a unique solution. Biologic variation within and between species can in this way be statistically evaluated.

The ability to predict the concentration–time curve of a chemical within a tissue not sampled or a metabolite concentration–time curve without measurements is a powerful tool. By manipulating the model, one can try various metabolic routes or tissue distribution patterns in an attempt to predict a toxic level of a chemical or combination of chemicals at a target site. Using all the available data, one can make an educated guess that should enable a better allocation of effort at the experimental level. After the pharmacokinetic parameters are established, they can be used to predict tissue levels after repeated administration in a long-term study. Therefore, instead of arbitrarily picking times for killing experimental animals and analysis of various effects, one can predict the time of most probable effects and concentrate the sampling around those times.

Models are derived in an attempt to describe the fate of a chemical in an intact animal in such a way that they can be easily converted into a set of differential equations, the solution of which results in a set of numerical constants which can be used to compare individuals within and between strains or species. The validity of the model is usually consistent among individuals within a strain, but may change when analyzing different strains or species (for example, different metabolic pathways). The rate constants describing the model are expected to vary from one individual to the other and can be used to describe the biologic variation among different individuals.

## I. One-Compartment Open Model

When choosing a model, the simplest model that is consistent with physiologic reality should be selected (GARRETT 1969). For example, suppose that a chemical is administered intravenously, is not metabolized, and is eliminated only through the urine. The simplest model representing elimination in this case is

$$B \xrightarrow{k_{BU}} U, \qquad \text{(Model I)}$$

where $B$ is the amount of chemical in the blood. $U$ is the amount of chemical eliminated in the urine, and $k_{BU}$ is the elimination rate constant.[1] Two assumptions made are that the volume of distribution of the chemical within the blood is a constant throughout the time course of the elimination, and elimination is a first-order (linear) process. A first-order process is one in which the rate of the reaction is proportional to the concentration of the chemical in question. In addition, body functions such as cardiac output, pH, renal clearance, etc., are assumed to remain constant throughout the duration of the elimination process. The constancy of each of these is questionable and should be considered in any pharmacokinetic analysis (WAGNER 1968 a, 1971). These first assumptions that are made in modeling are designed to facilitate analysis and may be modified as the experimental data dictate.

The differential equations for model I are

$$-\frac{dB}{dt} = k_{BU} B \qquad (1)$$

(the loss of the chemical from the blood with time is equal to the elimination constant multiplied by the amount of chemical in the blood); and

$$+\frac{dU}{dt} = k_{BU} B \qquad (2)$$

(the appearance of the chemical in the urine with time is equal to the elimination rate constant multiplied by the amount of chemical in the blood). By following a few rules, the differential equations for more complicated models may be formulated as follows:

1. Derive the proper signs (+ or −) from the directionality of the arrows.
   a) When expressing the loss (−) of chemical from blood with time $-dB/dt$, the rate constant $k_{BU}$ represents a process going away from $B$ and therefore is a positive factor (+) in the loss of chemical with time.
   b) When expressing the appearance (+) of chemical in urine with time $+dU/dt$, the rate constant $k_{BU}$ represents a process coming toward $U$ and therefore is a positive factor (+) in the appearance of chemical with time.
   c) Conversely, if expressing the formation of chemical in blood with time $+dB/dt$, the rate constant $k_{BU}$ now represents a negative factor (−) in the formation of chemical with time (i.e., is not contributing to formation, but rather to loss); therefore,

$$\frac{dB}{dt} = -k_{BU} B. \qquad (3)$$

2. Each term of the differential equation is comprised of a rate constant ($k_{XY}$) and an amount term $X$; the rate constant is that one associated with the arrow and

1 Throughout this article the rate constants subscripts will, for convenience, be described as a combination of both ends of the arrows, i.e., the first subscript will indicate from where the chemical is coming and the second subscript will indicate where the chemical is going. For more information on subscripts used for rate constants, see NOTARI (1973) and HULL (1979)

the amount term is taken from the back of the arrow or where the chemical is coming from.

3. The number of terms in the differential equation must equal the number of arrows associated with that term, both going to and coming from.

For graphic analysis, the equations need to be in some form of the equation for a straight line ($y=ax+b$). One transformation results from integration of Eq. (3);

$$\int_{B_0}^{B} \frac{dB}{B} = -k_{BU} \int_0^t dt, \tag{4}$$

where $B=B_0$ at $t=0$

$$\ln \frac{B}{B_0} = -k_{BU} t \tag{5}$$

$$\ln B = \ln B_0 - k_{BU} t. \tag{6}$$

Expressing Eq. (6) in its exponential form,

$$B = B_0 \exp - k_{BU} t. \tag{7}$$

The plot of $B$ versus $t$ results in a typical first-order decay curve (Fig. 1a). Equation (6) is the linear form of the first-order equation and the plot of ln $B$ versus $t$ results in a straight line with a slope of $-k_{BU}$ and an intercept of ln $B_0$ (Fig. 1b).

Since $U=0$ at $t=0$ and $U_\infty = B_0$, then $B = U_\infty - U$ at any time for Model (I); Eq. (2) can also be integrated to give

$$\int_0^U \frac{dU}{B} = \int_0^U \frac{dU}{U_\infty - U} = k_{BU} \int^t dt \tag{8}$$

$$\ln \frac{U_\infty}{U_\infty - U} = k_{BU} t \tag{9}$$

$$\ln (U_\infty - U) = \ln U_\infty - k_{BU} t. \tag{10}$$

Converting again to the exponential form

$$U = U_\infty - U_\infty \exp - k_{BU} t = U_\infty (1 - \exp - k_{BU} t). \tag{11}$$

The plot of accumulative $U$ versus $t$ from Eq. (11) is given in Fig. 1c. From Eq. (10), the plot of $\ln(U_\infty - U)$ versus $t$ will result in a straight line with an intercept of $\ln U_\infty$ and a slope of $-k_{BU}$ (Fig. 1d).

The volume of distribution ($V_B$) relates the amount $B$ of chemical in the blood or fluid compartment with the concentration $b$ of the chemical in that compartment (NOTARI 1973; FELDMAN 1974); i.e.,

$$B = V_B b \text{ or amount} = (\text{volume}) \times (\text{amount/volume}). \tag{12}$$

From this relationship some additional algebraic manipulation can be achieved which may be useful. In practice, the measurement of a chemical in the blood will result in a concentration term and Fig. 1a is more often plotted as $b$ versus $t$. The plot of $\ln b$ versus $t$ is also identical with Fig. 1b, the slope being the same, but the intercept being $\ln b_0$ or the natural logarithm of the concentration of chemical in the blood at time zero. Since one knows the amount injected into the system $B_0$,

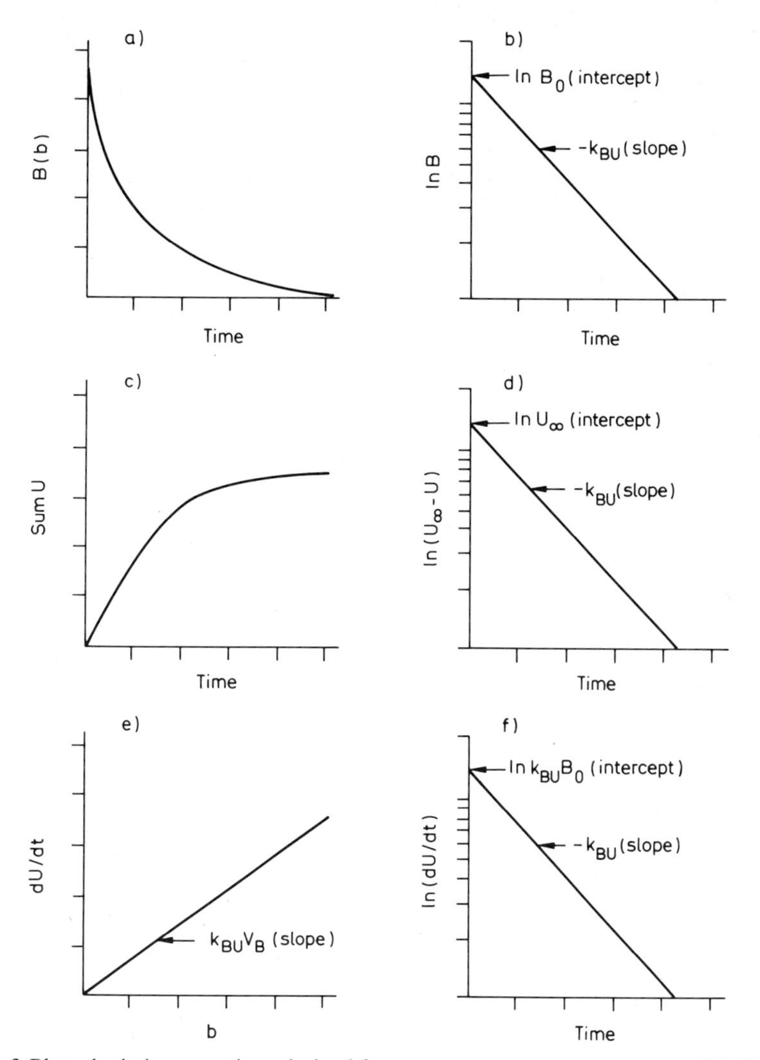


**Fig. 1 a–f.** Plots depicting equations derived from a one-compartment open model. See text for explanation

the volume of distribution $V_B$ can be calculated by rearranging Eq. (12),

$$V_B = B_0/b_0. \tag{13}$$

Another useful relationship results from the substitution of Eq. (12) into Eq. (2)

$$\frac{\mathrm{d}U}{\mathrm{d}t} = k_{BU} B = k_{BU} V_B b. \tag{14}$$

From the plot of $\mathrm{d}U/\mathrm{d}t$ versus $b$, a straight line going through the origin having a slope of $k_{BU} V_B$ will result (Fig. 1e). Care must be taken in data acquisition since the blood samples should fall at the midpoint of the urine collection to obtain the proper relationship between the rate of appearance of chemical in the urine and the chemical concentration in the blood. That is, one can see from Fig. 1c that the rate of change of $U$ (instantaneous slope) is not constant, and any calculation of $dU/dt$ must be an averaging effect. Therefore, if the blood sample is taken at the midpoint of the urine collection, the concentration of the chemical in the blood at that time more closely reflects the average concentration during this same time period.

Another relationship that may be utilized when only urine data is available, results from the substituting of Eq. (7) into Eq. (2),

$$\frac{dU}{dt} = k_{BU} B = k_{BU} B_0 \exp - k_{BU} t. \tag{15}$$

Taking the logarithm of both sides,

$$\ln \frac{dU}{dt} = \ln k_{BU} B_0 - k_{BU} t. \tag{16}$$

The plot of $\ln dU/dt$ versus $t$ is given in Fig. 1f and results in a straight line with a slope of $-k_{BU}$ and an intercept of $\ln k_{BU} B_0$ or $\ln k_{BU} V_B b_0$. However, without blood concentration data, the volume of distribution term can not be obtained in this manner.

The area under the blood concentration versus time curve (Fig. 1a) is often used when comparing bioavailability of one dosage form with another (Dost principle; DOST 1953, 1958). This area term is obtained by dividing Eq. (7) by the volume of distribution, substituting Eq. (12) after rearranging, and integrating; i.e.,

$$\frac{B}{V_B} = \frac{B_0}{V_B} \exp - k_{BU} t \text{ or } b = b_0 \exp - k_{BU} t \tag{17}$$

$$\int_0^\infty b(t) dt = A_1 = b_0 \int_0^\infty \exp - k_{BU} t \tag{18}$$

$$A_1 = b_0 \left[ \frac{-1}{k_{BU}} \exp - k_{BU} t \right]_0^\infty = \frac{-b_0}{k_{BU}} (0-1) \tag{19}$$

$$A_1 = \frac{b_0}{k_{BU}} = \frac{B_0}{V_B k_{BU}} = \frac{D_0}{V_B k_{BU}}, \tag{20}$$

where $A_1$ represents the area under the curve for an intravenous injection and first-order elimination, and $D_0$ equals the original dose or amount injected.

The half-life $t_{1/2}$ is the time it takes for one-half of the chemical to be eliminated from the blood, or that time for the blood level to go from $B$ to $B/2$ (WAGNER 1968a; RITSCHEL 1970). By making the substitution of $B = B_0/2$ and $t = t_{1/2}$ into Eq. 6,

$$\ln \left( \frac{B_0}{2} \right) = \ln B_0 - k_{BU} t_{1/2} \tag{21}$$

$$\ln \left( \frac{B_0}{2} \right) - \ln B_0 = \ln \left( \frac{B_0}{2 B_0} \right) = \ln 1/2 = -k_{BU} t_{1/2} \tag{22}$$

$$t_{1/2} = \frac{-\ln 1/2}{k_{BU}} = \frac{\ln 2}{k_{BU}} = \frac{2.303 \log 2}{k_{BU}} = \frac{0.693}{k_{BU}}. \tag{23}$$

Therefore, the half-life is independent of the blood concentration and dependent only on the elimination half-life. Caution is in order, however; Eq. (23) for half-life is only for first-order elimination. The half-life associated with both zero-order and second-order elimination are dependent on the initial dose of the chemical (i.e., for zero order $t_{1/2} = B_0/2k_0$ and for second order $t_{1/2} = 1/B_0k_2$, where $k_0$ and $k_2$ represent the zero-order and second-order rate constants, respectively).

## II. One-Compartment Model with Parallel Elimination

The simplest expansion of the first model is to add additional parallel pathways of elimination;

$$B \begin{array}{l} \nearrow U \\ \longrightarrow M, \\ \searrow F \end{array} \qquad \text{(Model II)}$$

where $M$ may represent a metabolite and $F$ elimination into the feces. By utilizing the rules outlined for forming differential equations,

$$-\frac{dB}{dt} = k_{BU}B + k_{BM}B + k_{BF}B = k_EB, \tag{24}$$

where

$$k_E = k_{BU} + k_{BM} + k_{BF} \tag{25}$$

Also,

$$\frac{dU}{dt} = k_{BU}B \tag{26}$$

$$\frac{dM}{dt} = k_{BM}B \tag{27}$$

$$\frac{dE}{dt} = k_{BF}B. \tag{28}$$

How does this expansion of the model affect the equations and plots? Integration of Eq. (24) results in

$$B = B_0 \exp - k_Et, \tag{29}$$

which can be seen to be identical to Eq. (7) except for the replacement of $k_{BU}$ by $k_E$. Therefore, plots in Fig. 1a, b should be the same, except the slope in Fig. 1b is now $-k_E$ (Fig. 2a) instead of $-k_{BU}$. Emphasis must be made of the potential hazard of mistaking $k_E$ for $k_{BU}$. The first-order plot for the blood level date ($\ln b$ versus $t$) resulting in a straight line does not assure one that the proper model has been chosen. Continuing the comparison, substitution of the volume of distribution relationship [Eq. (12)] into Eq. (26) results in an identical relationship [Eq. (14)] and, therefore, identical plots (compare Fig. 2b with Fig. 1e).

When considering the two mathematical relationships which resulted in Fig. 1d, f, additional calculations must be made for Model II. The substitution of $U_\infty - U$ for $B$ is no longer valid since $B$ is now equal to the sum of all the elimination products;

$$B_0 = U_\infty + M_\infty + F_\infty, \tag{30}$$

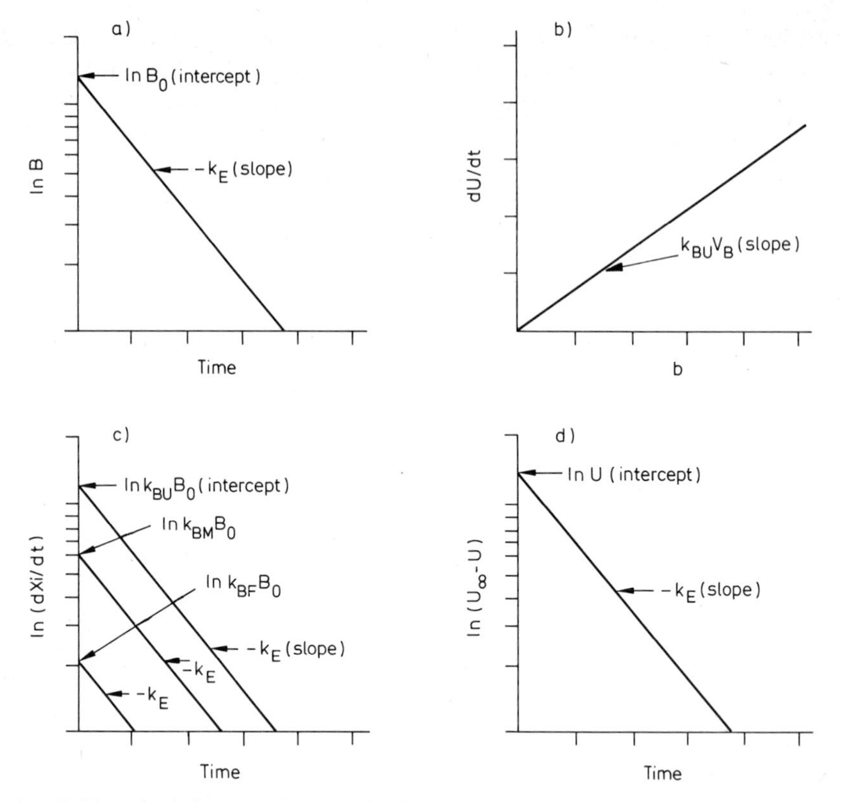


**Fig. 2 a–d.** Plots depicting equations derived from a one-compartment model with parallel elimination. See text for explanation

To obtain a similar plot as in Fig. 1f, Eq. (29) must be substituted into Eq. (26) for the proper comparison;

$$\frac{dU}{dt} = k_{BU} B_0 \exp - k_E t \tag{31}$$

$$\ln \frac{dU}{dt} = \ln k_{BU} B_0 - k_E t. \tag{32}$$

When comparing Eq. (32) with Eq. (15), the only difference is the slope which now becomes $k_E$ instead of $k_{BU}$ (compare Fig. 2c with Fig. 1f).

On integration of Eq. 31,

$$\int_0^U dU = k_{BU} B_0 \int_0^t \exp - k_E t \, dt \tag{33}$$

$$U = k_{BU} B_0 (-1/k_E)(\exp(-k_E t) - 1) = (k_{BU} B_0 / k_E)(1 - \exp - k_E t). \tag{34}$$

At $t = t_\infty$, $U = U_\infty$ and $\exp - k_E t_\infty$ approaches zero, Eq. (34) becomes

$$U_\infty = k_{BU} B_0 / k_E. \tag{35}$$

Substitution of Eq. 35 back into Eq. 34,

$$U = U_\infty(1 - \exp - k_E t) = U_\infty - U_\infty \exp - k_E t \tag{36}$$

$$\ln(U_\infty - U) = \ln U_\infty - k_E t. \tag{37}$$

Equation (37) now has the same form as Eq. (10) with the difference in the slope for Fig. 1c again becoming the substitution of $k_E$ for $k_{BU}$ (Fig. 2d).

Another useful relationship to be aware of is obtained by rearranging Eq. (35)

$$\frac{U_\infty}{B_0} = \frac{k_{BU}}{k_E}. \tag{38}$$

That is, the ratio of total amount excreted in the urine and initial dose is the same as the ratio of the rate constant $k_{BU}$ and the sum of all elimination rate constants.

Since $M$ and $F$ are parallel routes of elimination with $U$, identical equations and plots can be derived for each. The important relationship to obtain from this exercise is related to Eq. (38). Similar equations for $M$ and $F$ are

$$\frac{B_0}{k_E} = \frac{U_\infty}{k_{BU}} = \frac{F_\infty}{k_{BF}} = \frac{M_\infty}{k_{BM}}. \tag{39}$$

In the study where the chemical might fit this model, only the loss from the blood or the appearance of any one product plus the final amount of each elimination product needs to be obtained to be able to calculate all parameters. Caution must be taken, however, in that $t_\infty$ must have been obtained for the proper values to be evaluated. Another caution concerns the model itself; if the metabolite accumulates before elimination, this would not be the proper model as the metabolite is assumed to be excreted instantaneously in this example.

Hopefully, the reader has begun to formulate a solution to the earlier caution of mistaking $k_E$ for $k_{BU}$. From Eq. (32) and Fig. 2c, the intercept is seen to be $\ln k_{BU} B_0$; since $B_0$ is the initial dose, $k_{BU}$ can be calculated and compared with $k_E$. If $k_E = k_{BU}$, then Model (I) must hold, otherwise some form of Model (II) might be appropriate (GIBALDI 1971). It may appear unnecessary to be aware of all these intricacies in the mathematics when many sophisticated computer programs exist to analyze the data "automatically" and give the values of all the constants. However, there are limitations associated with any computer program. All computers must be supplied with some initial estimates of the constants and the limits around each to search for the "best fit" values. It is imperative to supply the computer with the proper model in most cases. (One digital computer program does exist for searching through several models, but considers only the blood level data; SEDMAN and WAGNER 1974c). If these initial estimates are not supplied, the efficiency of the computer is greatly decreased. The more complex the model, the better the initial estimates need to be to conserve computer time.

## III. One-Compartment Absorption Model

The most common route of administration of a chemical is the oral route. The simplest model which includes absorption from the gastrointestinal tract would be

$$G \xrightarrow{k_{GB}} B \xrightarrow{k_{BU}} U, \tag{Model III}$$

where $G$ represents the amount of chemical in the gut and $k_{GB}$ is the absorption rate constant. The differential equations are

$$-\frac{\mathrm{d}G}{\mathrm{d}t}=k_{GB}G \tag{40}$$

$$\frac{\mathrm{d}B}{\mathrm{d}t}=k_{GB}G-k_{BU}B \tag{41}$$

$$\frac{\mathrm{d}U}{\mathrm{d}t}=k_{BU}B. \tag{42}$$

Equation (40) is in the form of a simple first-order equation [identical in form to Eq. (1)] which on integration results in

$$G=G_0\exp-k_{GB}t. \tag{43}$$

The integration of Eq. (41) is slightly more involved: substitute Eq. (43) into Eq. (41) and rearrange to give

$$\frac{\mathrm{d}B}{\mathrm{d}t}+k_{BU}B=k_{GB}G_0\exp-k_{GB}t. \tag{44}$$

Since Eq. (44) is in the form of an exact integral, the integration factor of $\exp k_{BU}t$ is used

$$\exp k_{BU}t\left[\frac{\mathrm{d}B}{\mathrm{d}t}+k_{BU}B\right]=\frac{\mathrm{d}[B\exp k_{BU}t]}{\mathrm{d}t}=k_{GB}G_0\exp-k_{GB}t\exp k_{BU}t. \tag{45}$$

On integration

$$\int_0^B \mathrm{d}\,[B\exp k_{Bu}t]=\int_0^t k_{GB}G_0\exp(k_{BU}-k_{GB})t\,\mathrm{d}t \tag{46}$$

$$B\exp k_{BU}t=k_{GB}G_0\left(\frac{1}{k_{BU}-k_{GB}}\right)\{\exp((k_{BU}-k_{GB})t)-1\} \tag{47}$$

$$B=\frac{k_{GB}G_0}{k_{BU}-k_{GB}}(\exp-k_{GB}t-\exp-k_{BU}t). \tag{48}$$

A typical blood level versus time plot is given in Fig. 3a. The first-order plot (ln $B$ versus $t$) of Eq. (48) is given in Fig. 3b. If we make the assumption that absorption is complete in the latter stages of the concentration-time curve, $\exp-k_{GB}t$ is zero and Eq. (48) becomes

$$B'=-\frac{k_{GB}G_0\exp-k_{BU}t}{k_{BU}-k_{GB}}=\frac{k_{GB}G_0\exp-k_{BU}t}{k_{GB}-k_{BU}} \tag{49}$$

$$\ln B'=\ln\frac{k_{GB}G_0}{k_{GB}-k_{BU}}-k_{BU}t. \tag{50}$$

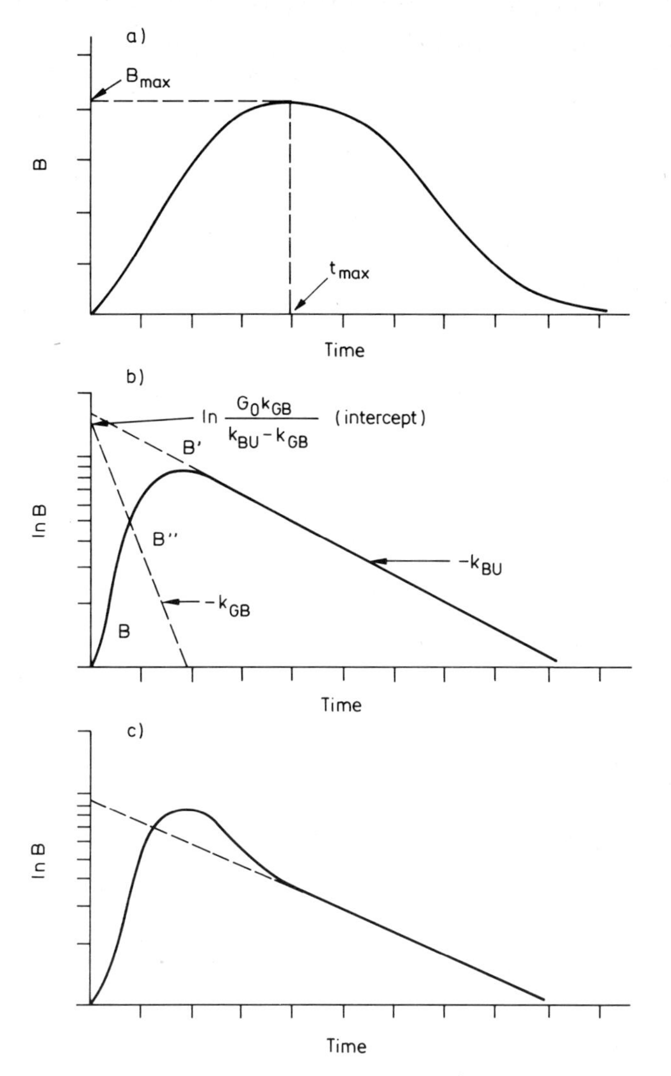


**Fig. 3 a–c.** Plots depicting equations derived from a one-compartment absorption model. See text for explanation

From Eq. (50) the slope in the latter stages of Fig. 3b can be seen to be $-k_{BU}$. By subtracting Eq. (49) from Eq. (48),

$$B - B' = B'' = \frac{k_{GB} G_0}{k_{BU} - k_{GB}} (\exp - k_{GB} t - \exp - k_{BU} t) + \frac{k_{GB} G_0}{k_{BU} - k_{GB}} \exp - k_{BU} t \tag{51}$$

$$B'' = \frac{k_{GB} G_0}{k_{BU} - k_{GB}} \exp - k_{GB} t \tag{52}$$

$$\ln B'' = \ln \frac{k_{GB} G_0}{k_{BU} - k_{GB}} - k_{GB} t. \tag{53}$$

By subtracting the projected curve $B'$ from the actual data curve $B$ and taking the logarithm of both sides of the equation, a new line may be drawn with a slope of $-k_{GB}$ or an estimate of the absorption rate constant. This technique of subtraction is often referred to as the "feathering technique" or method of residuals (GARRETT 1973). This technique is valid only when absorption is considered to be rapid and complete by the time of the maximum blood concentration. Graphically, this may be assumed if the projected line $B'$ does not intersect with the blood level curve $B$, as in Fig. 3b. However, if the projected line cuts through the blood level curve as in Fig. 3c, absorption is not complete and the feathering technique will not result in a valid estimate of the absorption rate constant.

Furthermore, until absorption is complete, a valid estimate of the half-life can not be made. However, if we assume that absorption is complete and that $k_{GB}$ is faster than $k_{BU}$ (about ten times is sufficient), then Eq. (49) can be reduced to

$$B' = \frac{k_{GB} G_0}{k_{GB}} \exp - k_{BU} t = G_0 \exp - k_{BU} t, \tag{54}$$

which is a simple first-order equation for which the half-life concept is valid.

To obtain the area under the blood level versus time curve (Fig. 3a), one must integrate Eq. (48) after dividing by $V_B$:

$$A_{11} = \int_0^\infty \frac{B(t)\,\mathrm{d}t}{V_B} = \frac{k_{GB} G_0 / V_B}{k_{BU} - k_{GB}} \left[ \int_0^\infty \exp - k_{BU} t\,\mathrm{d}t - \int_0^\infty \exp - k_{BU} t\,\mathrm{d}t \right], \tag{55}$$

where $A_{11}$ is the area under the blood concentration–time curve for two first-order processes (both absorption and elimination).

$$A_{11} = \frac{k_{GB} G_0}{V_B (k_{BU} - k_{GB})} \left[ \frac{(-1)}{k_{GB}} (0-1) - \frac{(-1)}{k_{BU}} (0-1) \right] =$$

$$A_{11} = \frac{k_{GB} G_0}{V_B (k_{BU} - k_{GB})} \left( \frac{1}{k_{GB}} - \frac{1}{k_{BU}} \right) \tag{56}$$

$$A_{11} = \frac{k_{GB} G_0}{V_B (k_{BU} - k_{GB})} \left( \frac{k_{BU} - k_{GB}}{k_{GB} k_{BU}} \right) = \frac{G_0}{k_{BU} V_B}. \tag{57}$$

Equation (57) assumes 100% absorption from an oral dosage. To cover those cases of incomplete absorption, let $\gamma$ be the fraction of the original dose ($D_0 = G_0$) that gets into the blood; Eq. (57) becomes

$$A_{11} = \frac{\gamma D_0}{k_{BU} V_B}. \tag{58}$$

Note that this area is dependent on the elimination rate constant and the fraction absorbed, but not the absorption rate constant. By comparing the area under the blood concentration–time curve from both an oral and intravenous dose of the same amount, the fraction of the dose absorbed may be calculated; i.e., divide Eq. (58) by Eq. (20):

$$\frac{A_{11}}{A_1} = \frac{\gamma D_0}{k_{BU} V_B} \div \frac{D_0}{k_{BU} V_B} = \gamma. \tag{59}$$

Caution must be exercised once again. Since individual variation is great, the comparison should be done only when both curves are from the same individual. Even within the same individual, consideration must be given to the location of the intravenous injection, and also to the extent of metabolism as both can influence the area under the blood concentration–time curve (GIBALDI and FELDMAN 1969; HARRIS and RIEGELMAN 1969; KAPLAN et al. 1973).

## C. Multicompartment Models

The first three models are considered to be one-compartment models (Sect. B); i.e., the chemical is distributed throughout a single hypothetical volume within the system, where it acts homogeneously in transport and transformation. Gut, urine, metabolite, and feces are not considered to be compartments. This conceptualization is based on the premises that the amount of chemical in the urine and feces has been eliminated from the system, the amount in the gut has not yet entered the compartment, and the amount metabolized is considered in a completely new compartmentalization system. As models become more complex, however, exceptions to this generalization take place. For instance, enterohepatic recirculation dictates that the gut be considered another compartment in the system, and renal tubular or bladder reabsorption of filtered chemical also dictates the consideration of an additional compartment.

Another way to view compartmentalization is to consider blood as a central compartment. No component of the system connected with the central compartment by a single arrow or unidirectionally would be considered an additional compartment. All components in free exchange with the central compartment through a pair of arrows would be considered additional compartments. When exchange between the blood compartment and an external compartment is fast and equilibrium between the two is rapidly achieved, both compartments can be considered and dealt with mathematically as a single fluid compartment.

The compartment concept may or may not be consistent with physiologic reality (WAGNER 1968b, 1971). The only limitation for the compartmental boundary is that the chemical acts homogenously. Therefore, the compartment might consist of one, two, or more actual physiologic units. For instance, in Model (I), the blood may act as a single compartment, limiting the distribution of the chemical to the plasma, or it could act as the total fluid of the body, with the chemical achieving a rapid equilibrium throughout. The calculated volume of distribution indicates the extent of distribution throughout the body.

### I. Two-Compartment Model

Compartmentalization concepts utilize two major terms, capacity and depth. Capacity is the term used to compare the volume of distribution of the secondary compartment with that of the central compartment. Depth of a compartment refers to the ability of the peripheral compartment to achieve equilibrium with the central compartment. A shallow compartment is one that has limited capacity and rapidly achieves equilibrium; a deep compartment is one that has a lage capacity and very slowly, if ever, achieves equilibrium.

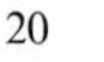

Consider the following two-compartment model

$$
\begin{array}{ccccc}
 & B & \underset{k_{TB}}{\overset{k_{BT}}{\rightleftharpoons}} & T, & \\
\swarrow k_{BF} & & & & \searrow k_{BU} \\
F & & & & U
\end{array}
\qquad \text{(Model IV)}
$$

where $B$ is the amount of chemical in the central compartment and $T$ is the amount of chemical in some peripheral or tissue compartment. The differential equations for this model are

$$-\frac{\mathrm{d}B}{\mathrm{d}t}=k_{BT}B-k_{TB}T+k_{BU}B+k_{BF}B \tag{60}$$

$$\frac{\mathrm{d}T}{\mathrm{d}t}=k_{BT}B-k_{TB}T \tag{61}$$

$$\frac{\mathrm{d}U}{\mathrm{d}t}=k_{BU}B \text{ and } \frac{\mathrm{d}F}{\mathrm{d}t}=k_{BF}B. \tag{62}$$

For shallow tissue compartments only, at some point in time after distribution is complete and a pseudoequilibrium has been achieved between $B$ and $T$, $T$ can be considered to be in a quasi-steady state (not a true steady state since elimination from $B$ is continuing, but sufficiently static for the assumption of $\mathrm{d}T/\mathrm{d}t \simeq 0$ to hold for a short period of time; LEVY 1974a). Equation 61 can be approximated by

$$\frac{\mathrm{d}T}{\mathrm{d}t}=k_{BT}B-k_{TB}T\simeq 0 \tag{63}$$

$$k_{BT}B\simeq k_{TB}T. \tag{64}$$

Substituting for the amount terms in Eq. (64) with Eq. (12) for the volume of distribution,

$$k_{BT}b\,V_B=k_{TB}t\,V_T. \tag{65}$$

Since the assumption of equilibrium has been made, the concentration of chemical in both compartments can be considered equal ($b=t$) and Eq. (65) can be rearranged to

$$\frac{V_T}{V_B}\simeq\frac{k_{BT}}{k_{TB}}, \tag{66}$$

i.e., the ratio of the volumes of distribution is equal to the inverse ratio of the respective rate constants. It is inherent within the definition that equilibrium be achieved before a value for the volume of distribution for the tissue compartment can be assigned.

The depth of the peripheral compartment is related to the elimination pathways of the central compartment. The depth of the peripheral ($T$) compartment is defined as the ratio of the rate constant going to that peripheral compartment and the sum of the elimination rate constants from the central compartment; i.e., from Model (IV)

$$\text{Depth}=\frac{k_{BT}}{k_{BU}+k_{BF}}. \tag{67}$$

Arbitrary limiting values are desirable to differentiate a shallow from a deep compartment. These may be set as follows:

a) Shallow compartment

$$\frac{k_{BT}}{k_{BU}+k_{BF}} > 10 \text{ and } V_T < 10\ V_B, \tag{68}$$

i.e., the rate of the chemical going into the peripheral compartment is ten times greater than the rate of the chemical being eliminated and the volume of distribution is somewhat limited. Equilibrium is rapidly achieved, and, if rapid enough, the two-compartment model ($B+T$) may revert to the one-compartment model and be considered as a single fluid compartment.

b) Deep compartment

$$\frac{k_{BT}}{k_{BU}+k_{BF}} < 10 \text{ and } V_T > 10\ V_B, \tag{69}$$

i.e., the rate of the chemical going into the peripheral compartment is less than ten times that of the rate of the chemical being eliminated and the volume of distribution of the peripheral compartment is relatively large. Equilibrium would not be readily achieved. The half-life of the chemical in the blood is no longer a constant since the decline is no longer a simple first-order process.

The rate of elimination is greatly affected by the peripheral compartment. If equilibrium is not achieved, the mathematics involved in the derivations becomes exceedingly complex and linear kinetics no longer apply. However, if equilibrium is achievable, Model (IV) may be approximated mathematically as,

$$-\frac{\mathrm{d}(B+T)}{\mathrm{d}t} \simeq k_{BU}B + k_{BF}B \tag{70}$$

substituting for $T$ from Eq. (64);

$$\frac{-\mathrm{d}\left[B+\dfrac{k_{BT}}{k_{TB}}B\right]}{\mathrm{d}t} \simeq (k_{BU}+k_{BF})\,B \tag{71}$$

$$-\frac{\mathrm{d}B}{\mathrm{d}t} \simeq \frac{k_{BU}+k_{BF}}{1+\dfrac{k_{BT}}{k_{TB}}}\,B = k_E B, \tag{72}$$

where $k_E = \dfrac{k_{BU}+k_{BF}}{1+\dfrac{k_{BT}}{k_{TB}}}$ (73)

and integration of Eq. (72) results in the same first-order equation for $B$ as before [Eq. (29)]

$$B = B_0 \exp - k_E t, \tag{74}$$

but with a much more complex $k_E$. Graphical representation would appear similar to Fig. 1 b and 2 a. However, if a deep compartment exists, a biphasic $\ln b$ versus $t$ plot will result (Fig. 4). The break will probably not be as distinct as this in practice, but two straight lines fit the curve better than a single line. The upper portion may

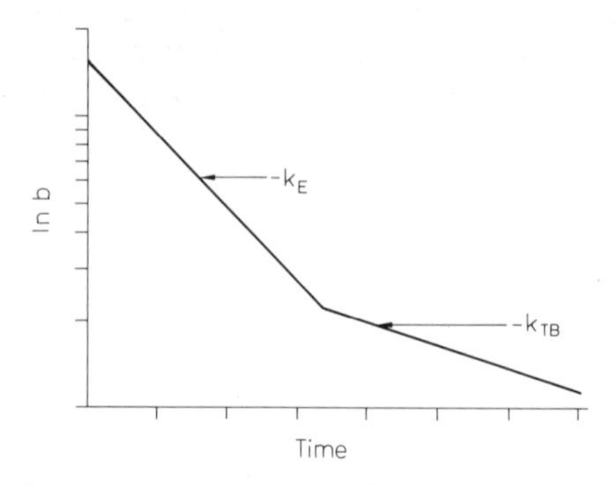


**Fig. 4.** First-order plot of a two-compartment model to illustrate the biphasic nature of the curve

usually be assigned a value of $k_E$ and the lower portion a value equal to the return from the deep compartment ($k_{TB}$). In these cases, $k_{TB} \ll k_E$.

In all cases so far, we have dealt only with first-order kinetics and a constant volume of distribution. These assumptions make the modeling and resultant mathematics relatively simple. However, real life does not always allow for such luxuries. The nonconstant volume of distribution can be visualized as occurring whenever a chemical is administered that causes either vasodilation or vasoconstriction. For example, as a vasodilator is administered, distribution occurs rapidly and quasi-steady state exists with its accompanying volume of distribution and elimination rate constant. However, as the chemical affects the active sites, vasodilation occurs, causing an increase in volume of distribution or an apparent decrease of the chemical concentration in the blood. Caution must be used in the correct interpretation of results, being sure to consider all known aspects of the chemical being tested.

## II. Protein Binding and Metabolism Models

Protein binding and metabolism are the two main examples of nonlinear or non-first-order kinetics used in pharmacokinetics (WAGNER 1973). The portion of a model that would cover protein binding is

$$B + P \underset{k_{BP,B}}{\overset{k_{B,BP}}{\rightleftharpoons}} BP, \qquad \text{(Model V)}$$

where $B$ is the amount of chemical in the blood, $P$ is the amount of protein that may bind to $B$ and $BP$ is the weak chemical–protein complex. The differential equations are written in the same manner as before, except both the concentration of the chemical and protein are involved.

$$-\frac{dB}{dt} = k_{B,BP}(B)(P) - k_{BP,B}(BP) = -\frac{dP}{dt} = \frac{d(BP)}{dt}. \tag{75}$$

The binding of a chemical to plasma proteins is usually a weak complex, where the equilibrium is very rapidly achieved and maintained. If the amount of protein is in sufficient excess to be considered a constant, Model V may revert to essentially a shallow compartment with first-order kinetics applying. The other end of the spectrum occurs when all the binding sites on the available protein are bound to the chemical or the protein is saturated with the chemical. In this case, the true equilibrium is not achieved and Eq. (75) no longer applies.

In all cases concerning protein binding, the analytic method for the chemical is important. If only the free unbound chemical is being analyzed in the blood, protein binding becomes of minor concern in the pharmacokinetic modeling. However, if total chemical, both bound and free, is being analyzed by the method (for instance, total radioactivity or whole blood) then the protein binding equations become very important and the fractional binding of the chemical must be known. As the amount of chemical administered into the system is increased, the protein will become saturated and the fractional binding will decrease. These saturation values may be obtained from independent in vitro studies by a variety of methods: ultrafiltration, equilibrium dialysis, and many others (ZETTNER 1973; ZETTNER and DULY 1974). The model for metabolism is similar to the protein binding model

$$B+E \underset{k_{BE,B}}{\overset{k_{B,BE}}{\rightleftharpoons}} BE \xrightarrow{k_{BE,M}} E+M\,, \qquad \text{(Model VI)}$$

where $E$ is the amount of enzyme available to interact with the chemical $B$ to form the equilibrium complex $BE$ which in turn forms the metabolite $M$ and regenerates the enzyme. When the metabolite is formed as rapidly as the complex is formed, (i.e., $k_{BE,M} \gg k_{B,BE} \gg k_{BE,B}$), model (VI) reverts to a simple first-order model,

$$B \xrightarrow{k_{BM}} M\,.$$

However, in those cases where this simplification is not valid, the second-order equations must be used. This is referred to as Michaelis–Menten kinetics (SEDMAN and WAGNER 1974a, b). An additional problem that may arise occurs in those cases where the enzyme reacting with the chemical can be induced or inhibited. In either case, the model will not hold throughout the time course of the study and appropriate compensations must be made.

## III. Drug-Chemical Interactions (Blood Protein and Tissue Binding)

Chemical interactions may occur at any level of pharmacokinetic interest: dissolution, absorption, distribution, metabolism, and/or elimination. The formation of complexes within a formulation which act to enhance or inhibit dissolution should be identifiable from in vitro tests. The absorption interactions can also be due to complexation, but more probably would result from direct competition for absorption sites or saturable carrier mechanisms. The distribution of a chemical and its interactions are closely related to the protein binding characteristics of the chemicals. Competition for protein binding sites is a well-documented phenomenon. However, enough emphasis has not been placed on the implications and far-reaching consequences of such a seemingly simple displacement reaction. The competition for a metabolizing enzyme or blockage of a metabolic pathway may be an important aspect of the toxicity of a chemical. The pH of the urine may influence the extent of elimination of a chemical and the pH may be easily altered by the injection of certain chemicals.

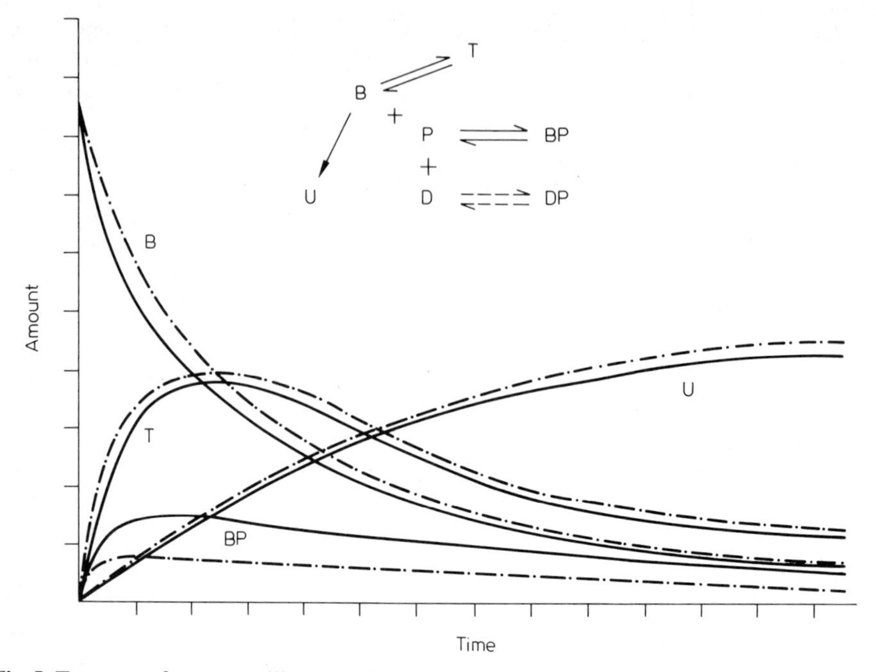


**Fig. 5.** Two sets of curves to illustrate the effects of competitive binding on a chemical. See text for explanation

Each of these areas of possible interactions has been reviewed intensively in the literature (BARR 1969; HOUSTON and LEVY 1976; LEVY 1976; WAGNER 1976). However, little has been published on the effects and implications of competitive protein binding. If we have a simple model, such as:

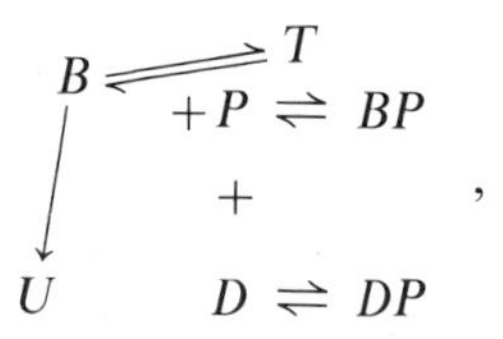


(Model VII)

where $B$ is the amount of chemical in the blood, $T$ the amount of chemical distributed into the tissues, $U$ the amount eliminated, $BP$ the amount bound to protein ($P$), and $DP$ the amount of competitive chemical ($D$) bound to protein, one might expect to get a set of curves as indicated in Fig. 5 (*full curves*). If a second chemical is introduced which competes for the same protein binding sites, the effects on the original chemicals are as indicated by the *broken curves* in Fig. 5. The amount of the original chemical in the blood increases since the amount bound decreases, provided that there is not an unlimited amount of protein for binding. As the amount of chemical in the blood increases, the amount available for distribution and elimination also increases, which results in higher tissue levels and in the amount eliminated. If total chemical is being measured in the blood (i.e., free plus bound), a problem in interpretation of the results may occur. For a highly bound chemical after the addition of the second chemical, the sum of free plus bound might easily result in a supposedly lower total blood level; however, this results from a higher free blood level followed by a redistribution and elimination and a much lower bound level. This can be visualized by mentally summing the curves for *B* and *BP* in Fig. 5 before and after the addition of the second chemical.

## D. Data Acquisition and Analysis

Once the model has been established and the graphical analysis has estimated the rate constants and volume of distribution, computer simulation of the experimental data is in order. Historically, the analysis of the equations was first accomplished using an analog computer (GARRETT et al. 1962, 1963; TAYLOR and WIEGAND 1962). Under this method, the differential equations were converted directly to analog form, and the manipulation of the parameters was done by hand until a satisfactory fit was obtained by the operator. This best fit was strictly an eye appeal fit; there was no statistical analysis or documenting involved. However, simulation by an analog computer is very fast, and with experience an operator can rapidly alter the model and parameters in order to obtain a satisfactory set of the pharmacokinetic parameters. The size or complexity of the model is of little concern since the simulation is a parallel operation by the analog computer; i.e., absorption, distribution, metabolism, and elimination are simulated simultaneously. With expansion of the model, however, problems may arise owing to limitations imposed by the operator's ability to make proper adjustments on the increasing number of parameters (GARRETT et al. 1974).

As more and more pharmacokinetic studies were made, an ever-increasing demand for statistical analysis and documentation led to the use of digital computers (LEVY et al. 1969; NOGAMI et al. 1969; NIEBERGALL et al. 1974; SEMAN and WAGNER 1974a, b, c, 1976; PEDERSEN 1977; LEFERINK and MAES 1979). These programs are fast, statistically validated, and documented. However, as the models become more and more complex, the serial solutions utilized by the digital computers become more and more time consuming. Hence, the usefulness of the digital computer by itself approaches a limit when complex models are employed.

Future needs for more complex pharmacokinetic models and predictions may necessitate the marriage of the best of the analog and digital computers in the form of a hybrid computer. Such a system would handle the simulation of the model directly by the analog portion of the hybrid; the control, statistical analysis, iterative techniques, and documentation would occur through the digital portion. Extremely complex models may be readily handled by this arrangement, with the predictive ability of the system being limited only by the imagination of the operator. Such a system has proven quite effective in preliminary investigations (YOUNG and HOLSON 1978; YOUNG et al. 1979; HOLSON et al. 1980; SMYTH and HOTTENDORF 1980).

Too often, the pharmacokinetic parameters are obtained, published, and forgotten (NOONEY 1966). Beyond this area lies "games people don't play, but should." For the toxicologist these games should become paramount. The real power of pharmacokinetics is the predictive ability of the model and modifications on the model (YOUNG and HALEY 1977; HALEY and YOUNG 1978; TILSTONE et al.

1979; RAMSEY and GEHRING 1980; WHITE et al. 1980). Modeling should be used to address questions such as: (1) what is the shape of the tissue concentration–time curve on multidosing? (2) can this curve be related to the toxicologic effect (RUNNER 1967; GIBALDI et al. 1971; JUSKO 1972)? (3) is there an accumulation of chemical or metabolite in a tissue? (4) what is the distribution picture when the dose is lowered to an environmental insult level and then multidosed for extended periods? At this early stage in the development of pharmacokinetic modeling for the toxicologist, these questions need not only to be addressed, but must be subsequently proven by experimental validation.

At present, state-of-the-art pharmacokinetics is being practiced in a few clinical–pharmacokinetic units around the country (LEVY 1974b). Individual drug therapy is being monitored and altered to suit an individual patient, based on that patient's own pharmacokinetic parameters for that particular drug. This is a long way from "two tablets, four times a day" for any and all patients; however, this idealized situation of individual patient monitoring is also a long way from being a universal practice.

A few comments and cautions on data acquisition and analysis need to be made for the budding pharmacokineticist:

a) Simplify the model as much as possible in your favor. Make the initial studies on intravenous administrations since this eliminates the absorption parameter. Even when the oral route is the most important, an initial intravenous study will prove invaluable.

b) Be sure to obtain sufficient early data points (GIBALDI 1971). To be able to simulate the distributive phase of the model, a large portion of the data points need to be concentrated early in the sampling schedule. Use an exponential type of sampling schedule; i.e., sample at 0, 1, 2, 4, 6, 9, 12, 16, 20, 25, 30... min from the blood.

c) Follow the decay for 6–7 half-lives, if possible. It is only in the latter stages that a deep compartment will appear (RITSCHEL 1970).

d) Always obtain blood, urine, and fecal samples throughout the study (unless of course, the chemical or its metabolites are eliminated exclusively by one route). The more data the better. With one, two, or three data points, one can fit any model chosen, no matter how simple or complex. However, as the number of experimental points increases, the fitting of the model becomes more difficult, but more exact. As the exactness of fit to good data increases, the ability to predict from the model also becomes more exact.

e) Do not average data among experimental subjects. The averaging of data points among individuals has often led to erroneous conclusions and interpretations. Individuals are different, even when homogeneous strains and littermates are considered. The only averaging that should occur is of the pharmacokinetic parameters themselves in order to get a statistical estimate of biologic variation.

f) Know your analytic method. What are you actually measuring? Free chemical? Free plus protein bound chemical? Chemical plus metabolite? In radioisotope studies, interpretation of the results may be drastically altered, depending on the analytic method.

g) Determine the extent to which the chemical is protein bound and metabolized. Is biliary excretion involved? What effect does pH play? After oral administration, is the amount of chemical in the feces due to the chemical not being absorbed or due to the biliary excretion of absorbed chemical? Intravenous administration will answer these questions as well as aid in the better calculation of the absorption and biliary rate constants.

h) Do not be satisfied with a poor fit of the data. As a rule of thumb, if more than three data points in succession lie on the same side of the predicted curve, keep trying for a better fit. Don't be afraid to expand or alter the model. A little more time invested in improving the initial fit will be rewarded by more accurate predictive ability.

i) Determine the half-life reported. Is it for blood? Elimination? Biologic? Was absorption complete and equilibria established with all peripheral compartments? The half-life concept is more involved than just measuring the time for the bood level to fall to one-half its original value. To report this type of "biologic half-life" is a cop-out. Radioisotope studies are infamous for this type of data reporting.

j) Validate your model. If accumulation in a compartment is predicted by your model, pick several times when the levels will be high, yet sufficiently different, for exclusion of biologic variation and sample at these limited number of specific times. This validation will usually be impossible when using human subjects.

Once you have obtained workable pharmacokinetic parameters from these pointers, begin to address the critical questions mentioned previously. Pharmacokinetics is an an area of paramount importance for the future of toxicology, and your continued interest is essential.

## References


Barr WH (1969) Factors involved in the assessment of systemic or biologic availability of drug products. Drug Inf Bull 3:27

Berlin NI, Berman M, Berk PD, Phang JM, Waldmann TA (1968) The application of multicompartmental analysis to problems of clinical medicine, Ann Intern Med 68:423

Cutler DJ (1978) On the definition of the compartment concept in pharmacokinetics. J Theor Biol 73:329

Dost FH (1953) Der Blutspiegel: Kinetic der Konzentrations-aublaute in der Kreislaufflüssigkeit. G Thieme, Leipzig

Dost FH (1958) Klin Wochschr 36:665

Feldman S (1974) Drug distribution, Med Clin North Am 58:917

Garrett ER (1969) Basic concepts and experimental methods of pharmacokinetics. Adv Biosci 5:7

Garrett ER (1970) Clinical significance of pharmacokinetics. In: Dengler HJ (ed) Pharmacological and clinical significance of pharmacokinetics, Symposia in medica Hoechst, F. K. Schaffauer-Verlag, Stuttgart New York pp. 5–21

Garrett ER (1973) Classical pharmacokinetics to the frontier. J Pharmacokinet Biopharm 1:341

Garrett ER, Johnston RL, Collins EJ (1962) Kinetics of steroid effects on $Ca^{47}$ dynamics in dogs with the analog computer. I. J Pharm Sci 51:1050

Garrett ER, Johnston RL, Collins EJ (1963) Kinetics of steroid effects on $Ca^{47}$ dynamics in dogs with the analog computer. II. J Pharm Sci 52:668

Garrett ER, Bres J, Schnelle K, Rolf LL Jr (1974) Pharmacokinetics of saturably metabolized amobarbital. J Pharmacokinet Biopharm 2:43

Gibaldi M (1971) Pharmacokinetic aspects of drug metabolism. Ann NY Acad Sci 179:19
Gibaldi M, Feldman S (1969) Pharmacokinetic basis for the influence of route of administration on the area under the plasma concentration-time curve. J Pharm Sci 58:1477
Gibaldi M, Levy G, Weintraub H (1971) Drug distribution and pharmacologic effects. Clin Pharmacol Ther 12:734
Haley TJ, Young JF (1978) A pharmacokinetic study of pentachlorophenol poisoning and the effects of forced diuresis. Clin Toxicol 12:41
Harris PA, Riegelman S (1969) Influence of the route of administration on the area under the plasma concentration-time curve. J Pharm Sci 58:71
Himmelstein KJ, Lutz RJ (1979) A review of the applications of physiologically based pharmacokinetic modeling. J Pharmacokin et Biopharm 7:127
Holson JF, Kimmel CA, Young JF (1980) The precision of pharmacokinetic parameters for predicting embryotoxicity endpoints. [Abstr] Presented at the 19th Annual Meeting of the Society of Toxicology, Washington DC, March 10, 1950
Houston J, Levy BG (1976) Effect of route of administration on competitive drug biotransformation interaction: salicylamide ascorbic acid interaction in rat. J Pharmacol Exp Ther 198:284
Hull CJ (1979) Symbols for compartmental models. Br J Anaesth 51:815
Jusko WJ (1972) Pharmacodynamic principles in chemical teratology: dose-effect relationships. J Pharmacol Exp Ther 183:469
Kaplan SA, Jack ML, Cotler S, Alexander K (1973) Utilization of area under curve to elucidate the disposition of an extensively biotransformed drug. J Pharmacokinet Biopharm 1:201
Leferink JG, Maes RAA (1979) STRIPACT, an interactive curve fit programme for pharmacokinetic analyses. Arzneim Forsch 29:1894
Levy G (1974a) Pharmacokinetic control and clinical interpretation of steady-state blood levels of drugs. Clin Pharmacol Ther 16:130
Levy G (1974b) An orientation to clinical pharmacokinetics. In: Levy G (ed) Clinical pharmacokinetics – a symposium. American Pharmaceutical Association, Academy of Pharmaceutical Sciences, Washington D. C. pp. 1–9
Levy G (1976) Pharmacokinetic approaches to the study of drug interactions. Ann NY Acad Sci 281:24
Levy G, Gibaldi M, Jusko WJ (1969) Multi-compartment pharmacokinetic models and pharmacologic effects. J Pharm Sci 58:422
Niebergall PJ, Sugita ET, Schnaare RL (1974) Calculation of plasma level versus time profiles for variable dosing regimens. J Pharm Sci 63:100
Nogami H, Hanano M, Awazu S, Moon HH (1969) Pharmacokinetic analysis on the disappearance of ethoxybenzamide from plasma. Statistical treatment of data of two compartmental model by a digital computer. Chem Pharm Bull (Tokyo) 17:2097
Nooney GC (1966) Mathematical models in medicine: a diagnosis. J Chronic Dis 19:325
Notari RE (1973) Pharmacokinetics and molecular modification: implications in drug design and evaluation. J Pharm Sci 62:865
Pedersen PV (1977) Curve fitting and modeling in pharmacokinetics and some practical experiences with NONLIN and a new program FUNFIT. J Pharmacokinet Biopharm 5:513
Ramsey JC, Gehring PJ (1980) Application of pharmacokinetic principles in practice. Fed Proc 39:60
Ritschel WA (1970) Biological half-lives of drugs. Drug Intell Clin Pharm 4:332
Runner MN (1967) Comparative pharmacology in relation to teratogenesis. Fed Proc 26:1131
Sedman AJ, Wagner JG (1974a) Quantitative pooling of Michaelis-Menten equations in models with parallel metabolite formation paths. J Pharmacokinet Biopharm 2:149
Sedman AJ, Wagner JG (1974b) Importance of use of appropriate pharmacokinetic model to analyze in vivo enzyme constants. J Pharmacokinet Biopharm 2:161
Sedman AJ, Wagner JG (1974c) AUTOAN manual. Publication Distribution Service, Ann Arbor, Michigan

Seman AJ, Wagner JG (1976) CSTRIP, a Fortran IV computer program for obtaining initial polyexponential parameter estimates. J Pharm Sci 65:1006
Smyth RD, Hottendorf GH (1980) Application of pharmacokinetics and biopharmaceutics in the design of toxicological studies. Toxicol Appl Pharmacol 53:179–195
Taylor JD, Wiegand RG (1962) The analog computer and plasma drug kinetics. Clin Pharmacol Ther 3:464
Tilstone WJ, Winchester JF, Reavey PC (1979) The use of pharmacokinetic principles in determining the effectiveness of removal of toxins from blood. Clin Pharmacokinet 4:23
Wagner JG (1968a) Pharmacokinetics. 3. Half-life and volume of distribution. Drug Intell 2:126
Wagner JG (1968b) Pharmacokinetics. 4. Body water compartments and the distribution of drugs. Drug Intell 2:158
Wagner JG (1971) "Biopharmaceutics and relevant pharmacokinetics." Drug Intelligence Publications, Hamilton, Illinois
Wagner JG (1973) A modern view of pharmacokinetics. J Pharmacokinet Biopharm 1:363
Wagner JG (1976) Simple model to explain effects of plasma protein binding and tissue binding on calculated volumes of distribution, apparent elimination rate constants and clearances. Eur J Clin Pharmacol 20:425
White CG, Young JF, Holson JF (1980) Pharmacokinetic approach to analysis of the "window effect" in teratologic sensitivity [Abstr]. Presented at the 19th Annual Meeting of the Society of Toxicology, Washington, D.C., March 10, 1980
Young JF, Haley TJ (1977) Pharmacokinetic study of a patient intoxicated with 2,4-dichlorophenoxyatic acid and 2-methoxy-3,4-dichlorobenzoic acid. Clin Toxicol 11:489
Young JF, Holson JF (1978) Utility of pharmacokinetics in designing toxicological protocols and improving interspecies extrapolation. J Environ Pathol Toxicol 2:169
Young JF, Kimmel CA, Holson JF (1979) Validation of a pharmacokinetic model for rat embryonal dosimetry of salicylates during a tertogenically susceptible period. Toxicol Appl Pharmacol 48:A21
Zettner A (1973) Principles of competitive binding assays (saturation analyses). I. Equilibrium techniques. Clin Chem 19:699
Zettner A, Duly PE (1974) Principles of competitive binding assays (saturation analyses). II. Sequential saturation. Clin Chem 20:5

CHAPTER 3

# Placental Drug Metabolism

S. T. CHAO and M. R. JUCHAU

## A. Introduction

The human placenta is an organ of metabolic interchange between the fetal and maternal circulations, and is clearly defined by the third month of gestation. After this time it grows, thickens, and spreads, developing along with the uterus. Both the placental structure and physiologic function are changing continually during the course of gestation. Numerous metabolic processes of vital importance are performed by the placenta during its short life, many of which have been considered necessary for optimal fetal development. For the fetus, the placenta serves as a combination gastrointestinal tract, kidney, lung, liver, spleen, thymus, and as a multifunctional endocrine organ with functions comparable to the anterior pituitary, ovarian follicle, and corpus luteum (SZABO and GRIMALDI 1970). In addition, the placenta transports nutrients such as amino acids, vitamins, carbohydrates, lipids, and minerals from the maternal to the fetal circulation, synthesizes and catabolizes proteins, carbohydrates, lipids, prostaglandins, nucleic acids, and steroid hormones.

During recent years, it has become increasingly appreciated that drugs given to the mother during pregnancy may harm the fetus. The grim evidence of the thalidomide tragedy, which resulted in the birth of many physically deformed children, and the occurrence of vaginal adenocarcinoma in some of the female offspring of mothers given diethylstilbestrol (HERBST et al. 1971) have given considerable impetus to the scientific study of drugs given during pregnancy. Recent studies have shown that pregnant women ingest between 3 and 29 drugs during their gestation, including labor and delivery medications (HILL 1973). This author has reported the mean number of drugs as 10.3. The drugs cited in her study do not include vitamins, iron, artificial sweeteners, cigarettes, environmental chemicals, or pesticides. While drugs administered during pregnancy have the mother as their principal target, the fetus is a corecipient in virtually all cases. Since nearly all drugs given during pregnancy cross the placenta and enter the fetal circulation, the placenta has been viewed as a determinant of the actions of drugs and foreign chemicals (xenobiotics) on the fetus, embryo, and mother.

Investigations in this area of research have become much more relevant owing to the increased recognition that many xenobiotics are metabolized by hepatic and extrahepatic tissue to reactive intermediates. The fact that many exogenous compounds, and perhaps even some endogenous compounds, can be metabolized to carcinogenic, cytotoxic, mutagenic, or teratogenic substances by normal enzymatic reactions is now generally accepted. However, this was not always the case. Current views on metabolic activation were developed extensively (MILLER and MILLER 1966; MILLER 1970) during studies on chemical carcinogenesis. These studies provided considerable impetus for recognition that metabolism of xenobiotics does not always result in the formation of polar, inactive metabolites, but can give rise to highly reactive metabolites which, acting as electrophiles, can subsequently interact to form covalent bonds with proteins, nucleic acids, and other critical cellular components. The presence of reactive metabolites in metabolizing or adjacent tissues poses a threat of a variety of toxic effects and stresses the importance of metabolic pathways leading to toxicity. Studies from various laboratories have provided evidence that chemically stable compounds can produce serious toxic reactions in humans and experimental animals, including hepatic and renal necrosis (NELSON 1977), teratogenesis (FANTEL et al. 1979), atherogenesis (BOND et al. 1979), bone marrow aplasia (GILLETTE et al. 1974), mutagenesis (HUBERMAN and SACHS 1977), carcinogenesis (HEIDELBERGER 1975), and several other pathologic abnormalities.

The capacity of various tissues to metabolize xenobiotics may be viewed as a function of the presence of enzyme systems that metabolize similar endogenous compounds (CONNEY 1967; CONNEY and KUNTZMAN 1971). Since the liver is involved in the catabolism of many endogenous compounds, it is not surprising that it can also metabolize a wide spectrum of xenobiotics. Many of the enzymes involved in the catalysis of xenobiotic biotransformation reactions are located in the liver, and for this reason most of the studies on drug metabolism have employed rat hepatic tissues as the model. However, xenobiotic metabolizing enzymes are also present to lesser and varying degrees in other organs such as the placenta, kidney, lung, adrenal gland, and gastrointestinal tract (GRAM 1980). It should be noted that a great many reviews on drug biotransformation in the placenta have appeared in the literature, several within the past few years (JUCHAU 1980a, b; JUCHAU et al. to be published; CHAO and JUCHAU 1980a). Studies of placental metabolism have both practical and theoretical implications. The placenta has been viewed as the lifeline of the fetus, any impairment of placental function may detrimentally influence the growth and development of the fetus.

Drug biotransformations occur via four principal processes: oxidation, reduction, hydrolysis, and conjugation with endogenous substances such as glucuronic acid. In terms of catalysis and regulatory control, these four reaction types involve oxidoreductases, hydrolases, and transferases. The oxidoreductases and hydrolases catalyze nonsynthetic reactions, also referred to as phase I reactions because they sometimes precede reactions catalyzed by transferase enzymes. Transferases catalyze synthetic reactions (conjugations) which may be referred to as phase II reactions although they do not always succeed nonsynthetic reactions.

## B. Oxidation Reactions

### I. Dehydrogenases

Oxidation of drug substrates can occur via reactions in which hydrogen atoms are removed from the drug substrate and transferred to an endogenous acceptor, monooxygenation (one atom of molecular oxygen is incorporated into the drug molecule and the other is reduced to water), dioxygenation (both atoms of molecular oxygen are incorporated into the substrate), and oxidations in which the oxygen is derived from $H_2O$. Of the dehydrogenases that catalyze drug oxidizing reactions, alcohol dehydrogenase (EC 1.1.1.1; HAGERMAN 1964, 1969; KRASNER et al. 1976) and aldehyde dehydrogenase are known to occur in rat and human placental tissues (SJOBLOM et al. 1978; KOURI et al. 1977). Acetaldehyde is thought to mediate the toxic effects of ethanol, therefore both activities are important to consider. Activities of the enzymes in both rat and human placentas were low when compared with rat liver. KOURI et al. (1977) suggested, however, that human placentas may not have sufficient aldehyde dehydrogenase to prevent acetaldehyde from diffusing into the fetal circulation. If this were the case, acetaldehyde could readily reach the fetal tissues, producing harmful effects on the metabolism of biogenic amines and protein synthesis (KOURI et al. 1977), and may perhaps also be involved in the fetal alcohol syndrome.

## II. Monoamine Oxidase

Placental tissue is very active in the metabolism of norepinephrine. Both monoamine oxidase (MAO; THOMPSON and TICKNER 1949) and catechol-o-methyltransferase (COMT; TISALO and CASTREN 1967) have been found in the human placenta. Placental MAO is believed to have an important role in protecting the fetus since MAO inhibitors have been found to cause death of the fetus and termination of pregnancy (KOREN 1965; POULSEN and ROBSON 1964). In placentas obtained from patients with toxemia of pregnancy, lower MAO activities and higher catecholamine levels were observed (DEMARIA and SEE 1966). It was suggested that the vasospasm in preeclampsia could be attributed to the higher levels of the pressor amines. Investigators have also suggested that placental MAO is involved in the regulation of blood flow through the uteroplacental–umbilical vasculature (JUCHAU 1973), and in the rate of transfer of norepinephrine and isoproterenol between maternal and fetal circulations (MORGAN et al. 1972).

## III. Monooxygenases

Of the oxidative reactions, the microsomal mixed function oxygenations have been the most intensively studied. The enzyme system which effects these reactions is located in the endoplasmic reticulum of hepatic parenchymal cells and also in the cells on the placenta, kidney, lung, and other tissues. It requires molecular oxygen and NADPH for its activity and is composed essentially of a hemoprotein known as cytochrome P-450 and a flavoprotein – cytochrome P-450 reductase in a phospholipid matrix. In general, the hepatic microsomal monooxygenase system is characterized by an apparent broad substrate specificity which includes endogenous substrates such as steroids and fatty acids as well as xenobiotics and drugs. From studies in vitro it was demonstrated that the relative reactivities and metabolite patterns varied markedly with species, age, diet, sex, or pretreatment of the animal with drugs, suggesting the presence of several P-450 cytochromes rather than a single monooxygenase. This suggestion has been confirmed by the isolation in hepatic tissues of several cytochrome P-450 species with different, but overlapping, substrate specificities (LU et al. 1972; HAUGEN et al. 1975; DEAN and COON 1977). The monooxygenase reactions are also those most heavily implicated in the generation of reactive intermediates. Two pathways of toxicity considered here are the epoxide–dihydrodiol pathway and the catechol–O-quinone pathway.

It now seems generally established that the mutagenic and carcinogenic effects of polycyclic aromatic hydrocarbons (PAH) are due to the oxidative conversion of the parent compounds to electrophilic metabolites such as epoxides or diolepoxides which react readily with tissue macromolecules and form covalent bonds (JERINA et al. 1971). The hydroxylation of PAH, using benzo[*a*]pyrene (BaP) as a substrate, is one of the most extensively studied drug-oxidizing reactions in the microsomal fraction of the liver and placenta. The main metabolites of BaP are epoxides which are further transformed to several secondary metabolites via spontaneous rearrangement to phenols, catalytic conversion to dihydrodiols by epoxide hydrolase, conjugation to glutathione conjugates occuring both nonenzymatically and enzymically via glutathione *S*-epoxide transferase, or reduction to the parent compound catalyzed by epoxide reductase or occurring spontaneously. The hydroxylation of BaP is catalyzed by a cytochrome P-450-dependent enzyme system which is also termed aryl hydrocarbon hydroxylase (AHH) or BaP hydroxylase (EC 1.14.1.1). Its requirement for molecular oxygen and NADPH categorizes it as a monooxygenase or mixed function oxidase.

PAH are widespread environmental contaminants that are generated by the combustion of organic matter. Interest in these compounds stems from their presence in tobacco smoke, smoked foods, emissions from motor vehicles, etc. The concern over their prevalence arises from the evidence that a significant number is known to be carcinogenic and mutagenic.

Much of the interest in human placental monooxygenase activities and their implications for fetal welfare grew from the findings that human placental tissues could catalyze the hydroxylation of BaP (WELCH et al. 1968; NEBERT 1974). While higher than normal levels of AHH activity can be induced in various tissues of experimental animals, it is of considerable interest that the human placenta also possesses AHH activity with a high degree of inducibility. BaP hydroxylation reactions were observed to proceed at much more rapid rates in placentas from women who smoke (WELCH et al. 1968). Studies from several independent laboratories have confirmed these observations (WELCH et al. 1969; JUCHAU 1971; PELKONEN et al. 1972). This increased hydroxylation has been attributed to induction of the monooxygenase system (or systems) by PAH present in cigarette smoke.

Several laboratories (PELKONEN and KÄRKI 1975; JUCHAU et al. 1976; BERRY et al. 1977; WANG et al. 1977; JUCHAU et al. 1978; VAUGHT et al. 1979) have studied the placental metabolism of BaP. Conflicting results were reported regarding the spectrum of BaP metabolites formed. JUCHAU et al. (1976, 1978) found considerable quantities of phenolic metabolites formed in placentas obtained from mothers who smoke, but only small quantities of dihydrodiols. Results from other investigators (WANG et al. 1977; PELKONEN and KÄRKI 1975; VAUGHT et al. 1979) indicated that large quantities of diols, especially BaP-7,8-diol, were formed in placental preparations. This discrepancy is of interest since the 7,8-diol metabolite has been implicated as a proximate carcinogen. Further studies on this aspect of BaP metabolism were conducted by NAMKUNG and JUCHAU (1980). Their work demonstrated that the use of high substrate concentrations resulted in concentration-dependent increases in ratios of phenols : diols formed. By employing high substrate concentrations (200 μ*M*) in earlier experiments, only minimal quantities of diols appeared in the metabolite profiles. Other laboratories employed much lower BaP concentrations (2.7–63 μ*M*), thus explaining the presence of high quantities of diols in the metabolite profiles. The results are of importance since BaP-7,8-diol generated in placental tissues could be transferred to the fetus and there converted to the highly reactive diolepoxide via P-450 or arachidonate-dependent systems.

While cigarette smoking does result in apparent induction of human placental enzymes which can catalyze conversion of a known carcinogen to reactive metabolites, there is insufficient data as to whether cigarette smoking during pregnancy contributes to the susceptibility to cancer after birth. PELKONEN et al. (1972, 1979) reported that maternal cigarette smoking had no effect on fetal hepatic drug metabolism, but that offspring from pregnancies with elevated AHH weighed about 400 g less and were over 1 cm shorter than offspring from mothers whose placentas exhibited very low AHH activities. The exact causal relationship between cigarette smoking and the birth of smaller infants, however, remains obscure.

In addition to BaP, JUCHAU et al. (to be published) demonstrated that placental monooxygenases can catalyze the hydroxylation of several PAH, including benz[*a*]anthracene, 7,12-dimethylbenz[*a*]anthracene, 7,12-dimethylbenz[*a*]anthracene (DMBA), 3-methylcholanthrene, benzo[*e*]pyrene, chrysene, and dibenz[*a,h*] anthracene. The placental monooxygenases responsible for the hydroxylation of these compounds appeared to be similar to those responsible for the aromatic ring hydroxylations of BaP and *N*-2-fluorenylacetamide (FAA) inasmuch as all activities were elevated in placentas from women who smoke.

Enzymes present in placental tissues also catalyzed the conversion of BaP to metabolites that bound covalently to DNA (BERRY et al. 1977; VAUGHT et al. 1979). Placentas with high AHH activity possessed the greatest capacity to catalyze covalent binding of BaP to DNA. In experiments with *Salmonella typhimurium*, JONES et al. (1977) showed that placental microsomes from smokers catalyzed the formation of mutagenic metabolites of BaP, DMBA, and FAA. Placentas obtained from nonsmokers did not catalyze the conversion of PAH to metabolites mutagenic to strains of *S. typhimurium*. Catechol formation is a route of metabolism for many exogenous aromatic compounds and for many endogenous phenolic compounds (HORNING et al. 1978). Much attention has been directed at this pathway because most natural and synthetic estrogens are known to be metabolized through catechol formation.

The hepatic metabolism of estrogens involves oxidation–reduction of hydroxy or keto groups in ring D, methylations, and conjugations to produce sulfate, glucuronides, or mercapturic acid derivatives, and hydroxylation reactions primarily in positions 2, 4, $6\alpha$, $6\beta$, $7\alpha$, $15\alpha$, and $16\alpha$ (KRAYCHY and GALLAGHER 1957, WILLIAMS et al. 1974). Hydroxylation of $17\beta$-estradiol at positions 2 or 4 yields 2-hydroxyestradiol or 4-hydroxyestradiol, also referred to as catechol estrogens. They undergo further transformation to their *O*-methyl monoethers via COMT. A P-450 cytochrome (or cytochromes) is believed to function in the formation of catechol estrogens (NELSON et al. 1976; SASAME et al. 1977; PAUL et al. 1977; NUMAZAWA et al. 1979). However, it is unknown whether the same cytochrome P-450 is responsible form the formation of both 2- and 4-hydroxyestrogens, or if separate cytochromes are involved.

The catechol estrogens have been regarded as reactive metabolites of estrogens and potentially capable of producing adverse reactions. Although 4-hydroxyestradiol has been demonstrated to have about 10% of the activity of 17 β-estradiol, and 2-hydroxyestradiol has been reported to have weak estrogenic properties, the endocrinologic significance of catechol estrogen formation remains to be determined. The presence of both 2- and 4-hydroxyestrogens has been reported in human tissues and urine (KRAYCHY and GALLAGHER 1957; WILLIAMS et al. 1974). Both 2-and 4-hydroxyestrogens have been found to be excellent inhibitors of the *O*-methylation of catecholamines by COMT, with 2-hydroxyestradiol as the perferred substrate for the enzyme (BALL et al. 1972). 2-Hydroxyestradiol has been reported to inhibit lipid peroxidation, demethylation of mestranol (BOLT and KAPPUS 1976), and to decrease plasma levels of the anterior pituitary luteinizing hormone (PARVIZI and ELLENDORFF 1980).

Placental, as well as fetal enzymes from tissues of humans, stump-tailed macaques (*Macaca arctoides*), rats, and rabbits catalyzed the formation of catechol estrogens when 17 β-estradiol was employed as the substrate (HOFFMAN et al. 1980; CHAO et al. 1980). While the administration of Aroclor 1254 (a mixture of polychlorinated biphenyls) or 3-methylcholanthrene (3-MC) to pregnant rats induced BaP hydroxylase activity in the placenta and fetus (ALVARES and KAPPAS 1975; OMIECINSKI et al. 1980), pretreatment of pregnant rats with phenobarbital, Aroclor 1254, or 3-MC-enhanced catechol estrogen formation in placental microsomes (CHAO et al. 1980). Specific activities of catechol estrogen formation in human and rat placental preparations were considerably less than those observed in adult rat liver preparations; human placental microsomes exhibited consistently much higher activities than rat placental microsomes (Table 1). Phenobarbital and related inducing agents reportedly have no effect on placental drug metabolism

**Table 1.** Catechol estrogen formation in placental microsomes of control and 3-MC-pretreated rats ultilizing the method of PAUL and AXELROD (1977a)

| Experiment[a] | Specific activity (pmol/mg protein/10 min)[b] | |
|---|---|---|
| | Control[c] | 3-MC |
| 1 | 2.1 | 2.8 |
| 2 | 0.9 | 1.2 |
| 3 | 1.9 | 3.8 |
| 4 | 2.2 | 3.1 |
| 5 | ND | 0.8 |
| 6 | 0.3 | 1.0 |
| 7 | ND | 2.6 |
| 8 | 0.1 | 1.8 |
| Mean | $0.94 \pm 0.26$ | $2.14 \pm 0.38$ |

[a] Each experiment was conducted with pooled placental tissues from 3–4 rats

[b] Values expressed are the mean of 2 separate experiments

[c] ND indicates that activity was not detectable. For methods, see CHAO et al. 1980

**Table 2.** Catechol estrogen formation in male and pregnant female rat liver microsomes[a]

| Treatment | Specific activity (pmol/mg protein/10 min)[b] | |
|---|---|---|
| | Male | Pregnant female |
| Experiment 1 | | |
| Control | 1,021 | 74 |
| 3-MC | 873 | 54 |
| Experiment 2 | | |
| Control | 1,049 | 92 |
| 3-MC | 605 | 60 |

[a] Each value is derived from experiments with pooled hepatic tissues from 3–4 rats

[b] Values expressed are the mean of 2 separate experiments

(PELKONEN et al. 1973; TRAEGER et al. 1972; PAPARELLA et al. 1977; JUCHAU 1980a, b). However, pretreatment of pregnant rats with phenobarbital was observed to enhance catechol estrogen formation (CHAO et al. 1980). The extent of induction with phenobarbital, however, was much less pronounced as that seen following pretreatment of pregnant rats with 3-MC or Aroclor 1254.

Exposure to cigarette smoke did not affect human placental aromatase activity (CONNEY and KUNTZMAN 1971; ZACHARIAH and JUCHAU 1977), but did induce catechol estrogen formation as well as BaP monooxygenation in human placentas (CHAO et al. 1980). Pretreatment with 3-MC also produced increases in both parameters in rat placental microsomes. In marked contrast, pretreatment with 3-MC did not increase estrogen hydroxylation in adult rat liver microsomes (Table 2). In fact, in both male and pregnant female livers, pretreatment with 3-MC consistently produced a decrease in catechol estrogen formation at the doses utilized. This suggests that rat hepatic and placental catechol estrogen formation are catalyzed by a separate spectrum of P-450 cytochromes or are under separate regulatory control.

All human placental microsomes studied catalyzed the formation of catechol estrogens. More extensive catechol estrogen formation was observed in placentas that also exhibited high BaP hydroxylase activity. Hematin, which is known to enhance rates of BaP monooxygenation in extrahepatic tissues (OMIECINSKI et al. 1978, 1980), also stimulated catechol estrogen formation in placental tissues (CHAO et al. 1980). These data suggested that various regulatory factors affect the aromatic hydroxylation of 17$\beta$-estradiol and BaP in a similar fashion. However, preliminary studies in our laboratory indicated that, although 17$\beta$-estradiol inhibits BaP monooxygenation, BaP exerted only a slight inhibitory effect on catechol estrogen formation even when concentrations were 100 times greater than that of substrate. This apparent lack of mutual inhibition, as well as quantitative differences in the responses of the two systems to inducing and activating agents, would suggest that the two reactions may be catalyzed by separate cytochrome P-450 enzyme systems.

One indicator for the production of reactive intermediates has been the irreversible (covalent) binding of compounds to cellular macromolecules. Several lab-

**Table 3.** Catechol estrogen formation, BaP hydroxylation and covalent binding of estradiol $^{3}H$ to calf thymus DNA catalyzed by placental microsomes[a]

| Tissue | Catechol estrogen formation (pmol/mg protein/10 min) | BaP hydroxylation (pmol/mg protein/10 min) | Estradiol $^{3}H$ binding to calf thymus DNA (fmol/mg DNA/mg protein/30 min) |
|---|---|---|---|
| Human placental microsomes | | | |
| Nonsmoker | 9.8±2.1 (11) | 40.7± 17.1 (8) | 314.1±62.8 (6) |
| Smoker | 18.1±5.7 ( 8) | 686.9±176.8 (8) | 178.8±71.1 (3) |
| Rat placental microsomes | | | |
| Control | 2.2 | 60.1 | 559.5 |
| 3-MC pretreated | 3.1 | 219.5 | 2,731.7 |
| Rat liver supernatant (9,000 g) | | | |
| Aroclor 1254 pretreated | 99.00 | 827.0 | 4,771.0 |

[a] Specific activities represent the mean±standard error of 2–3 experiments; figures in parentheses give the number of measurements

oratories (MARKS and HECKER 1969; REMMER et al. 1977; TSIBRIS and MCGUIRE 1977) have reported catalysis of the conversion of catechol estrogens by microsomal enzymes to highly reactive electrophilic compounds that bind covalently to hepatic microsomal protein. Estrone, ethinylestradiol, and catechol estrogens reportedly bind covalently to rat liver DNA and proteins in vitro and in vivo (MARKS and HECKER 1969; KAPPUS et al. 1973; JAGGI et al 1978). MARKS and HECKER (1969) have reported that 2-hydroxylation of estrone was required for the binding to occur. They postulated that the reactive intermediate was an *ortho*-semiquinone of 2-hydroxyestrone. However, no studies have employed placental tissues as the enzyme source to catalyze the conversion of estrogenic compounds to intermediates that bind covalently to DNA. Preliminary studies in our laboratory (Table 3) revealed that tritiated 17$\beta$-estradiol would bind covalently to calf thymus DNA when incubated with human placental microsomes or rat placental microsomes as well as with male rat liver 9,000 g supernatant fractions. In rat placentas and liver, the binding to DNA was markedly enhanced by pretreatment of the animals with 3-MC and Aroclor 1254, respectively.

Placental microsomal preparations from both smokers and nonsmokers were capable of bioactivating estradiol $^{3}H$ to intermediates that bound irreversibly to calf thymus DNA. Interestingly however, no correlations were observed between binding to DNA and BaP hydroxylating activity in these human placental preparations. The binding measured was roughly equal in magnitude to the binding oberserved for DMBA to calf thymus DNA with epidermal homogenates of mouse skin as the enzyme source (DIGIOVANNI et al. 1978).

Since estrogens are endogenous compounds, it may be assumed that some covalent binding of estrogens to macromolecules may occur during the normal course of events. REMMER et al. (1977) have calculated that for ethinylestradiol, not more than three microsomal protein molecules in a million are altered by covalent binding. These calculations suggest that the amounts of protein altered by endogenous estrogen would be very small. The existence of protective mechanisms, such as glutathione, glutathione transferring enzymes, enzymic methylation of 2-hydroxyestrogens, etc., is suggested by the decreased protein binding in vivo as compared with the situation in vitro (MARKS and HECKER 1969). However, the extent to which these protective mechanisms occur remains unknown. Further studies should elucidate the significance of reactive estrogen metabolites in human placental tissues.

Spectral studies with human placental microsomes indicated that, although various substances can interact with human placental microsomal cytochrome P-450 to produce type I, type II, and reverse type I spectral changes, most drugs and xenobiotics do not produce type I binding spectra. Steroids, especially those with structures closely similar to androstenedione, produce very intense type I binding spectra and display very high affinities for the placental cytochrome (BERGHEIM et al. 1973; SYMMS and JUCHAU 1973; JUCHAU 1975; JUCHAU and ZACHARIAH 1975). Spectral binding studies by ZACHARIAH et al. (1976) revealed that androstenedione binds either to two separate sites on the same cytochrome, or to two separate cytochromes. Studies with the estrogenic hormones, 17*β*-estradiol, estrone, and estriol also suggested the existence of multiple sites for estrogen binding, or of multiple cytochromes (JUCHAU and CHAO 1977; CHAO and JUCHAU 1980b).

At least five functionally distinct P-450 cytochromes have been postulated to exist in human placental tissues (JUCHAU 1980a) based on indirect data obtained so far. Separate cytochromes are thought to be involved in the aromatization of androstenedione, the hydroxylation of BaP, side chain cleavage of cholesterol, *N*-hydroxylation of *N*-2-fluorenylacetamide, and hydroxylation of 17*β*-estradiol to form catechol estrogens. Research from this laboratory (ZACHARIAH and JUCHAU 1977; JUCHAU and ZACHARIAH 1975; HODGSON and JUCHAU 1977) suggests that virtually all of the spectrally visible cytochrome P-450 in human placental microsomes is functional in the conversion of androgens to estrogen and that the P-450 functional in xenobiotic monooxygenation is spectrally invisible with techniques commonly employed.

Human placental microsomal cytochrome P-450 participates in steroid hydroxylations, and has been identified as a terminal oxygenase in the placental conversion of androgens to estrogens (THOMPSON and SIITERI 1974; CANICK and RYAN 1978; ZACHARIAH and JUCHAU 1977). The aromatization reaction was not increased in placental microsomes obtained from smokers which exhibited increased AHH activity (JUCHAU et al. 1974; CONNEY and KUNTZMAN 1971), suggesting that separate P-450 cytochromes mediate these two reactions. No positive correlations were found between smoking habits and aromatase activity or with cholesterol side chain oxidase activity (JUCHAU et al. 1972). The latter occurs in the mitochondrial fractions of the placenta. An inverse correlation was observed between AHH activity and mitochondrial cholesterol side chain cleavage activities (JUCHAU et al. 1972). CONNEY and KUNTZMAN (1971) also reported no correlation betwen placental aromatase and BaP hydroxylase. Differing sensitivities to CO inhibition, lack of significant reciprocal competitive inhibition by respective substrates, lack of correlations between concentrations and/or spectral properties of human placental cytochrome P-450 (ZACHARIAH et al. 1976; JUCHAU et al. 1974) and lack of capacity of either androsteredione or 19-norandrostenedione to alter the inhibitory effect of CO on human placental AHH activity (ZACHARIAH and JUCHAU 1977) together suggest very strongly that separate cytochromes function in these placental monooxygenase reactions.

Studies from our laboratory (JUCHAU et al. 1975; NAMKUNG et al. 1975) indicated that enzymes in placental tissues of humans and pig-tailed macaques (*Macaca nemestrina*) could catalyze *C*-hydroxylation of FAA at positions 1, 3, 5, and 7 as well as *N*-hydroxylation. Human placental tissues possessed all the necessary enzymes for bioactivation of FAA (NAMKUNG et al. 1977) although activities were lower than those obtained with adult rat liver. While *N*-hydroxylation of FAA was observed to increase in placentas from cigarette smokers, no correlation was noted between 7,3- or 5-hydroxylation of FAA and *N*-hydroxylation of FAA (JUCHAU et al. 1975; JUCHAU 1980a, b), suggesting separate P-450 cytochromes for the *N*- and *C*-hydroxylating reactions. JUCHAU et al. (1978) have also demonstrated both biotransformation and bioactivation of DMBA in human placental tissues.

With regard to the apparent substrate specificity of placental monooxygenation of xenobiotics, positive results have been reported for the *C*-hydroxylations of several PAH, FAA, zoxazolamine, and biphenyl; the *O*-deethylation of 7-ethoxycoumarin, the *N*-demethylations of 3′-methyl-4-monomethylaminoazobenzene, *N*-methylaminobenzoic acid, *N*-methylaniline, and 4-chloromethylaniline, and for the *N*-hydroxylation of FAA. References for each of these reactions have been provided in a recent reviews (JUCHAU 1980a, b; JUCHAU et al. to be published) and evidence for placental catalysis of these reactions is very good. Negative results have been reported with respect to catalysis of oxidative *N*-demethylations of aminopyrine (JUCHAU and DYER 1972), ethylmorphine (CHAKRABORTY et al. 1971), meperidine (VAN PETTEN et al. 1968), and a large number of other substrates in human placental homogenates. In general, substances whose oxidative metabolism in hepatic tissues is increased by phenobarbital pretreatment do not appear to be substrates for placental monooxygenases.

## C. Reduction Reactions

Catalysis of the reduction of several substrates in human placental preparations has been observed in our laboratory (JUCHAU 1968; JUCHAU et al. 1968; JUCHAU and YAFFE 1969). Reduction of aromatic nitro groups to the corresponding primary amines has been studied in placental preparations, and the activities have been very low in comparison with rat liver unless flavin is added to the incubation mixture (JUCHAU and ZACHARIAH 1975). 3-MC or phenobarbital pretreatment of experimental animals did not produce any observable effect on the placental nitroreductase activity.

Data from studies on the reduction of aromatic nitro groups indicated that reduced pyridine nucleotide plus a flavin plus any one of several purified heme-containing compounds (hemoglobin, catalase, peroxidase methemoglobin, cytochromes c, $b_5$, P-450, P-420, and even hematin per se) would catalyze the reduction of nitro groups to primary amines (SYMMS and JUCHAU 1972). This indicated that any tissue possessing such components would catalyze the reaction, provided that the oxygen tension was sufficiently low.

JUCHAU and ZACHARIAH (1975) found, in studies on the enzymatic catalysis of the azo linkage reduction of neoprontosil, that activity was very low or negligible in microsomal fractions of human placentas. Additional studies utilizing 3′-methyl-4-monomethylaminoazobenzene or 4-dimethylaminoazobenzene also revealed that no detectable reductive cleavage of the azo linkages of these two compounds occurred in placental particulate preparations (JUCHAU 1973). It has also been noted that intestinal bacterial play a major role in the reduction of both azo linkages and aromatic nitro groups in vivo, and that placental tissues probably play only a very minor role in these processes (JUCHAU 1980a). Other reduction reactions, such as aldehyde reduction, sulfoxide reduction, dehydroxylation, reductive dehalogenation, and others have not been studied with regard to placental xenobiotic metabolism to our knowledge. The generation of reactive metabolites via reduction pathways in placental tissues, and the significance regarding their possible toxicity, therefore, remain to be determined.

## D. Hydrolytic Reactions

Hydrolases are quite ubiquitous in mammalian tissues, and frequently display less substrate specificity than other enzyme classes. Hypothetically, placental hydrolases may play an important role in the regulation of the endocrinology of pregnancy. Since placental hydrolases can catalyze hydrolysis of several endogenous compounds, their function in the metabolism of drugs and xenobiotics with hydrolyzable moieties is of interest.

Hydrolysis of drugs and xenobiotic substrates in placental tissues has not been investigated systematically, and the toxicologic significance of these reactions is not understood at present. Xenobiotics which have been reported to undergo hydrolysis in human placental preparations include meperidine (VAN PETTEN et al. 1968), acetylsalicylic acid, procaine (JUCHAU and YAFFE 1969), naphthyl phosphates, phenyl phosphates phenolic and catechol sulfates (HAGERMAN 1969), naphthyl acetate, norethindrone acetate, 5-bromoindoxyl acetate, choline esters, and naphthol-$\beta$-*D*-glucuronide (HAGERMAN 1969). However, the extent to which contaminating plasma esterases catalyzed these reactions was not ascertained.

Neutral arylamidases (EC 3.4.11.2) are present in placental tissues (HIWADA et al. 1977) and catalyze the hydrolysis of neutral amino acid arylamides. They also catalyze the hydrolysis of xenobiotics such as L-alanyl-$\beta$-naphthylamide and L-leucyl-$\beta$-naphthylamide. Aminopeptidase activity has been found in human placentas, and studies by OYA et al. (1976) indicate that aminopeptidase activities are distributed in three subcellular sites: lysosomal–mitochondrial, microsomal, and supernatant fractions. Multiple molecular forms of aminopeptidase are postulated to exist within the human placenta. Aminopeptidase are involved in the hydrolysis of oxytocin, and it is generally believed that oxytocinase is identical with cystine aminopeptidase (EC 3.4.11.3; MELANDER 1965). Oxytocinase catalyzes hydrolysis of the peptide bond between $NH_2$-terminal cystine and adjacent tyrosine, resulting in the loss of the biologic effect of oxytocin. Since oxytocin is an important hormone in the control of parturition, placental oxytocinase activity may play a major role in pregnancy outcome.

Possibly the most interesting of the hydrolytic enzymes are the epoxide hydrolases, a group of enzymes that catalyzes the conversion of alkene and arene oxides to their corresponding dihydrodiols. For the great majority of cases, the reaction represents a detoxification mechanism since the diols exhibit far less biologic activity than the epoxides. In the case of polycyclic aromatic hydrocarbons with bay-region epoxides, however, expoxide hydrolases can catalyze the conversion of epoxides to diols that are proximate mutagens and carcinogens. The best example is the conversion of BaP-7,8-oxide to BaP-7,8-diol which, upon subsequent monooxygenation, is converted to the very highly reactive 7,8-diol-9,10-epoxide. Placentas of both humans (JUCHAU and NAMKUNG 1974; VAUGHT et al. 1979) and experimental animals (BEND et al. 1975; BERRY et al. 1977) exhibit very low epoxide hydrolase activities and preexposure to inducing agents such as 3 MC does not increase the activities. This scenario would appear to predispose to the generation of reactive intermediates in placental tissues, except, perhaps, in the case of PAH with bay-regions.

## E. Conjugation Reactions

Conjugation of xenobiotics with water-soluble endogenous compounds has been regarded as important in the prevention and/or termination of toxic effects. The presence of various transferase enzymes which catalyze these conjugation reactions plays an important role in preventing the toxic effects of xenobiotics.

Uridine diphosphoglucuronyl transferase (UDPGT, EC 2.4.1.17) catalyzes the transfer of the glucuronic acid moiety from uridine diphosphoglucuronic acid (UDPGA) to a variety of acceptor groups on drug molecules. Steroids and bilirubin are some of the more important endogenous acceptors. Attempts to demonstrate glucuronidation of these substrates in placental preparations have indicated either very low or negligible activity (TROEN et al. 1966). JUCHAU and YAFFE (1969) were unable to demonstrate glucuronidation of p-aminophenol placental homogenates from early gestation or term. Glucuronide conjugation of bilirubin, estrogens, or p-nitrophenol could not be observed in placentas of humans and experimental animals (DUTTON 1966). Glucuronidation reactions are thus generally not considered to be extensively catalyzed by placental tissues.

Nevertheless, BERTE et al. (1966) and AITIO (1974) have reported UDPGT activity in placentas of rats, rabbits, and guinea pigs. Activities, in most instances, were extremely low when compared with those obtained with hepatic preparations. Pretreatment of pregnant rats with 2,3,7,8-tetrachlorodibenzo-p-dioxin (TCDD), a potent inducing agent of the 3-MC type, reportedly increased the rate of placentally catalyzed glucuronidation a p-nitrophenol (LUCIER et al. 1975).

The placental catalysis of sulfate transfer via aryl sulfotransferase from 3′-phosphoadenosine-5′-phosphosulfate (PAPS) to various steroid acceptors has been reported (HAGERMAN 1969). Human placentas wre found to be less active than bovine placentas. Catalysis of the sulfonation of many phenolic substrates (7-hydroxy-*N*-2-fluorenylacetamide, 17$\beta$-estradiol, diethylstilbestrol, and morphine) was detectable in preparations of placental tissues form humans and guinea pigs (NAMKUNG et al. 1977). These reactions proceeded at relatively rapid rates, but placental sulfonation of *N*-hydroxy-FAA was low to negligible in humans and guinea pigs.

Several laboratories have reported acylation of xenobiotics possessing primary amino groups (VAN PETTEN et al. 1968; JUCHAU and YAFFE 1969; BERTE et al. 1969).

Among the acylation reactions (acetylation, glycine conjugation, and glutamine conjugation) involving xenobiotics, placental acetylations have received the most attention. However, the possible contribution of contaminating blood in placental homogenate fractions should not be overlooked since blood is known to contain acetyl transferase activity.

In terms of chemical toxicity, glutathione conjugation is now recognized as an extremely important reaction. Reduced glutathione can form covalent bonds with reactive, electrophilic methabolites, and is regarded as a prime detoxification mechanism. JUCHAU and NAMKUNG (1974) observed that human placental tissues would catalyze the conversion of epoxides to glutathione conjugates at relatively rapid rates. Glutathione *S*-transferase has also been detected in the placentas of guinea pigs (BEND et al. 1975) and rabbits (JAMES et al. 1977). These investigators also reported relatively rapid reactions.

Other conjugation reactions studied include conjugation of glycine with p-aminobenzoic acid (JUCHAU and YAFFE 1969) and methylation. Methylation seems to be a possible mechanism for placental xenobiotic metabolism since several endogenous substrates undergo methylation in placental tissues. For example, *N*-methylation of the imidazole ring of histamine and O-methylation of the 2-hydroxyl group of estrogens proceed within the placenta. Foreign acceptor molecules, however, have not been studied to our knowledge. Human placental COMT has been isolated and partially characterized in a purified form (GUGLER er al. 1970). α-Methyldopa, L-dopa, epinephrine, and norepinephrine are also substrates for placental COMT. Important drug conjugation reactions which remain to be studied in placental tissues include glutamine conjugation, glucoside formation, mercaturic acid formation, riboside formation, and thiocyanate formation.

## References


Aitio A (1974) UDP-glucuronosyl-transferase of the human placenta. Biochem Pharmacol 23:2203–2205

Alvares AP, Kappas A (1975) Induction of aryl hydrocarbon hydroxylase by polychlorinated biphenyls in the foeto-placental unit and neonatal livers during lactation. FEBS Lett 50:172–174

Ball P, Knuppen R, Haupt M, Breuer H (1972) Interactions between estrogens and catecholamines III. Studies on the methylation of catechol estrogens, catecholamines and other catechols by the catechol-o-methyltransferase of human liver. J Clin Endocrinol Metab 34:736–746

Bend JR, James MO, Devereux TR, Fouts JR (1975) Toxication-detoxication systems in hepatic and extrahepatic tissues in the perinatal period. In: Morselli PL, Garattini S, Sereni F (eds) Basic and therapeutic aspects of perinatal pharmacology. Raven Press New York

Bergheim P, Rathgen GH, Netter KJ (1973) Interaction of drugs and steroids with human placental microsomes. Biochem Pharmacol 22:1633–1645

Berry DL, Zachariah PK, Slaga TJ, Juchau MR (1977) Analysis of the biotransformation of benzol[a]pyrene in human fetal and placental tissues with high pressure liquid chromatography. Eur J Cancer 13:667–675

Berte F, Manzo L, DeBernardi M, Benzi G (1969) Ability of the placenta to metabolize oxazepam and aminopyrine before and after drug stimulation. Arch Int Pharmacodyn 182:182–188

Bolt HM, Kappus H (1976) Interaction by 2-hydroxyestrogens with enzymes of drug metabolism. J Steroid Biochem 7:311–313

Bond JA, Omiecinski CJ, Juchau MR (1979) Kinetics, activation and induction of aortic monooxygenases: analysis of the mixed function oxidation of benzo[a]pyrene with high pressure liquid chromatography. Biochem Pharmacol 28:305–312
Canick JA, Ryan KS (1978) Properties of the aromatase system associated with the mitochondrial fraction of the human placenta. Steroids 32:499–509
Chakraborty J, Hopkins R, Parke DV (1971) Biological oxygenation of drugs and steroids in the placenta. Biochem J 125:15–16
Chao ST, Juchau MR (1980a) Cytochrome P-450 mixed function oxygenases in placental tissue: metabolism of endogenous and exogenous compounds. Proc West Pharmacol Soc 23:3–7
Chao ST, Juchau MR (1980b) Interactions of endogenous and exogenous estrogenic compounds with human placental microsomal cytochrome P-450 (P-450 hpm) J Steroid Biochem 13:127–133
Chao ST, Omiecinski CJ, Namkung MJ, Nelson SD, Dvorchik BH, Juchau MR (1981) Catechol estrogen formation in placental and fetal tissues of humans, macaques, rats and rabbits. Dev Pharmacol Ther 2:1–17
Conney AH (1967) Pharmacological implications of enzyme induction. Pharmacol Rev 19:317–366
Conney AH, Kuntzman R (1971) Metabolism of normal body constituents by drug metabolizing enzymes in liver microsomes. In: Brodie BB, Gillette JR (eds) Concepts in chemical pharmacology. 2. Springer, Berlin Heidelberg New York
Dean WL, Coon MJ (1977) Immunological studies on two electrophoretically homogenous forms of rabbit liver microsomal P-450, P-450LM$_2$ and P-450 LM$_4$. J Biol Chem 252:3255–3261
DeMaria FJ, See HYC (1966) Role of the placenta in pre-eclampsia. Am J Obstet Gynecol 94:471–476
DiGiovanni J, Slaga TJ, Viaje A, Berry DL, Harvey RG, Juchau MR (1978) Effects of 7,8-benzoflavone on skin tumor-initiating activities of various 7- and 12-substituted derivatives of 7,12-dimethylbenz[a]anthracene in mice. J Natl Cancer Inst 67:135–140
Dutton GJ (1966) The biosynthesis of glucuronides. In: Dutton GJ (ed) Glucuronic acid: free and combined. Chemistry, biochemistry, pharmacology, and medicine. Academic Press New York
Fantel AG, Greenaway JC, Shepard TH, Juchau MR (1979) Cytochrome P-450 dependent teratogenic action of cyclophosphamide. Fed Proc 38:473A
Gillette JR, Mitchell JR, Brodie BB (1974) Biochemical mechanisms of drug toxicity. Annu Rev Pharmacol 14:271–288
Gram TE (ed) (1980) Extrahepatic metabolism of drugs and other foreign compounds. Spectrum, New York
Gugler R, Knuppen R, Breuer H (1970) Reinigung und Charakterisierung einer S-Adenosyl-methionine: Catechol-O-methyltransferase der menschlichen Placenta. Biochim Biophys Acta 220:10–21
Hagerman DD (1964) Enzymatic capabilities of the placenta. Fed Proc 23:785–790
Hagerman DD (1969) Enzymology of the placenta. In. Klopper A, Diczfalusy E (eds) Foetus and placenta. Blackwell, Oxford
Haugen DA, Van der Hoeven JA, Coon MJ (1975) Purified liver microsomal cytochrome P-450: separation and characterization of multiple forms. J Biol Chem 250:3567–3570
Heidelberger C (1975) Chemical carcinogenesis. Annu Rev Biochem 44:79–121
Herbst AL, Ulfelder H, Poskanzer DC (1971) Adenocarcinoma of the vagina. Association of maternal stilboestrol therapy with tumor appearance in young women. N Engl J Med 284:878–881
Hill RM (1973) Drugs ingested by pregnant women. Clin Pharmacol Ther 14:654–659
Hiwada K, Terao M, Nishimura K, Kokubu T (1977) Comparison of human membrane-bound neutral arylamidases from small intestine, lung, kidney, liver and placenta. Clin Chim Acta 76:267–275
Hodgson E, Juchau MR (1977) Ligand binding to human placenta cytochrome P-450: interaction of steroids and heme-binding ligands. J Steroid Biochem 8:669–677
Hoffman AR, Paul SM, Axelrod J (1980) Estrogen-2-hydroxylase in the rat. Distribution and response to hormonal manipulation. Biochem Pharmacol 29:83–87

Horning EC, Thenot JP, Helton ED (1978) Toxic agents resulting from the oxidative metabolism of steroid hormones and drugs. J Toxicol Environ Health 4:341–361
Huberman E, Sachs L (1977) DNA binding and its relationship to carcinogenesis by different polycyclic hydrocarbons. Int J Cancer 19:122–127
Iisalo E, Castren O (1967) The enzymatic inactivation of noradrenaline in human placental tissue. Ann Med Exp Biol Fenn 45:253–257
Jaggi W, Lutz WK, Schlatter C (1978) Covalent binding of ethinylestradiol and estrone to rat liver DNA in vivo. Chem Biol Interact 23:13–18
James MO, Foureman GL, Law FC, Bend JR (1977) The perinatal development of epoxide-metabolizing enzyme activities in liver and extrahepatic organs of guinea pig and rabbit. Drug Metab Dispos 5:19–28
Jerina DM, Kaubisch N, Daly JW (1971) Arene oxides as intermediates in the metabolism of aromatic substrates: alkyl and oxygen migrations during isomerization of alkylated arene oxides. Proc Nat Acad Sci USA 68:2545–2548
Jones AH, Fantel AG, Kocan RA, Juchau MR (1977) Bioactivation of procarcinogens to mutagens in human fetal and placental tissues. Life Sci 21:1831–1836
Juchau MR (1969) Studies on the reduction of aromatic nitro groups in human and rodent placental homogenates. J Pharmacol Exp Ther 165:1–8
Juchau MR (1971) Human placental hydroxylation of 3,4-benzpyrene during early gestation and term. Toxicol Appl Pharmacol 18:665–675
Juchau MR (1973) Placental metabolism in relation to toxicology. CRC Crit Rev Toxicol 2:125–159
Juchau MR (1978) Mixed-function oxidation in the human placenta. In: Morselli PL, Garrattini S, Sereni F (eds) Basic therapeutic aspects of perinatal pharmacology. Raven, New York, pp 29–39
Juchau MR (1980a) Extra-hepatic drug metabolism: The placenta. In: Gram TE (ed) Monographs in drug metabolism: extra-hepatic metabolism of drugs and other foreign compounds. Spectrum Publications, Holliswood, NY, pp 211–239
Juchau MR (1980b) Drug biotransformation in the placenta. Pharmacol Ther 8:501–524
Juchau MR, Chao ST (1977) Interactions of contraceptive steroids with human placental cytochrome P-450 (P-450hpm). Fed Proc 36:1034
Juchau MR, Dyer DC (1972) Pharmacology of the placenta. Pediatr Clin North Am 19:65–79
Juchau MR, Namkung MJ (1974) Studies on biotransformation of naphthalene-1,2-oxide in fetal and placental tissues of humans and monkeys. Drug Metab Dispos 2:380–386
Juchau MR, Yaffe SJ (1969) Biotransformation of drug substrates in placental homogenates. In: Pecile A, Finzi C (eds) The foeto-placental unit. Int Congr Ser No 183. Excerpta Med Found, Amsterdam, pp 260–271
Juchau MR, Zachariah PK (1975) Comparative studies on the oxidation and reduction of drug substrates in human placental versus rat hepatic microsomes. Biochem Pharmacol 24:227–233
Juchau MR, Krasner J, Yaffe SJ (1968) Studies on reduction of azo linkages in human placental homogenates. Biochem Pharmacol 17:1969–1979
Juchau MR, Lee QH, Blake PH (1972) Inverse correlation between aryl hydrocarbon hydroxylase activity and conversion of cholesterol to pregnenolone in human placentas at term. Life Sci 11:949–956
Juchau MR, Symms KG, Zachariah PK (1974) Drug metabolizing enzymes in the placenta. In: Dancis J, Hwang JC (eds) Perinatal pharmacology, Raven, New York, pp 89–101
Juchau MR, Namkung MJ, Berry DL, Zachariah PK (1975) Oxidative biotransformation of 2-acetylaminofluorene in fetal and placental tissues of humans and monkeys: Correlations with aryl hydrocarbon hydroxylase activities. Drug Metab Dispos 3:494–502
Juchau MR, Berry DL, Zachariah PK, Namkung MJ, Slaga TJ (1976) Prenatal biotransformation of benzo[a]pyrene and N-2-fluorenylacetamide in human and subhuman primates. In: Jones PW, Freudenthal R (eds) Carcinogenesis: a comprehensive survey, vol 1. Raven, New York, pp 23–35
Juchau MR, Namkung MJ, Jones AH, DiGiovanni J (1978) Biotransformation and bioactivation of 7,12-dimethylbenz[a]-anthracene in human fetal and placental tissues. Drug Metab Dispos 6:273–281

Juchau MR, Chao ST, Namkung MJ (to be published) Metabolism of polycyclic aromatic hydrocarbons in the placenta. In: Jollow DJ, Parke DV, Snyder R (eds) Biological reactive intermediates, vol 2. Plenum, New York

Kappus H, Bolt H, Remmer H (1973) Irreversible protein binding of metabolites of ethynylestradiol in vivo and in vitro. Steroids 22:203–225

Koren Z (1965) The significance of monoamine oxidase in amniotic fluid in human foetal development. J Obstet Gynaecol Br Common 72:775–777

Kouri M, Koivula T, Koivusalo M (1977) Aldehyde dehydrogenase activity in human placenta. Acta Toxicol 40:460–463

Krasner J, Tischler F, Yaffe SJ (1976) Human placental alcohol dehydrogenase. J Med 7:323–332

Kraychy S, Gallagher TF (1957) 2-Methoxyestrone, a new metabolite of estradiol-17 in man. J Biol Chem 229:519–526

Lu AYH, Kuntzman R, West S, Jacobson M, Conney AH (1972) Reconstituted liver microsomal enzyme system that hydroxylates drugs, other foreign compounds and endogenous substrates. J Biol Chem 247:1727–1734

Lucier GW, Sonawane BR, McDaniel OS, Hook GER (1975) Postnatal stimulation of hepatic microsomal enzymes following administration of TCDD to pregnant rats. Chem Biol Interact 11:15–26

Marks F, Hecker E (1969) Metabolism and mechanism of action of estrogens. XII. Structure and mechanism of formation of water soluble and protein-bound metabolites of oestrone in rat liver microsomes in vitro and in vivo. Biochim Biophys Acta 187:250–265

Melander S (1965) Plasma oxytocinase activity. Acta Endocrinol [Suppl 48] (Copenh) 96:1–94

Miller EC, Miller JA (1966) Mechanisms of chemical carcinogensis:nature of proximate carcinogens and interactions with macromolecules. Pharmacol Rev 18:805–838

Miller JA (1970) Carcinogenesis by chemicals: an overview. Cancer Res 30:559–576

Morgan CD, Sandler M, Panigel M (1972) Placental transfer of catecholamines in vitro an in vivo. Am J Obstet Gynecol 112:1068–1074

Namkung MJ, Juchau MR (1980) On the capacity of human placental enzymes to catalyze the formation of diols from benzo[a]pyrene. Toxicol Appl Pharmacol in press

Namkung MJ, Berry DL, Zachariah PK, Juchau MR (1975) Biotransformation of 2-acetylaminofluorene (AFF) and benzo[a]pyrene (BP) in fetal and placental tissues of humans and monkeys. The Pharmacologist. 17:208–209

Namkung M, Zachariah PK, Juchau MR (1977) O-Sulfonation of N-hydroxy-2-fluorenylacetamide or 7-hydroxy-N-2-fluorenyl-acetamide in fetal and placental tissues of humans and guiena pigs. Drug Metabl Dispos 5:288–294

Nebert DW (1974) Genetic and environmental factors affecting placental and fetal metabolism of xenobiotics. In: Moghissi KS, Hafez ESE (eds) The placenta. Thomas, Springfield, IL, pp 207–238

Nelson SD, Mitchell JR, Dybing E, Sasame HA (1976) Cytochrome P-450 mediated oxidation of 2-hydroxy-estrogens to reactive intermediates. Biochem Biophys Res Commun 70:1157–1165

Nelson SD, Boyd MR, Mitchell JR (1977) Role of metabolic activation in chemical-induced tissue injury. In: Jerina DM 8ed) Drug metabolism concepts. Proc. 172nd meeting American chemical society held in San Francisco, Calif; ACS Symposium Series, Washington, DC, pp 155–188

Numazawa M, Soeda N, Kuyono Y, Nambara T (1979) Properties of estradiol 2-hydroxylase and 2-hydroxy-3-deoxyestradiol 3-hydroxylase in rat liver. J Steroid Biochem 10:227–233

Omiecinski CJ, Bond JA, Juchau MR (1978) Stimulation by hematin of monooxygenase activity in extra-hepatic tissues from rats, rabbits and chickens. Biochem Biophys Res Commun 83:1004–1011

Omiecinski CJ, Chao ST, Juchau MR (1980) Modulation of monooxygenase activities by hematin and 7,8-benzoflavone in fetal tissues of rats, rabbits and humans. Dev Pharmacol Ther 1:90–100

Oya M, Wakabayashi T, Yoshino M, Mizutami S (1976) Subcellular distribution and electrophoretic behavior of aminopeptidase in human placenta. Physiol Chem Phys 8:327–335

Paparella P, Castaldo F, Terranova T, Romor R, Bompiani A (1977) The behavior of microsomal monoelectron carriers in adult and fetal liver and placenta throughout pregnancy. Acta Obstet Gynecol Scand 56:173–178

Parvizi N, Ellendorff E (1980) Recent views on endocrine effects of catecholestrogens. J Steroid Biochem 12:331–335

Paul SM, Axelrod J, Diliberto EJ (1977) Catechol estrogen-forming enzyme of brain: demonstration of a cytochrome P-450 monooxygenase. Endocrinology 101:1604–1610

Pelkonen O, Karki NT (1975) Epoxidation of xenobiotics in the human fetus and placenta: A possible mechanism of transplacental drug-induced injuries. Biochem Pharmacol 24:1445–1448

Pelkonen O, Jouppilla P, Karki NT (1972) Effect of maternal cigarette smoking on 3,4-benzpyrene and N-methylaniline metabolism in human fetal liver and placenta. Toxicol Appl Pharmacol 23:399–407

Pelkonen O, Jouppila P, Karki NT (1973) Attempts to induce drug metabolism in human fetal liver and placenta by the administration of phenobarbital to mothers. Arch Int Pharmacodyn Ther 202:288–297

Pelkonen O, Karki NT, Koivisto M, Tuimala R, Kauppila A (1979) Maternal cigarette smoking, placental aryl hydrocarbon hydroxylase and neonatal size. Toxicol Lett (Amst) 3:331–335

Poulsen E, Robson JM (1964) Effect of phenelzine and some related compounds on pregnancy and sexual development. J Endocrinol 30:205–215

Remmer H, Schenlen M, Kappus H, Bolt HM (1977) The significance of covalent binding of catechols to proteins in vivo. Arch Toxicol 39:31–39

Sasame HA, Ames MA, Nelson SC (1977) Cytochrome P-450 and NADPH cytochrome C reductase in rat brain: Formation of catechol and reactive catechol metabolites. Biochem Biophys Res Commun 78:919–926

Sjoblom M, Pilstrom L, Morland J (1978) Activity of alcohol dehydrogenase and acetyldehyde dehydrogenases in the liver and placenta during the development of the rat. Enzyme 23:108–115

Symms KG, Juchau MR (1972) Mechanism of aromatic nitro group reduction in the soluble fraction of human placenta. Biochem Pharmacol 21:2519–2527

Symms KG, Juchau MR (1973) Stabilization, solubilization, partial purification and some properties of cytochrome P-450 present in $CaCl_2$-precipitated human placental microsomes. Life Sci 13:1221–1230

Szabo AJ, Grimaldi RD (1970) The metabolism of the placenta. Adv Metab Disord 4:185–228

Thompson EA Jr, Siiteri PK (1974) The involvement of human placental microsomal P-450 in aromatization. J Biol Chem 249:5373–5378

Thompson RHS, Tickner A (1949) Observations on the monoamine oxidase activity of placenta and uterus. Biochem J 45:125–130

Traeger A, Hoffman H, Franke H, Gunther M (1972) Untersuchungen über den Einfluß von Phenobarbital auf arzneimittelabbauende Enzyme in der menschlichen Placenta, auf die Feinstruktur der Chorionzotten und den Verlauf der Serumbilirubin-Konzentration Neugeborener. Z. Geburtshilfe Perinatol 176:397–402

Troen P, DeMiguel M, Alonso C (1966) Perfusion studies of the human placenta. IV. Conjugation of estriol-16-$^{14}C$. Biochemistry 5:332–337

Tsibris JCM, McGuire PM (1977) Microsomal activation of estrogens and binding to nucleic acids and proteins. Biochem Biophys Res Commun 78:411–417

Van Petten GR, Hirsch GH, Cherrington AD (1968) Drug metabolizing activity of the human placenta. Can J Biochem 46:1057–1064

Vaught JB, Gurtoo HL, Parker NB, LeBoeuf R, Doctor G (1979) Effects of smoking on benzo[a]pyrene metabolism by human placental microsomes. Cancer Res 39:3177–3183

Wang IY, Rasmussen RE, Creasey R, Crocker TT (1977) Metabolites of benzo[a]pyrene produced by placental microsomes from cigarette smokers and non-smokers. Life Sci 20:1265–1272

Welch RM, Harrison YE, Conney AH, Poppers PJ, Finster J (1968) Cigarette smoking: stimulatory effect on metabolism of 3,4-benzpyrene by enzymes in humans placenta. Sciencie 160:541–542

Welch RM, Harrison YE, Gomni BW, Poppers PJ, Finster M, Conney AH (1969) Stimulatory effects of cigarette smoking on the hydroxylation of 3,4-benzpyrene and the N-demethylation of 3-methyl-4-monomethylaminoazobenzene by enzymes in human placentas. Clin Pharmacol Ther 10:100–115

Williams JB, Longcope C, Williams KIH (1974) 4-hydroxyestrone: a new metabolite of estradiol-17 from humans. Steroids 24:687–701

Zachariah PK, Juchau MR (1977) Inhibition of human placental mixed-function oxidations with carbon monoxide: Reversal with monochromatic light. J Steroid Biochem 8:221–228

Zachariah PK, Lee OP, Symms KG, Juchau MG (1976) Further studies on the properties of human placental microsomal cytochrome P-450. Biochem Pharmacol 25:793–800

CHAPTER 4

# Genetic Differences in Drug Metabolism: Proposed Relationship to Human Birth Defects

D. W. NEBERT

## A. Introduction

Pharmacogenetics research involves the attempt to understand the hereditary basis for two individuals (with the possible exception of identical twins) responding differently to drugs or other foreign chemicals. These responses include therapeutic effects (e.g., control of seizures), but also undesirable effects (e.g., increased risk of drug toxicity or cancer). The experimental model to be examined in detail in this chapter represents principally a genetic difference in receptor concentration. Because of this defect, there are large genetic differences in the biotransformation and pharmacokinetics of certain drugs and other environmental pollutants, resulting in important variations in risk toward birth defects, drug toxicity, mutation, and certain types of cancer.

First the general characteristics of the drug-metabolizing enzymes are described. Second, the genetic differences in this model system in mice are examined. How these differences are associated with increased risk toward birth defects and other intrauterine toxicity is then presented. Last, the presence of this same genetic system in humans is discussed briefly.

### I. Phase I and Phase II Drug-Metabolizing Enzymes

Most drugs and other environmental pollutants are so fat soluble that they would remain in the body indefinitely were it not for the metabolism resulting in more water-soluble derivatives. These enzyme systems, located principally in the liver (but also present to some degree in virtually all tissues of the body), are usually divided into two groups: phase I and phase II. During phase I metabolism, one or more water-soluble groups (such as hydroxyl) are introduced into the fat-soluble parent molecule, thus allowing a "handle", or a position, for the phase II conjugating enzymes to attack. Many phase I products, but especially the conjugated phase II products, are sufficiently water soluble so that these chemicals are excreted readily from the body [(detoxication); WILLIAMS 1959].

### II. Fundamental Aspects of Cytochrome P-450

The majority of all phase I oxidations[1] is performed by cytochrome P-450. Cytochrome, derived from Greek, literally means "colored substance in the cell." The color is derived from the subatomic properties of the iron in this hemoprotein, and, indeed, cytochromes appear reddish in color when sufficient concentrations exist in the test tube. P-450 denotes a reddish pigment with the unusual property of having its major optical absorption peak (Soret maximum) at about 450 nm, when the material has been reduced and combined with carbon monoxide (OMURA and SATO 1964). Although the name P-450 was intended to be temporary, until more knowledge about this substance was known, the terminology has persisted for almost two decades now, because of the increasing complexity of this enzyme system which is revealed with each passing year, and because of the lack of agreement on any better nomenclature.

## III. Assessment of Substrates Metabolized by Cytochrome P-450

Cytochrome P-450 represents a large family of an unknown number of isozymes possessing catalytic activity toward thousands of substrates. This collection of enzymes is known to metabolize: almost all drugs and laboratory reagents; small chemicals, such as benzene, thiocyanate, or ethanol; polycyclic aromatic hydrocarbons, such as benzo[a]pyrene (BaP) (ubiquitous in city smog, cigarette smoke and charcoal-cooked foods) and biphenyl; halogenated hydrocarbons, such as polychlorinated and polybrominated biphenyls, defoliants, insecticides, and ingredients in soaps and deodorants; certain fungal toxins and antibiotics; many of the chemotherapeutic agents used to treat human cancer; strong mutagens, such as *N*-methyl-*N′*-nitro-*N*-nitrosoguanidine and nitrosamines; aminoazo dyes and diazo compounds; many chemicals found in cosmetics and perfumes; numerous aromatic amines, such as those found in hair dyes, nitroaromatics, and heterocyclics; *N*-acetylarylamines and nitrofurans; wood terpenes; epoxides; carbamates; alkyl halides; safrole derivatives; antioxidants, other food additives, and many ingredients of foodstuffs, fermentative alcoholic beverages, and spices; both endogenous and synthetic steroids; prostaglandins; and other endogenous compounds, such as biogenic amines, indoles, thyroxine, and fatty acids.

The evidence now is very convincing that metabolism to reactive intermediates (toxification) by the cytochrome P-450-mediated enzymes is a prerequisite for toxicity, teratogenesis, mutagenesis, and carcinogenesis caused by numerous drugs, polycyclic hydrocarbons, and other environmental pollutants. These reactive intermediates bind covalently to numerous cellular macromolecules. Most of this binding is probably random. The steady-state levels of these reactive intermediates and, consequently, the rates at which they interact with critical subcellular targets are dependent upon a delicate balance between toxification and detoxication. Changes in this balance in any particular tissue of an individual may therefore affect the risk of toxicity or tumorigenesis. An important mechanism of action of toxic, teratogenic, or carcinogenic foreign chemicals is related to the genetic control of enzymes which metabolize these substrates to reactive intermediates.

---

1 In this chapter, cytochrome P-450 is defined as all forms of CO-binding hemoproteins associated with membrane-bound NADPH-dependent monooxygenase activities; cytochrome $P_1$-450 is defined as all forms of CO-binding hemoprotein that increase in amount concomitantly with rises in induced aryl hydrocarbon hydroxylase activity following polycyclic aromatic inducer treatment. In view of the existence of more than one such form of $P_1$-450 (LANG and NEBERT 1981; LANG et al. 1981), it is emphasized that this definition of $P_1$-450 is simplistic

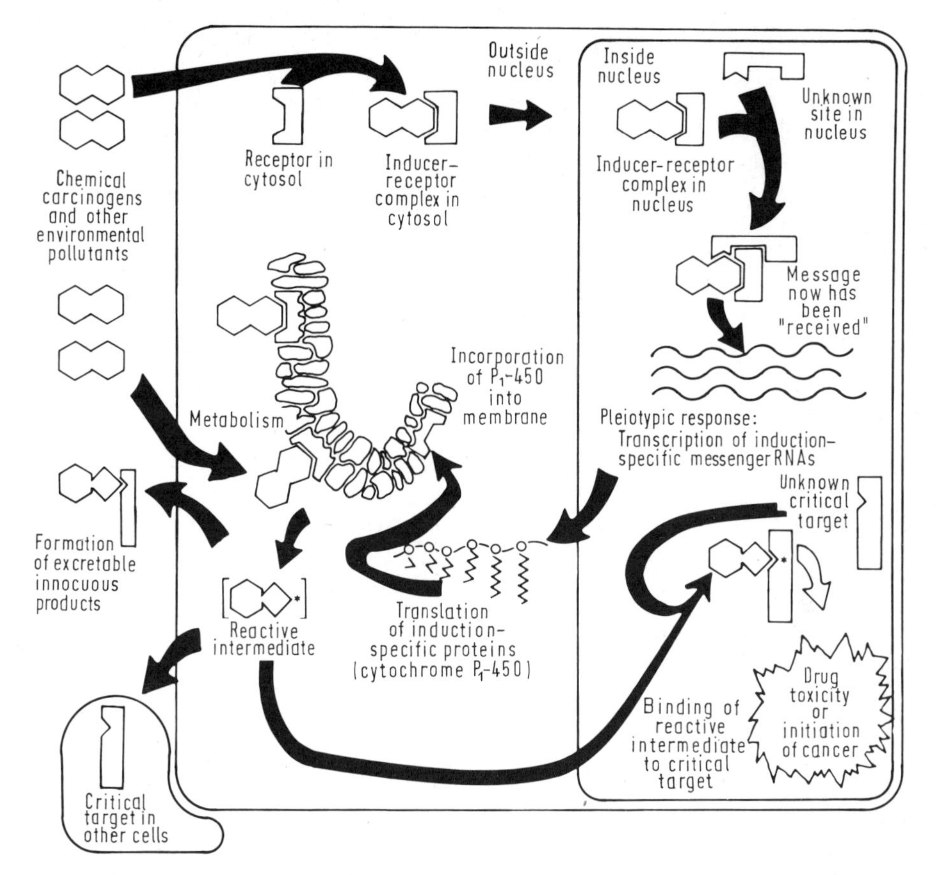


**Fig. 1.** Diagram of a cell and the hypothetical scheme by which a cytosolic receptor, a product of the regulatory *Ah* gene, binds to inducer. The resultant "pleiotypic response" includes greater amounts of cytochrome $P_1$-450 (and numerous other forms of P-450 still being characterized), leading to enhanced steady-state levels of reactive intermediates, which are associated with genetic increases in drug toxicity, teratogenesis, or chemical carcinogenesis. Depending upon the half-life of the reactive intermediate, important binding may occur in the same cell in which metabolism took place, or in some distant cell. Although the unknown critical target is illustrated here in the nucleus, there is presently no experimental evidence demonstrating unequivocally the subcellular location of a critical target, or targets, required for the initiation of toxicity or cancer or, for that matter, whether the target is nucleic acid or protein. NEBERT (1979)

## B. The *Ah* Locus

### I. Genetics

The *Ah* locus (Fig. 1) represents a group of genes controlling the induction of numerous drug-metabolizing enzyme activities by polycyclic aromatic compounds such as 3-methylcholanthrene (3-MC) and 2,3,7,8-tetrachlorodibenzo-p-dioxin (TCDD). The *Ah* system comprises numerous regulatory, structural, and perhaps temporal genes which may or may not be linked (NEBERT et al. 1982). Numerous studies indicate that the major product of the *Ah* regulatory genes is a cytosolic re-

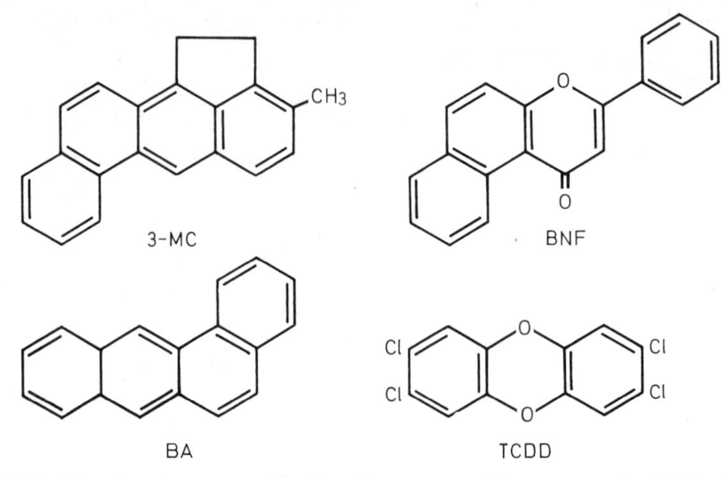


**Fig. 2.** Molecules that interact with the *Ah* receptor (NEBERT et al. 1981). 3-MC, 3-methylchloanthrene; BA, benz[*a*]anthracene; BNF, *β*-naphthoflaone; and TCDD, 2,3,7,8-tetrachlorodibenzo-p-dioxin. NEBERT et al. (1981)

ceptor capable of binding to certain polycyclic aromatic inducers (Fig. 1). To our knowledge, only foreign chemicals bind with a high degree of specificity (Fig. 2). The inducer-receptor complex translocates into the nucleus and in some manner activates structural genes, thereby leading to increases in enzymes ($P_1$-450) which metabolize these inducers (and other polycyclic aromatic noninducing compounds). In addition to innocuous products, reactive metabolites may also be generated. These reactive metabolites in mice have been shown (NEBERT and JENSEN 1979) to be correlated with genetically determined increases in birth defects, toxicity, cancer, mutation, and detoxification, depending on the experimental conditions employed.

Certain inbred strains of mice, as well as many individuals in the human population, lack sufficiently high levels of the *Ah* receptor and therefore are relatively nonresponsive to the $P_1$-450 induction process. This ability to respond to aromatic hydrocarbons was designated the *Ah* locus (NEBERT et al. 1982); the allele $Ah^b$ stands for the B6 mouse having ample amounts of receptor and the allele $Ah^d$ represents the D2 mouse having nondetectable levels of cytosolic receptor (Fig. 3). The heterozygote ($Ah^b/Ah^d$) is phenotypically similar to the responsive homozygote ($Ah^b/Ah^b$). Hence, the trait of having the *Ah* receptor and therefore the maximal $P_1$-450 induction response is autosomal dominant, in much the same way that red color of garden peas is dominant over with color. Moreover, the same genetic expression of *Ah* responsiveness exists in virtually all tissues of any given individual (NEBERT and JENSEN 1979; NEBERT et al. 1982).

## II. Pleiotypic Response of the *Ah* System

Recent studies have shown that the induction of more than two dozen enzyme activities is closely associated with the $Ah^b$ allele. These 3-MC-inducible activities include the metabolism of: BaP and other polycyclic hydrocarbon carcinogens, zox-

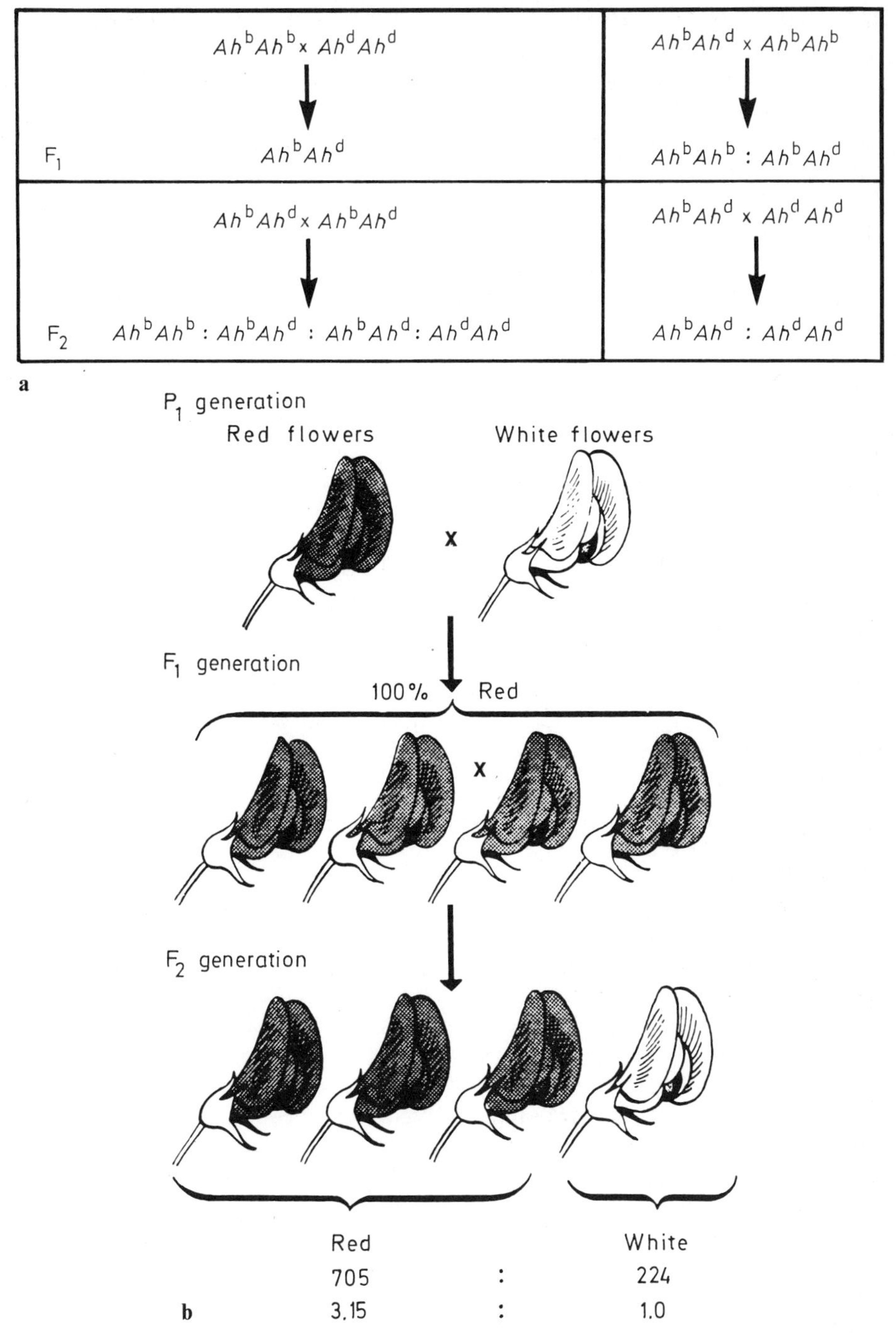


**Fig. 3. a** Simplified genetic scheme for aromatic hydrocarbon "responsiveness" in the mouse. It should be noted that the genetics of *Ah* responsiveness can be much more complicated than this, depending on the strains of mice studied (NEBERT et al. 1982). **b** Illustration of genetic differences in flower color of the garden pea

azolamine, biphenyl, acetanilide, naphthalene, aflatoxin $B_1$, 2-acetylaminofluorene, acetaminophen, p-chloroacetanilide, 7-ethoxycoumarin, phenacetin, ethoxyresorufin, p-nitroanisole, several aminoazobenzene dyes, theophylline, *N,N*-dimethylnitrosamine, $\beta$-naphthoflavone, $\alpha$-naphthoflavone, ellipticine, lindane, niridazole, caffeine, and theobromine. P-450-mediated activities known *not* to be associated with the *Ah* locus include the induced metabolism of: aminopyrine, (+)-benzphetamine, phenytoin, hexobarbital, aniline, benzene sulfonanilide, chlorcyclizine, ethylmorphine, pentobarbital, cyclophosphamide, halothane, enfluorane, carbon tetrachloride, chloroform, estrogen 2-hydroxylation, and testosterone $7\alpha$-, $16\alpha$-, and $6\beta$-hydroxylations (NEBERT and JENSEN 1979; NEBERT et al. 1982).

In addition to the multiple forms of P-450 induced by 3-MC or TCDD (NEGISHI and NEBERT 1979; LANG et al. 1981; LANG and NEBERT 1981), polycyclic aromatic compounds also compete with $^{125}$I-labeled epidermal growth factor (EGF) for its cell surface receptor (IVANOVIC and WEINSTEIN 1981) in much the same order as that seen for compounds competing with TCDD $^3$H for the cytosolic *Ah* receptor (BIGELOW and NEBERT 1982). These inducers also cause porphyria (JONES and SWEENEY 1980), immunosuppression (reviewed in NEBERT 1979; NEBERT et al. 1982), epidermal keratinization (KNUTSON and POLAND 1980), and birth defects (SHUM et al. 1979; POLAND and GLOVER 1980). The cytosolic *Ah* receptor and the $P_1$-450 induction process apparently occur very early in gestation, even before implantation of the mouse embryo (GALLOWAY et al. 1980; FILLER and LEW 1981). All these data therefore suggest that the *Ah* system may be involved in certain growth processes, including differentiation and promotion of cancer, in addition to the previously discovered phenomenon of induction of drug-metabolizing enzymes.

## C. Genetic Influences on Drug-Induced Birth Defects

Numerous drugs have been implicated in causing birth defects in humans, although experimental proof is, of course, difficult. Most notably, "drug-induced syndromes" have been described for phenytoin, warfarin, trimethadione, and alcohol exposure; the clinical features of one syndrome often overlap with those of another, though some investigators maintain that clear-cut distinctions exist for each of these syndromes (SMITH 1976). Several investigators have reported a human pharmacogenetic difference that involves the metabolism of phenytoin (KUTT 1971; VASKO et al. 1980; SLOAN et al. 1981). It is of interest to note that only one child may be afflicted with a drug-induced syndrome when the mother has received the same medication for two or more pregnancies. There have also been cases of one fraternal (dizygotic) twin being affected but not the other, and cases of both identical (monozygotic) twins being affected with a drug-induced syndrome. The situation clearly sounds like a complicated combination of genetic and environmental factors.

About 10 years ago, workers in this laboratory wondered if the importance of a genetic component could be demonstrated with the use of the *Ah* locus and inbred strains of mice. For example, could the genetic predisposition of a particular embryo be more important than maternal influences in causing or preventing a birth defect?

## D. Use of *Ah* Locus for Teratogenesis Studies

3-MC-inducible aryl hydrocarbon hydroxylase (AHH) activity is commonly used as a biochemical marker for the $Ah^b$ allele and therefore ample amounts of the *Ah* receptor (NEBERT et al. 1982). Figure 4 shows that AHH induction by 3-MC can be present or relatively absent among different fetuses in the same uterus. In the experiment illustrated, the enzyme in seven of ten (B6D2)$F_2$ fetuses in the same uterus of a 3-MC-treated (B6D2)$F_1$ mother is about 5–15 times greater than that found in the placenta, fetal bowel, or fetal liver of the three genetically nonresponsive individuals or of control $F_2$ mice (NEBERT 1973). If AHH activity is increased in the placenta, the enzyme is also increased in fetal liver and bowel of that individual, and vice versa. The fact that the *Ah*-responsive mother and responsive individuals in the uterus do not influence AHH induction in the *Ah*-nonresponsive fetuses or their placentas in the same uterus indicates that no humoral agent circulating in the pregnant animal is able to "derepress" AHH induction in $Ah^d/Ah^d$ fetuses (NEBERT 1973).

### I. Genetic Differences in BaP Teratogenicity

One *Ah*-responsive (B6) and one *Ah*-nonresponsive (AK) inbred strain was chosen and the dosage of BaP and the day of gestation on which the BaP is given was varied. Combined stillbirths, resorptions, and malformations were about four-fold greater in B6 than in AK, whether the BaP was given on gestational day 7, 10, or

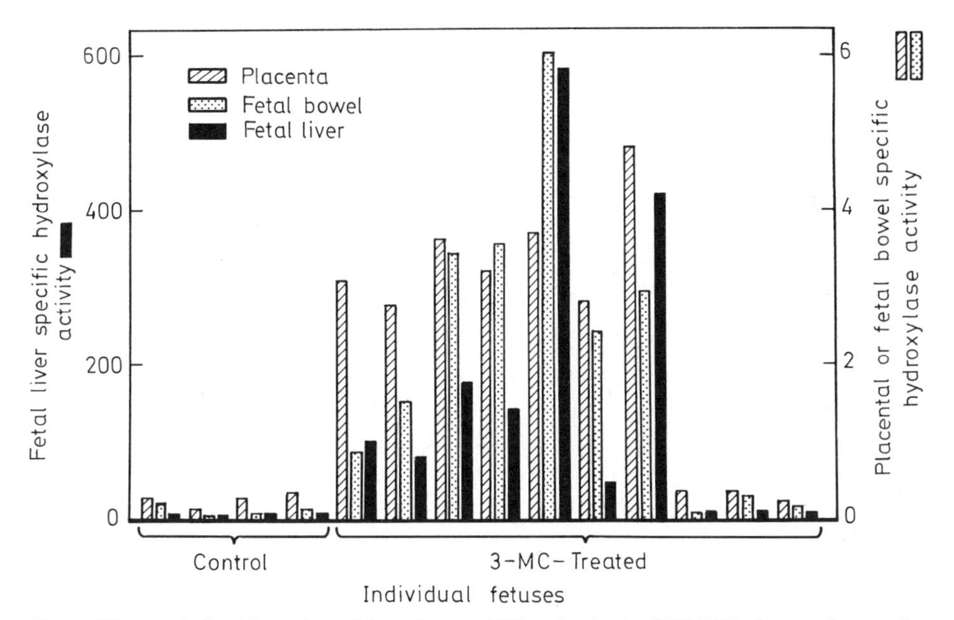


**Fig. 4.** Placental, fetal bowel, and fetal liver AHH activities in (B6D2)$F_2$ fetuses from a 3-MC-treated (B6D2)$F_1$ mother. 3-MC was administered intraperitoneally (80 mg/kg) at about 19 days gestational age, and enzyme activities on individual fetal mice were determined 24 h later. A control (B6D2)$F_1$ mother at about 19 days gestation received corn oil alone. NEBERT (1973)

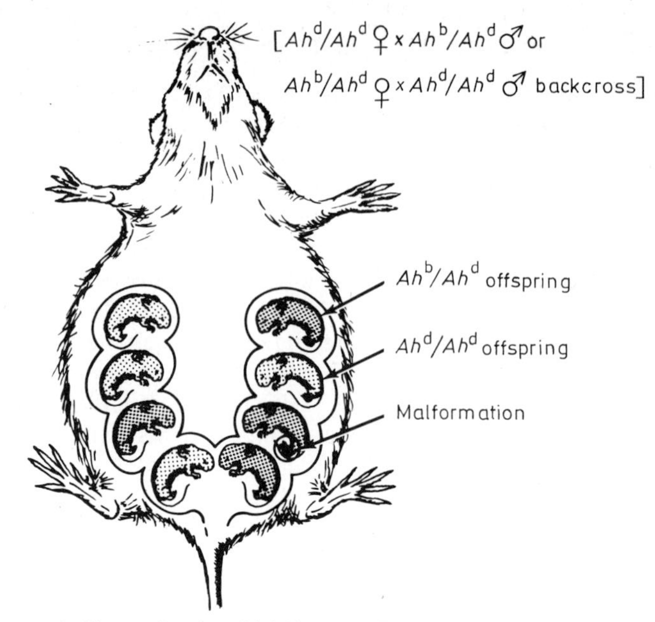


**Fig. 5.** Diagrammatic illustration in which fetuses of two distinct phenotypes reside in the uterus from a mother of either one or the other phenotype. With either backcross, the expected ratio of responsive to nonresponsive fetuses is 1:1. NEBERT et al. (1977)

12. This study (LAMBERT and NEBERT 1977) does not, however, demonstrate a strict correlation with the $Ah^b$ allele, since these inbred strains vary by thousands of genes. Some other strain dissimilarity between B6 and AK may account for our observed differences in teratogenesis. Only after the phenotype of offspring from the $F_1$ × recessive parent backcross (Fig. 5) is examined, can one be certain whether the $Ah^b$ allele is correlated specifically with dysmorphogenesis. There are two ways to generate progeny from the backcross: one is with a nonresponsive $Ah^d/Ah^d$ mother; the other is with a responsive $Ah^b/Ah^d$ mother.

## II. Correlation of BaP-Induced Stillbirths and Resorptions with the *Ah* Allele

β-Naphthoflavone-inducible AHH activity in 18-day-old fetuses was chosen as the best marker for determining allelic differences at the *Ah* locus. From inbred B6 and inbred AK individuals (Fig. 6a, b), it was determined with 95% confidence that specific AHH activities of 25 or greater represent *Ah*-responsive fetuses and those of less than 25 represent *Ah*-nonresponsive fetuses. This hypothesis is supported by the expected equal distribution ($P = 0.50$) of AHH activity among progeny of the AK × B6AK backcross [2] (Fig. 6, c). In other words, approximately half of the individuals ($Ah^d/Ah^d$) had AHH specific activities of less than 25 and approximately half ($Ah^b/Ah^d$) had specific activities of greater than 25.

Treatment of the AK mother with BaP on day 7 or 10 (Fig. 6d, e) results in more apparent nonresponsive than responsive viable fetuses. This finding is highly

2 The accepted order for expressing genetic crosses is the female parent first and the male parent second (female × male)

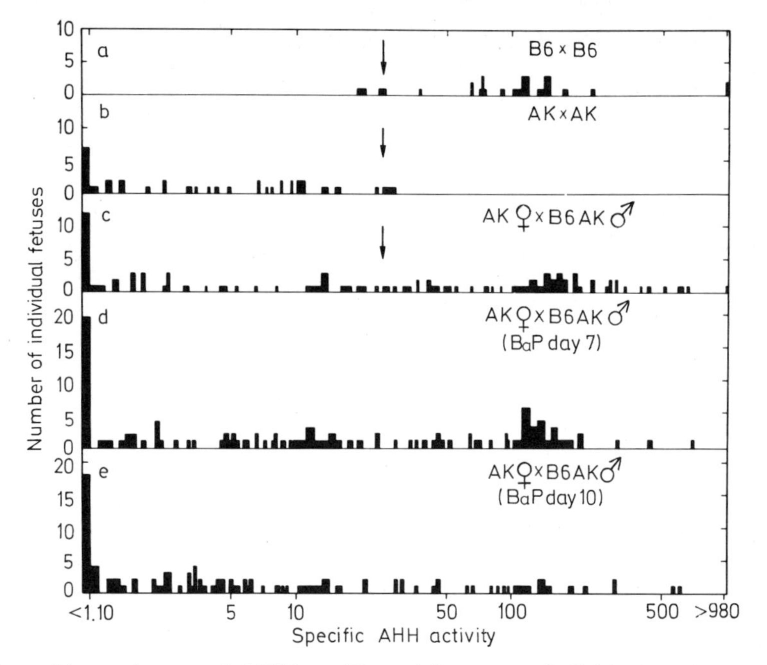


**Fig. 6 a–e.** Liver microsomal AHH specific activity among individual 18-day-old fetuses whose mother on day 16 had received intraperitoneal $\beta$-naphthoflavone (200 mg/kg). From **a** inbred B6 (5 litters); **b** inbred AK (10 litters); **c** progeny of the AK × B6AK backcross (19 litters), **d** progeny of the same backcross (20 litters) whose mother had received BaP (200 mg/kg) on day 7, **e** progeny of the same backcross (23 litters) whose mother had received BaP (200 mg/kg) on day 10. The *arrows* at 25 units/mg microsomal protein denote the arbitrarily assigned value: fetuses with a specific AHH activity of 25 or more are likely ($P<0.05$) to be responsive ($Ah^b/Ah^b$ or $Ah^b/Ah^d$); fetuses having a specific AHH activity below 25 are likely ($P<0.05$) to be nonresponsive ($Ah^d/Ah^d$). SHUM et al. (1979)

**Table 1.** Statistical analysis of phenotype of 18-day-old fetuses whose mother had received BaP (200 mg/kg) earlier in the pregnancy (SHUM et al. 1979)

| Backcross | Day of gestation | | Phenotype | | $\chi^2$ | $P$ |
|---|---|---|---|---|---|---|
| | | | $Ah^b/Ah^d$ | $Ah^b/Ah^d$ | | |
| AK mother × B6AK father | 7 | Observed: | 44.0 | 71.0 | 6.33 | 0.01–0.02 |
| $(Ah^d/Ah^d) \times (Ah^b/Ah^d)$ | | Expected: | 57.5 | 57.5 | | |
| | 10 | Observed: | 25.0 | 79.0 | 28 | $<0.0001$ |
| | | Expected: | 52.0 | 52.0 | | |
| B6AK mother × AK father | 7 | Observed: | 16.0 | 18.0 | 0.118 | $>0.70$ |
| $(Ah^b/Ah^d) \times (Ah^d/Ah^d)$ | | Expected: | 17.0 | 17.0 | | |
| | 10 | Observed: | 23.0 | 16.0 | 1.26 | $>0.20$ |
| | | Expected: | 19.5 | 19.5 | | |

statistically significant (Table 1), especially when BaP was given on day 10. It is thus concluded that $Ah^b/Ah^d$ fetuses, owing to greater amounts of inducible $P_1$-450 and AHH and therefore higher steady-state levels of toxic BaP metabolites, are more prone than $Ah^d/Ah^d$ fetuses to stillbirths and resorptions. Hence, an increased number of viable $Ah^d/Ah^d$ are found on day 18 when the AHH assay was per-

**Table 2.** Effect of BaP (200 mg/kg on day 10) on weight and AHH activity in fetuses from either the AK × B6AK or the B6AK × AK backcross (SHUM et al. 1979)

| Backcross | Phenotype | Number of fetuses | Fetal weight[a] (mg) | Specific AHH activity[a] (units/mg liver microsomal protein) |
|---|---|---|---|---|
| AK mother × B6AK father[b] | $Ah^b/Ah^d$ | 20 | 680 ± 57 | 155 ± 157 |
| $(Ah^d/Ah^d) \times (Ah^b/Ah^d)$ | $Ah^d/Ah^d$ | 26 | 820 ± 105[c] | 4.09 ± 2.68 |
| B6AK mother × AK father[d] | $Ah^b/Ah^d$ | 19 | 640 ± 61 | 208 ± 191 |
| $(Ah^b/Ah^d) \times (Ah^d/Ah^d)$ | $Ah^d/Ah^d$ | 14 | 700 ± 91 | 3.70 ± 3.01 |

[a] Mean values ± standard deviations
[b] Seven litters
[c] $P < 0.001$ by $Z$ score (critical ratio) analysis
[d] Five litters

formed. When backcross progeny from the B6AK mother × AK father were studied, however, this difference in stillbirths and resorptions between responsive and nonresponsive fetuses is not statistically significant.

## III. Association of BaP-Induced Embryotoxicity with the *Ah* Allele

Among fetuses in the same rodent uterus, it is well known that fetal weights can vary considerably because of uterine position, probably owing to variation in nutrients offered by the uterine blood supply. In spite of this variation, there was a trend among progeny from the AK × B6AK backcross for a negative correlation between fetal weight and AHH specific activity. This correlation between BaP-induced decreases in fetal weight and the $Ah^b$ allele is highly statistically significant (Table 2) among progeny of the AK × B6AK backcross, but is not statistically significant among progeny of the B6AK × AK backcross.

## IV. Correlation of BaP-Induced Teratogenesis with the *Ah* Allele

Table 3 shows that when the mother is *Ah* nonresponsive, a statistically significant increase in the number of malformations is found. When the mother is *Ah* responsive, however, this significant increase is not seen. We conclude that the $Ah^b$ allele and therefore the induced $P_1$-450 and enhanced production of toxic BaP metabolites in fetal tissues (or fetal placenta) are associated with BaP teratogenesis, if the mother is nonresponsive at the *Ah* locus. If the mother is responsive at the *Ah* locus, however, these genetic differences among the fetuses are overridden by the higher amounts of $P_1$-450 in the mother and therefore higher levels of toxic BaP metabolites generated by the mother.

Higher steady-state levels of toxic BaP metabolites generated by the B6AK mother's tissues are believed to be readily transferred via the placenta to the fetus. An increased amount of BaP metabolites is observed bound covalently to DNA and especially protein in $Ah^b/Ah^d$ fetuses, more so than in $Ah^d/Ah^d$ fetuses when the AK mother was used. This genetic difference in covalent binding of metabolites is not seen when the B6AK mother was used. Further, α-naphthoflavone (a relatively specific inhibitor of $P_1$-450 metabolism), given concomitantly with radiolabeled BaP to the pregnant mother, decreases considerably the amount of BaP metabolites that bind covalently (SHUM et al. 1979).

**Table 3.** Statistical analysis of phenotype of malformed fetuses[a] whose mother had received BaP (200 mg/kg) on day 7 of gestation

| Backcross | | Phenotype | | $\chi^2$ | $P$ |
|---|---|---|---|---|---|
| | | $Ah^b/Ah^d$ | $Ah^d/Ah^d$ | | |
| AK mother × B6AK father | Observed: | 55.0 | 28.0 | 4.4 | 0.02–0.05 |
| $(Ah^d/Ah^d) \times (Ah^b/Ah^d)$ | Expected: | 41.5 | 41.5 | | |
| B6AK mother × AK father | Observed: | 14.0 | 17.0 | 0.5 | 0.7 |
| $(Ah^b/Ah^d) \times (Ah^d/Ah^d)$ | Expected: | 15.5 | 15.5 | | |

[a] Malformations observed include anophthalmia, open eyelids, hypoplastic mandible, short nose, cleft palate and/or lip, ectopia cordis, morphological changes in liver, hypoplastic and/or aplastic kidney and ureter, malformed uterus, clubfoot, curly tail, hemangioendothelioma or red nevus of the skin, abnormal pigmentation or white nevus of the skin, scalp defect, scoliosis, parietal mass, and gastroschisis (SHUM et al. 1979)

## V. Developmental Expression of *Ah* Allele in the Mouse Embryo

Mouse embryos explanted at gestational day $3^1/_2$, $5^1/_2$, $7^1/_2$, and $8^1/_2$ have been cultured in medium containing BaP and supplemented with 5-bromodeoxyuridine to allow detection of sister chromatid exchanges (Fig. 7). This technique (LATT et al., 1977; GALLOWAY et al., 1980) was chosen because of its exquisite sensitivity in detecting toxicity, in this case presumably caused by BaP metabolites formed by the induced AHH activity. A strong correlation was seen between increased sister chromatid exchanges (SCE) and the $Ah^b$ allele among five inbred strains, one outbred strain, and two recombinant inbred strains (GALLOWAY et al., 1980). These data suggested that genetically responsive mouse embryos (late preimplantation

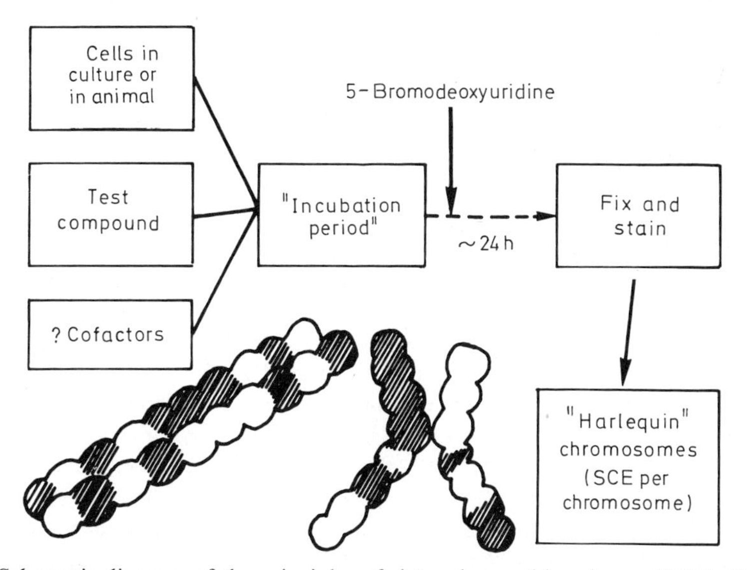


**Fig. 7.** Schematic diagram of the principles of sister chromatid exchange (SCE). Cells can be exposed in culture to a test compound, with or without cofactors. Cells (e.g., lymphocytes) can also be removed from the animal and cultured, following exposure of the animal to a test compound. NEBERT (1981)

and early postimplantation stages) possess the subcellular processes necessary for induction of enzymes that metabolize BaP to its chemically teratogenic/toxic form of forms. More recently, TCDD-induced metabolites of BaP were found in the cultured $3^1/_2$-day embryo; the *Ah*-responsive B6 displayed more metabolites than the *Ah*-nonresponsive D2 (FILLER and LEW 1981). Both the *Ah* regulatory gene product (in other words, the cytosolic receptor) and the structural gene product (inducible $P_1$-450) therefore appear to be functional from a very early embryonic age (NEBERT and SHUM 1980).

Thus, we believe that the genetic predisposition for the metabolism of a drug or other chemical *in a given tissue of an individual fetus*, rather than in tissues of the mother can be important in the etiology of certain birth defects. This could explain why a birth defect is found in one child, for example, when the mother had received the same dose of the same drug during each of two or more pregnancies. Other chemicals and drugs, known or suspected to interact with cytochrome $P_1$-450, should also be examined with this experimental model system.

## E. Extrapolation of Data to the Human

With the use of inbred strains of mice and the appropriate genetic crosses, it is therefore possible to demonstrate that a single allelic difference, or a very small number of genes, can have a profound influence on an individual's increased susceptibility to several types of toxicity, cancer, and mutation produced by environmental chemicals (NEBERT and JENSEN 1979). Certainly the mechanisms of these effects are complex and may also involve modifying genes other than the *Ah* system. There is also evidence for the *Ah* locus in the human (NEBERT 1980; KOURI et al. 1982), and there is no reason to believe that the *Ah* phenotype does not play some clinical role in certain types of birth defects, drug toxicity, and environmentally related cancers.

Clinicians should therefore keep in mind that birth defects might vary among siblings in the same family, because embryonic and fetal differences in drug metabolism can be regulated by a relatively small number of genes. For each drug, it also remains to be determined whether a reactive metabolite or the parent nonmetabolized drug is important in the mechanism of teratogenesis. A study with phenytoin in the mouse (ATLAS et al. 1980), for example, suggests no correlation between genetic differences in phenytoin metabolism and susceptibility to tertogenicity.

Finally, what impact should pharmacogenetics have on the practicing physician? The *Ah* locus is most likely one of a large number of genetic systems which control the drug-metabolizing enzymes. Whereas there may exist an "estimated normal dose" for a given drug, such a dose administered to any particular patient may be ineffective, or may be toxic, depending upon the pharmacogenetic makeup of that patient. This result might occur with *any* drug, whether the patient is being treated for a bacterial infection or seizure disorder, or is receiving chemotherapy for cancer. More and more assays for blood, saliva, or urine concentrations of drugs or metabolites are being developed each year. As these assays become less expensive, less time consuming, and more popular, physicians will be able to monitor much more successfully the *effective* drug dosage for each individual patient. In other words, the genetic constitution of drug-metabolizing enzymes in each patient will begin to be appreciated. At all times, however, the physician should be aware that drug idiosyncrasies will occasionally occur, and that there may be 2-fold, 20-fold, or even 100-fold differences in drug response, even among members of the same family. The physician should be aware that, just as the patient has genetically determined color of hair and eyes and unique fingerprints, most likely the patient also has a unique genetically determined drug-metabolizing capability.

## F. Summary

A study of genetic differences in the metabolism of certain drugs can be made quite simple with the use of inbred mouse strains. Highly inducible levels of a drug-metabolizing enzyme activity (called aryl hydrocarbon hydroxylase) reflect a Mendelian dominant trait over low inducible levels. This system is called the *Ah* locus and is known to exist in many mammalian species, including humans.

It is shown in these mice that the tendency to develop birth defects (and other intrauterine toxicity) depends upon the genetic predisposition of the individual embryo, rather than that of the maternal tissues. The experimental model system presented here provides an example that might explain clinically why sometimes only one child is affected with an apparently drug-induced syndrome, although the mother has taken the same dose of the particular drug during each of two or more pregnancies. Of special interest in this study is the fact that the mother and the father both must be of a particular phenotype before differences in birth defects among fetuses (due to *each fetus*' phenotype) will be expressed. Most likely the *Ah* locus is just one of a large number of genetic systems which regulate various enzymes that metabolize drugs, chemical carcinogens, and other environmental pollutants and teratogens.

*Acknowledgment.* The expert secretarial assistance of Ms. INGRID E. JORDAN is greatly appreciated.

## References

Atlas SA, Zweier JL, Nebert DW (1980) Genetic differences in phenytoin pharmacokinetics. *In vivo* clearance and *in vitro* metabolism among inbred strains of mice. Dev Pharmacol Ther 1:281–304

Bigelow SW, Nebert DW (1982) The *Ah* regulatory gene product: survey of fifteen polycyclic aromatic compounds' and fifteen benzo[a]pyrene metabolites' capacity to bind to the cytosolic receptor. Toxicol Lett (Amst) 10:109–118

Filler R, Lew KJ (1981) Developmental onset of mixed-function oxidase activity in preimplantation mouse embryos. Proc Nat Acad Sci USA 78:6991–6995

Galloway SM, Perry PE, Meneses J, Nebert DW, Pedersen RA (1980) Cultured mouse embryos metabolize benzo[a]pyrene during gestation: genetic differences detectable by sister chromatid exchange. Proc Nat Acad Sci USA 77:3524–3528

Ivanovic V, Weinstein IB (1981) Benzo[a]pyrene and other inducers of cytochrome $P_1$-450 inhibit binding of epidermal growth factor (EGF) to cell surface receptors [Abstr] J Supramol Struct Cell Biochem [Suppl] 5:232

Jones KG, Sweeney GD (1980) Dependence of the porphyrogenic effect of 2,3,7,8-tetrachlorodibenzo(p)dioxin upon inheritance of aryl hydrocarbon hydroxylase. Toxicol Appl Pharmacol 53:42–49

Knutson JC, Poland A (1980) Keratinization of mouse teratoma cell line XB produced by 2,3,7,8-tetrachlorodibenzo-*p*-dioxin: an *in vitro* model of toxicity. Cell 22:27–36

Kouri RE, McKinney D, Slomiany DJ, Snodgrass DR, Wray NP, McLemore TL (1982) Positive correlation between high aryl hydrocarbon hydroxylase activity and primary lung cancer–Analysis in cryopreserved lymphocytes. Cancer Res (in press)
Kutt H (1971) Biochemical and genetic factors regulating dilantin metabolism in man. Ann NY Acad Sci 179:705–722
Lambert GH, Nebert DW (1977) Genetically mediated induction of drug-metabolizing enzymes associated with congenital defects in the mouse. Teratology 16:147–153
Lang MA, Nebert DW (1981) Structural gene products of the *Ah* locus. Evidence for many unique P-450-mediated monooxygenase activities reconstituted from 3-methylcholanthrene-treated C57BL/6N mouse liver microsomes. J Biol Chem 256:12,058–12,067
Lang MA, Gielen JE, Nebert DW (1981) Genetic evidence for many unique liver microsomal P-450-mediated monooxygenase activities in heterogeneic stock mice. J Biol Chem 256:12,068–12,075
Latt SA, Allen JW, Stetten G (1977) *In vitro* and *in vivo* analyses of chromosome structure, replication, and repair using BrdU-33258 Hoechst techniques. In: Brinkley BR, Porter KR (eds) Proceedings of the first international congress on cell biology. Rockefeller University Press, New York, pp 520–527
Nebert DW (1973) Use of fetal cell culture as an experimental system for predicting drug metabolism in the intact animal. Clin Pharmacol Ther 14:693–699
Nebert DW (1979) Multiple forms of inducible drug-metabolizing enzymes. A reasonable mechanism by which any organism can cope with adversity. Mol Cell Biochem 27:27–46
Nebert DW (1980) The *Ah* locus. A gene with possible importance in cancer predictability. Arch Toxicol [Suppl] 3:195–207
Nebert DW (1981) Birth defects and the potential role of genetic differences in drug metabolism. In: Bloom AD, James LS (eds) Birth defects: original article series, vol XVII. AR Liss, New York, pp. 51–70
Nebert DW, Jensen NM (1979) Genetic regulation of the metabolism of carcinogens, drugs, and other environmental chemicals by cytochrome P-450-mediated monooxygenases. In: Fasman GD (ed) CRC critical reviews in biochemistry, vol 6. CRC Press, Cleveland, pp 410–437
Nebert DW, Shum S, (1980) Reply to the letter of Doctors Shepard and Fantel. Teratology 22:349–350
Nebert DW, Levitt RC, Jensen NM, Lambert GH, Felton JS (1977) Birth defects and aplastic anemia: differences in polycyclic hydrocarbon toxicity associated with the *Ah* locus. Arch Toxicol 39:109–132
Nebert DW, Eisen HJ, Negishi M, Lang MA, Hjelmeland LM, Okey AB (1981) Genetic mechanisms controlling the induction of polysubstrate monooxygenase (P-450) activities. Annu Rev Pharmacol Toxicol 21:431–462
Nebert DW, Negishi M, Lang MA, Hjelmeland LM, Eisen HJ (1982) The *Ah* locus, a multigene family necessary for survival in a chemically adverse environment: comparison with the immune system. Adv Genet 21:1–52
Negishi M, Nebert DW (1979) Structural gene products of the *Ah* locus. Genetic and immunochemical evidence for two forms of mouse liver cytochrome P-450 induced by 3-methylcholanthrene. J Biol Chem 254:11,015–11 023
Omura T, Sato R (1964) The carbon monoxide-binding pigment of liver microsomes. I. Evidence for its hemoprotein nature. J Biol Chem 239:2370–2378
Poland A, Glover E (1980) 2,3,7,8-Tetrachlorodibenzo-p-dioxin: Segregation of toxicity with the *Ah* locus. Mol Pharmacol 17:86–94
Shum S, Jensen NM, Nebert DW (1979) The *Ah* locus: *In utero* toxicity and teratogenesis associated with genetic difference in benzo[a]pyrene metabolism. Teratology 20:365–376
Sloan TP, Idle JR, Smith RL (1981) Influence of $D^H/D^L$ alleles regulating debrisoquine oxidation on phenytoin hydroxylation. Clin Pharmacol Ther 29:493–497
Smith DW (ed) (1976) Recognizable patterns of human malformation, 2nd edn. WB Saunders, Philadelphia
Vasko MR, Bell RD, Daly DD, Pippenges CE (1980) Inheritance of phenytoin hypometabolism: a kinetic study of one family. Clin Pharmacol Ther 27:96–103
Williams RT (ed) (1959) Detoxication mechanisms, 2nd edn. Wiley & Sons, New York

# Mechanisms of Teratogenesis

CHAPTER 5

# Viruses as Teratogens

J. L. SEVER

## A. Introduction

Many viruses can be transmitted to the fetus and cause infection and tissure damage. Five viruses are known to be teratogenic in humans: cytomegalovirus, rubella, herpes simplex, Venezuelan equine encephalitis, and varicella viruses. Other viruses which can infect and produce disease in the fetus are influenza, rubeola, Western equine encephalitis, variola, vaccinia, hepatitis B, echoviruses, and poliovirus. This chapter summarizes some of the newer findings for the five teratogenic viruses.

## B. Discussion

### I. Epidemiology

The frequency of viral infections in pregnant women and their children has been determined from a number of clinical, virologic, and serologic studies. Some of the current estimates are given in Table 1. Factors which influence the frequency of these infections include: (1) the type of population sampled; (2) the occurrence of epidemics; (3) the method of diagnosis used; (4) the use of vaccines for rubella; (5) delivery by cesarean section when maternal herpes infection is present; and (6) the increasing use of therapeutic abortions.

Fortunately, rubella has decreased to low levels, and no major epidemics have occurred in the United States since 1964 (PREBLUD et al. 1980). At present, however, approximately 20% of women of childbearing age are at risk for this infection in this country. This is actually twice the number which were at risk before the 1964

**Table 1.** Frequency of viral infections in pregnant women and their children

| | Mother/10,000 | Child/10,000 |
|---|---|---|
| 1. Rubella virus | | |
| Epidemic | 200–400 | 20 – 40 |
| Nonepidemic | 10– 20 | 1 – 2 |
| Current United States | < 1 | < .1 |
| 2. Cytomegalovirus | 300–500 | 50 –150 |
| 3. HSV-1 and HSV-2 | 50–150 | 0.5 – 5 |
| 4. Venezuelan equine encephalitis virus | With epidemics | |
| 5. Varicella virus | 1– 2 | < 0.01– 1 |

epidemic. Since the majority of children are immunized, and we have not had a major epidemic, we are fortunate that this high proportion of women who are currently at risk are rarely or very infrequently exposed to rubella. As a result, there are now less than 25 reported cases of congenital rubella each year. When "mini" epidemics occur or if suceptible women travel to other countries, the opportunity for risk of infection is great. For this reason, immunization programs must continue to emphasize the use of rubella vaccine for women at risk in this age group.

Maternal infections with cytomegalovirus are surprisingly frequent. In most studies, 3%–5% of women shed this virus at term (HILDEBRANDT et al. 1967). Almost all of these women are asymptomatic. About one-third of the children of infected women are also infected at birth, and many more acquire this infection in the first months of life. Severe damage due to congenital cytomegalovirus infection occurs at a rate of about 1/5,000–1/20,000 births. Studies of asymptomatic infected, newborns, however, suggest that as many as 5%–10% of these children have some damage due to this infection. The most frequent problems are low intelligence and some degree of deafness.

Herpes infections have become increasingly frequent. At present it is estimated that there are over 300,000 new cases each year in the United States, and because of recurrences with herpes, over 5,000,000 people experience genital herpes each year. In addition to the pain and discomfort associated with the infection, virus present in the vagina at term can be transmitted to the child during the birth process. In over 50% of cases, this leads to severe, often fatal disease in the newborn. The use of cesarean section for delivery significantally reduces the frequency of infections in the newborn.

Venezuelan equine encephalitis can be transmitted to humans during epidemics. This in turn can result in spread of the virus to the baby where severe infection of the brain and eyes can occur. The affected children may have hydrocephaly, porencephalic cysts, and cataracts (WENGER 1967). Most of the epidemics occur in the Caribbean, or Central and South America.

Varicella (chickenpox) is now recognized as a teratogen (WILLIAMSON 1975). Infection of the mother prior to term can lead to severe skeletal and brain damage of the child in approximately 1%–10% of cases. In addition, varicella at term can be transmitted intravenously to the child. This direct infection in the last few days of gestation may result in generalized varicella which is fatal for approximately one-third of the children.

## II. Rubella Virus

The defects due to congential rubella are associated primarily with infection during the first 5 months of pregnancy (Table 2). The frequency of abnormal children following maternal infection is highest with rubella in the first month of gestation (50%) and this decreases to 22% in the second month, 10% in the third month, and 6% in the fourth and fifth month. In the United States, approximately 15%–20% of the women of childbearing age are at risk for rubella infection. With infections, clinical manifestations occurs in approximately two-thirds of women of this age group (SEVER et al. 1969). The most useful laboratory test has been the hemagglutination inhibition (HI) method for antibody determination. With this

**Table 2.** Congenital rubella

| | |
|---|---|
| Defects | Malformations of heart and great vessels<br>Microcephaly, deafness, catarcts, mental retardation<br>Newborn bleeding, hepatosplenomegaly, pneumonitis hepatitis, encephalitis<br>Death |
| Detection | |
| Mother | Exposure, rash, nodes<br>Lab tests – antibody response (hemagglutination inhibition and other tests, IgM specific antibody); virus isolation from nasopharynx |
| Child | Congenital rubella syndrome<br>Lab tests – rubella-specific IgM; persisting rubella antibody after 6 months of age; virus isolation from nasopharynx or cerebrospinal fluid |
| Prevention | Rubella vaccine<br>Abortion |

method, susceptible individuals can be identified on the basis of absence of antibody, and seroconversions can be documented. New enzyme-linked immunosorbent assay (ELISA) tests are also available and correlate with HI results (GRAVELL et al. 1977). Several other new methods are now available for general use. IgM rubella-specific antibody is also detectable for a number of weeks following infection, and this determination can be used to document recent infection.

The usual manifestations of congenital rubella include malformations of the heart and great vessels, deafness, cataracts, microcephaly, and mental retardation. The newborns may also exhibit hepatosplenomegaly, hepatitis, pneumonitis, and encephalitis. Most infected newborns have rubella-specific IgM antibody which persists for a number of months. Rubella virus can be isolated from throat swabs and urine of congenitally infected children for a period of several months. The children are infectious and contact with pregnant women should be avoided.

Rubella virus is spread hematogenously from the mother through the placenta to the baby. Maternal infection in the first months of pregnancy almost always results in placental infection. Only about one-third of the fetuses, however, show evidence of the virus. The virus in the fetus may be localized to one or a few organs, or it may be widely disseminated. Chronic infection of the fetus and child persists, even in the presence of high titers of specific antibody. The shedding of virus, however, ceases in almost all infants between approximately 6 months and 1 year of age, suggesting that some change in the immune status of the child has taken place. The nature of the immune deficiency in congenital infections is not known, but it may be related to absence of specific cellular immune responses. In rare cases, in the second decade of life, the persisting virus spreads slowly throughout the brain causing progressive rubella panencephalitis, which is fatal.

Rubella vaccines have now been administered to more than 80,000,000 individuals in the United States. All of these vaccines produce a low incidence of side reactions, primarily arthritis and arthralgia, most marked in women of childbearing age. Immunity produced by the vaccines appears to be permanent. There is no satisfactory animal for the teratogenic effects of congential rubella.

## III. Cytomegalovirus

The most common cause of congenital infections is cytomegalovirus (CMV; Table 3). Several serologic surveys in the United States have shown that approximately one-third to two-thirds of adult women have antibody to this group of closely related viruses (SEVER 1966). In addition CMV generally can be isolated from the cervix or urine of from 3%–5% of pregnant women (HILDEBRANT et al. 1967; STARR and GOLO 1968). The great majority of infected women are asymptomatic. Occasionally, cervicitis and illness resembling infectious mononucleosis are caused by infection with these viruses. Infection can be documented by isolation of the virus from the urine or cervical area, or by the production of antibody. The hemagglutination, fluorescent, and ELISA tests appear to be the most practical and reliable methods for detecting antibody and seroconversions (FUCCILLO et al. 1971; CASTELLANO et al. 1977).

Congential infection with CMV occurs in 0.5%–1.5% of births (BIRNBAUM et al. 1969). Present information indicates that as much as 5%–10% of these children exhibit permanent damage in the form of mental and/or motor retardation, occasionally accompanied by microcephaly and deafness. Children with normal neurologic findings at 2 years of age generally have a good prognosis. The severe form of cytomegalic inclusion disease occurs in 1/5,000–1/20,000 live births. Congential infection can be documented by isolation of the virus from the nasopharynx and urine. Specific IgM cytomegalovirus antibody is also present in many of the infected newborns.

Fetal infection apparently results from hematogenous spread from the mother. The infection is usually widely disseminated and the virus can be isolated from many tissues. Damage to the brain includes direct tissue destruction with the formation of calcified areas. Similarly, chorioretinitis is associated with direct infection by the virus. Infected children shed the virus for many months, and spread of infection from the baby to other members of the family has been well documented.

Therapy with adenine arabinoside has been tried but is not useful. Vaccines are not yet available for use in women, but are being tested in special populations. In

**Table 3.** Congenital Cytomegalovirus infection

| | |
|---|---|
| Birth Defects | Microcephaly, choriorentinitis, deafness<br>Mental retardation, hepatosplenomegaly<br>Epilepsy, hydrocephalus, cerebral palsy<br>Death |
| Detection | |
| Mother | No clinical symptoms (rarely, infectious mononucleosis-like symptoms)<br>Virus isolation from urine and cervix<br>Seroconversion (indirect hemagglutination, fluorescence, ELISA) |
| Chlid | Wide spectrum of clinical findings (listed above)<br>Only severely affected are usually recognized<br>Lab tests – CMV-specific IgM; virus isolation from nasopharynx and urine; large cells in tissues |
| Prevention | Avoid contact<br>Chemotherapy (?)<br>Vaccines (?) |

many hospitals, pregnant women (nurses, doctors, and hospital employees) who do not have antibody to CMV are advised to avoid close contact with newborns with congenital CMV disease. It is assumed that this may decrease the risk of intense exposure to this virus. Unfortunately, no satisfactory animal model is available for the study of human CMV.

## IV. Herpes Simplex Virus

Congential herpes simplex virus (HSV) infections usually are acquired at birth (Table 4. Maternal infection is transmitted as a venereal disease, and 90% of such infections are due to HSV-2 (NAHMIAS et al. 1970). HSV-1, on the other hand, usually affects the mouth, face, or upper part of the trunk. The congenital infections studied in detail in the Collaborative Perinatal Project Study were all related to primary HSV-2 infection occurring late in gestation (SEVER 1966). Other studies, however, have shown that HSV-1 can also result in severe fetal damage. Prior maternal infection with either strain does not completely protect the child; however, the severity of lesions is often reduced (YEAGER et al. 1980). Most women with vaginal HSV infection do not exhibit lesions; thus infection is underreported. The diagnosis can be made by recognition of the typical inclusions in the cells of Papanicolaou smear, fluorescent staining, or by direct virus isolation.

The child with congenital infection usually appears normal at birth, but signs and symptoms of the disease develop during the first 1–3 weeks of life. The disease is manifested in three general forms: (a) vesicular lesions of the skin or throat with or without conjunctivitis (15% of cases); (b) central nervous system involvement, characterized by spinal fluid pleocytosis, elevated pressure, increased protein content, and convulsions (15% of cases); (c) systemic disease, manifested by hepatitis,

**Table 4.** Perinatal herpes simplex infection

| | |
|---|---|
| Defects | Three groups:<br>a) Limited – vesicular lesions on skin, throat, and sometimes conjunctivitis<br>b) Central nervous system – convulsions<br>c) Systemic – hepatitis, jaundice, hepatomegaly, thrombocytopenia, petechiae, hemolytic anemia, pulmonary disease |
| Detection | |
| Mother | Many asymptomatic and no herpetic lesions<br>Virus isolation most sensitive<br>Vaginal-cervical infection; some ulcerative lesions; husband may also have infection<br>Lab tests – Papanicolaou smear often shows cells with inclusions; fluorescent tests often positive; virus isolation from cervix |
| Child | Often difficult to recognize initially<br>Skin lesions present in about 50% of cases; most later develop severe brain or systemic disease (listed above)<br>Lab tests – isolation of virus from skin lesions, throat, eyes, or tissues; specific herpes IgM antibody |
| Prevention | Delivery by cesarean section<br>Chemotherapy, particularly for limited infections (vidarabine)<br>Vaccines (?) |

jaundice, pulmonary disease, hemolytic anemia, petechiae, hepatomegaly, and thrombocytopenia (70% of cases). The prognosis in children with localized vesicular lesions (and conjunctivitis) is good, although about 50% of them progress to more extensive disseminated infection. Systemic infection is fatal in over 90% of cases (NAHMIAS et al. 1970). Laboratory tests useful in the diagnosis of HSV infection are the isolation of virus from lesions, the pharynx or conjunctiva, or the presence of specific HSV IgM antibody.

Chemotherapy for congenital infection, using adenine arabinoside (vidarabine) has been reported (WHITELY et al. 1980). While this drug reduces the frequency of fatalities, many survivors have permanent neurologic sequelae. If there is only limited infection, however, the drug significantly recudes the number of permanent neurologic sequelae. Vaccines are not presently available, but are being investigated. Delivery by cesarean section is recommended in order to avoid contact of the child with the infected vaginal lesions if these are found to be present near term.

The prevalence of HSV infections appears to be increasing. The infection is transmitted as a veneral disease. Primary infection of the mother at term is of greatest importance in the production of congenital disease. Only rarely is there evidence of intrauterine infection, and when this occurs it is usually limited to the last few days of gestation.

## V. Venezuelan Equine Encephalitis Virus

Venezuelan equine encephalitis is a member of the group A arborviruses. Epidemics have occurred in South America, Central America, Mexico, Texas, and Florida. The infection can be transmitted by mosquitoes of many different species, and is both endemic and epidemic. There are many hosts among wild animals, including monkeys, rats, mice, opossums, jackrabbits, foxes, and bats. Domestic animals other than horses, which have been infected include cattle, pigs, goats, and sheep. In humans, infection results in a mild febrile illness, usually without neurologic complications. There is no age or sex predominance. The incubation period is approximately 2–5 days. The primary symptoms are headache, fever, malaise, and myalgia. Occasionally patients have seizures, mental confusion, coma, tremors, and ancephalitis (Table 5). The symptoms usually last 3–8 days and the virus can be isolated from the serum or spinal fluid.

In 1962 an epidemic in Venezuela resulted in over 6000 officially registered cases, 389 of which were severe, and 43 individuals died (WENGER 1967). Frequent abortions were noted among pregnant women who suffered encephalitis in the first 3 months of pregnancy. In addition, women with encephalitis between the 13th and 36th week of pregnancy were found to have children with severe central nervous system damage. In three cases in which encephalitis occurred at 13–20 weeks gestation, the newborns had microphthalmia, no cerebellum, and the cranial cavities were filled with fluid. Only small rests of nervous tissue were found. In four cases of maternal encephalitis at about the eight months of pregnancy, the infant's central nervous system showed massive necrosis, softening, and hemorrhage in the cerebrum, and to a lesser degree in the cerebellum. Experimental studies have been reported in which pregnant rhesus monkeys were inoculated with live Venezuelan equine encephalitis virus vaccine by the direct intracerebral route of approximately

**Table 5.** Congenital Venezuelan equine encephalitis infection

| | |
|---|---|
| Defects | Abortion<br>Micropthalmia<br>Absent cerebrum<br>Massive CNS necrosis<br>Hydrocephalus |
| Detection | |
| Mother | Exposure (epidemic) in area)<br>Fibrile illness<br>Myalgia<br>Encephalitis<br>Specific antobody |
| Child | Micropthalmia, hydrocephalus, severe brain damage<br>Specific antibody |
| Prevention | Vaccines to animals<br>Possible danger of vaccines to pregnant women |

100 days gestation. The offspring of these pregnancies also had congenital microcephaly, hydrocephalus cataracts, and porencephaly (LONDON et al. 1977).

Venezuelan equine encephalitis can be controlled by immunization of animals and quarantine. Vaccines for this virus have also been used in human beings. When administered directly the rhesus fetuses, however, the vaccines produced severe damage to the brain and eyes. This should be considered if the vaccine virus is being advocated for administration to women of childbearing age.

## VI. Varicella Virus

Varicella (chickenpox) and herpes zoster (shingles) are caused by the same virus. In the United States, approximately 15% of women of childbearing age are susceptible to varicella infection, and some of those infected during pregnancy have produced children with congenital defects (Table 6). In the tabulation of defects in 11 cases from the literature cataracts, microphthalmia, Horner's syndrome, anisocornia, optic atrophy, nystagmus, and chorioretinitis were reported in 9 infants; brain damage was seen in 7, and skin scars and hypoplasia of specific parts could have been due to the degeneration of the nerve supply to that particular area (WILLIAMSON 1975).

Varicella very late in pregnancy is often manifested at birth or in the newborn by the presence of the characteristic chickenpox skin lesion or severe pneumonia with other complications. Maternal infection 5–10 days before delivery may produce disease in the infant and symptoms usually develop within 4 days of delivery. These infants usually escape severe effects of infection, presumably due to maternal antibody conferring some protection. However, maternal infection 0–4 days before delivery may result in infection of the infant, and approximately 30% of infected children die of disseminated disease. The use of high titered varicella zoster immune globulin (VZIG) shortly after birth prevents the disseminated disease.

**Table 6.** Congenital varicella

| | |
|---|---|
| Defects | Cataracts |
| | Micropthalamus |
| | Horner's syndrome |
| | Aniscornia |
| | Optic atrophy |
| | Nystagmus |
| | Chorioretinitis |
| | Mental retardation |
| | Skin scarring |
| | Hypoplasia of limbs |
| Detection | |
| Mother | Rash, antibody response (fluorescence, ELISA) |
| Child | Defects (listed above) |
| | Specific IgM antibody to varicella |
| Prevention | Avoid exposure |
| | Vaccines (?) |
| | Abortion (?) |

## C. Summary

Five viruses are recognized to be causes of fetal infections and malformation. These are: rubella virus, cytomegalovirus, herpesvirus, Venezuelan equine encephalitis virus, and varicella virus. Fortunately, rubella can now be prevented through the use of safe and effective vaccines. Clinical approaches for the prevention and treatment of congenital herpesvirus infections are already being used in many parts of the world. These include the use of cesarean section delivery to avoid exposure of the child to the virus and treatment with vidarabine. The use of immune globulin at the time of birth prevents disseminated varicella in the newborn. New methods for the detection of several other virus teratogens now provide opportunities for the study of the frequency and pathogenesis of these diseases. Hopefully, this will aid us in the control of these infections. Intensive utilization of vaccines and other methods of prevention are needed for the control of congenital infections. New studies are also needed to develop methods to prevent congenital cytomegalovirus, Venezuelan equine encephalitis, and congenital varicella infections, and to detect new, unrecognized agents of importance in humans.

## References


Birnbaum G, Lynch JI, Margileth AM, Lonergan WM, Sever JL (1969) Cytomegalovirus infections in newborn infants. J Pediatr 75:789

Castellano GA, Hazzard GT, Madden DL, Sever JL (1977) Comparison of the enzyme-linked immunosorben assay and the indirect hemagglutination test for detection of antibody to cytomegalovirus. J Infect Dis 136:337–342

Fuccillo DA, Moder FL, Traub RG, Henson S, Sever JL (1971) Micro indirect hemagglutination test for cytomegalovirus. Appl Microbiol 21:104

Gravell M, Dorsett PH, Gutenson O, Ley AC (1977) Detection of antibody to rubella virus by enzyme-linked immunosorbent assay. J Infect Dis 136:300–304

Hildebrandt RJ, Sever J, Margileth AM (1967) Cytomegalovirus in the normal pregnant female. Am J Obst Gynecol 98:1125
London WT, Levitt NH, Kent SG, Wang VG, Sever JL (1977) Congenital cerebral and ocular malformations induced in rhesus monkeys by Venezuelan equine encephalitis virus. Teratology 16:285
Nahmias JJ, Alford CA, Korones SB (1970) Infection of the newborn with herpesvirus hominis. In: Schulman I (ed) Advances in pediatrics, vol I. Year Book Medical, Chicago, p 185
Preblud SR, Serdula MK, Frank JA, Hinman AR (1980) Current status of rubella in the United States 1969–1979. J Infec Dis 142:776–779
Sever JL (1966) Perinatal infections affecting the developing fetus and newborn. In: National institute of child health and human development conference on the prevention of mental retardation through the control of infectious disease. US Public Health Service, Washington DC, Publ 1692
Sever JL, Hardy JB, Nelson RB, Gildeson MR (1969) Rubella in the collaborative perinatal research study. II. Clinical and laboratory findings in children through 3 years of age. Am J Dis Child 118:123
Starr JG, Gold E (1968) Screening of new born infants for cytomegalovirus infections. J Pediatr 73:830
Wenger F (1967) Massive cerebral necrosis of the fetus in cases of Venezuelan equine encephalitis. Invest Clin (Maracaibo) 21:13
Whitely RJ, Nahmias AJ, Seng-Jau S, Galasso GG, Fleming CL, Alford CA (1980) Vidarabine therapy of neonatal herpes simplex infection. Pediatrics 66:495–501
Williamson A (1975) The varicella-zoster virus in the etiology of severe congenital defects. Clin Pediatr (Phila) 14:553–558
Yeager AS, Arvin AM, Urbani JL, Kempf JA (1980) Relationship of antibody to outcome in neonatal herpes simplex virus infections. Infect Immun 29:532–538

CHAPTER 6

# Hormonal Involvement in Palatal Differentiation

R. M. GREENE

## A. Introduction

Development of the mammalian secondary palate has been the object of intense research interest. Palatal development in a variety of laboratory animals has served as a model system with which to investigate possible mechanisms of palatal clefting. These studies have thus used the developing secondary palate as an *object* of research, emphasizing the study of teratogens that induce cleft palatal (BAXTER and FRASER 1950; KOCHHAR 1968; WILK et al. 1978). More recently, this system has been used as a *tool* which has enabled extensive investigation of a wide variety of developmental phenomena occuring during palatal ontogenesis. Morphogenetic movements (WEE et al. 1976; WEE and ZIMMERMAN 1980; KUHN et al. 1980), epithelial mesenchymal interaction (TYLER and KOCH 1977 a, b; TYLER and PRATT 1980), cellular adhesion (GREENE and PRATT 1977), and programmed cell death (PRATT and GREENE 1976; GREENE and PRATT 1979 a) have all been examined during palatal development.

Recent evidence suggests that glucocorticoids, prostaglandins, and cyclic AMP (cAMP) all appear to play a role in normal growth and differentiation of the developing orofacial region, and may be specifically required for proper modulation of palatal differentiation. This chapter deals with recent progress made toward understanding some mechanisms of hormonal control of development of the secondary palate. Attention will be focused on the putative role of cyclic nucleotides and prostaglandins in normal palate development. Involvement of glucocorticoids has recently been discussed in an excellent review (SALOMON and PRATT 1979).

## B. Developmental Aspects of Secondary Palate Formation

Mammalian palatal shelves arise as outgrowths from the oral aspect of the maxillary processes, and orient vertically on each side of the tongue (Fig. 1). Each shelf consists of mesenchymal cells derived from the neural crest and embedded in a hyaluronate-rich (PRATT et al. 1973) extracellular matrix enclosed by epithelium several cell layers thick.

During the seventh week of gestation in humans (FULTON 1957), and corresponding gestational ages in a variety of laboratory mammals (COLEMAN 1965; WALKER and FRASER 1956; SHAH and CHAUDHRY 1974), the palatal shelves reorient into a horizontal position between the tongue and nasal septum. Anteriorly, the shelf reorients by a process resembling rotation around a hinge (COLEMAN 1965; DIEWERT 1974). This morphogenetic movement proceeds, however, along most of

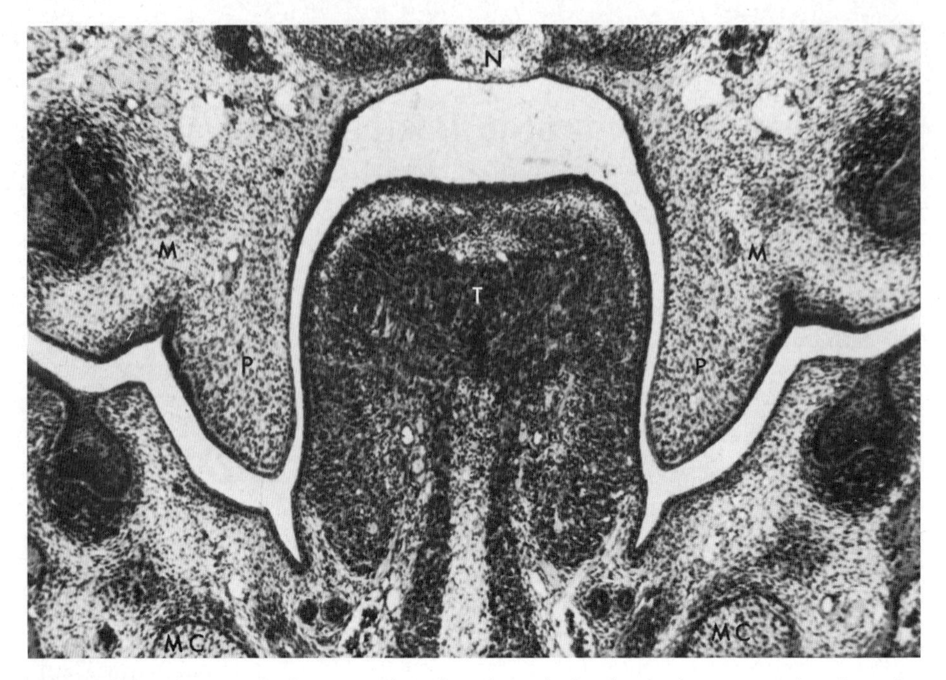


**Fig. 1.** Light micrograph of a coronal section through the developing oronasal region of a mouse fetus prior to reorientation of the palatal processes. Note that each palatal process (*P*), and outgrowth from the maxillary region (*M*), is vertically oriented laterally on either side of the tongue (*T*). Meckel's cartilage (*MC*); nasal septum (*N*). × 50

the length of the shelf by means of a "remodeling" of the vertical shelf (Fig. 2), despite the obstructive nature of the intervening tongue (WALKER and PATTERSON 1974; BRINKLEY et al. 1978).

Many factors have been implicated as being responsible for this palatal shelf movement (see GREENE and PRATT 1976 for review). Synthesis of palatal extracellular matrix components (LARSSON 1961; WALKER 1961, ANDERSON and MATHIESSEN 1967; PRATT and KING 1972; PRATT et al. 1973; HASSELL and ORKIN 1976; WILK et al. 1978) and palatal nonmuscular contractile systems (LESSARD et al. 1974; BABIARZ et al. 1975; KRAWCZYK and GILLON 1976; WEE and ZIMMERMAN 1980; KUHN et al. 1980) have been most frequently and recently cited as playing a role in shelf elevation.

Although most investigators support the concept of factors intrinsic to the palatal shelves as playing a critical role in shelf elevation, the interrelationships between these various factors with each other and with other orofacial components is largely speculative. Difficulty with determining the relative importance of these factors to shelf elevation in vivo has led to the development of various in vitro procedures to facilitate direct observation of shelf movement (WALKER and PATTERSON 1974; BRINKLEY et al. 1978; WEE et al. 1976; LEWIS et al. 1980; FERGUSON 1981). Refinement of these systems should facilitate clarification of the possible role, or roles, of embryonic movement (WALKER 1969; WALKER and PATTERSON 1974), the

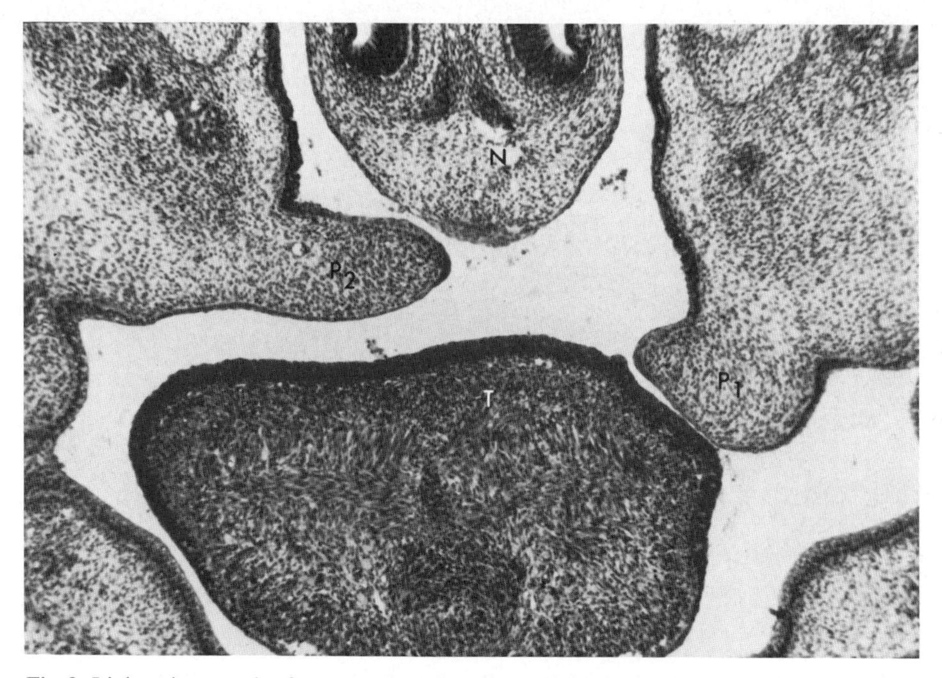


**Fig. 2.** Light micrograph of a coronal section through the developing oronasal region of a mouse fetus during the period of palatal process reorientation. Note that one process ($P_1$) is undergoing reorientation into a horizontal plane between the tongue ($T$) and nasal septum ($N$) while the homologous palatal process ($P_2$) has already assumed a horizontal orientation above the tongue. × 50

tongue (WALKER and QUARLES 1976; WALKER and PATTERSON 1974), the cranial base (BRINKLEY et al. 1978; BRINKLEY and VICKERMAN 1978), extracellular matrix components (HASSELL and ORKIN 1976; WILK et al. 1978), intracellular contractile elements (WEE et al. 1976; BRINKLEY and VICKERMAN 1979; WEE and ZIMMERMAN 1980), or putative neurotransmitter substances (WEE et al. 1979, 1980) in palatal shelf movement.

Soon after elevation, the surfaces of the medial edge epithelium (MEE) of apposing palatal shelves contact and quickly adhere to one another (DEANGELIS and NALBANDIAN 1968; FARBMAN 1968). Palatal MEE synthesizes cell surface glycoconjugates (GREENE and KOCHHAR 1974; DEPAOLA et al. 1975; PRATT and HASSELL 1975; MELLER and BARTON 1978) which facilitate initial adhesion to the opposite shelf (GREENE and PRATT 1977) until more permanent desmosomal attachments are established (SMILEY 1970) in the formation of a palatal midline epithelial seam (Fig. 3). This epithelial seam undergoes autolysis (MATO et al. 1966; FARBMAN 1968; HAYWARD 1969; CHAUDHRY and SHAH 1973), allowing mesenchyme from the two originally separate palatal shelves to merge and form the secondary palate.

Physiologic cell death is a common occurrence during embryogenesis of a variety of tissues and organ systems (SAUNDERS 1966; DORGAN and SCHULTZ 1971; GOLDIN and FABIAN 1971; BROADDUS 1970; ILIES 1970; FALLON and SIMANDL 1978) including, as noted, the developing rodent and human palatal epithelial cells

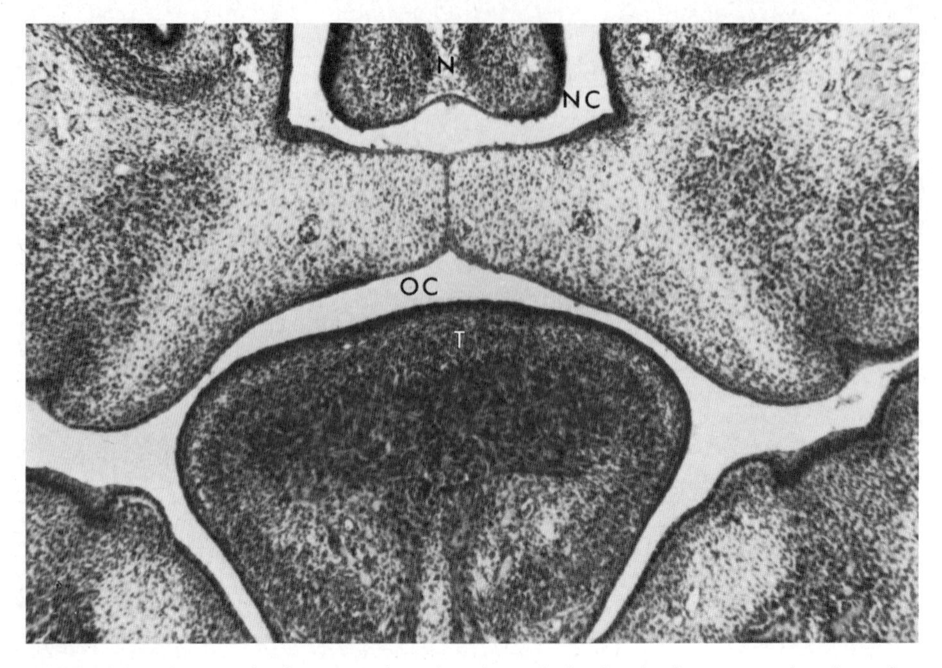


**Fig. 3.** Light micrograph of a coronal section through the developing oronasal region of a mouse fetus after both palatal processes have reoriented into a position between the tongue (*T*) and nasal septum (*N*). Note that the two shelves have merged into a single definitive secondary palate separating the nasal cacity (*NC*) from the oral cavity (*OC*). × 50

(SMILEY 1970; MATO et al. 1972; SMILEY and KOCH 1972; WATERMAN and MELLER 1974; PRATT and GREENE 1976). Cellular alterations accompanying palatal MEE degeneration have been well documented and include cessation of MEE DNA synthesis (HUDSON and SHAPIRO 1973; PRATT and MARTIN 1975) and a requirement for the synthesis by MEE of lysosomal enzymes (MATO et al. 1967; HAYWARD 1969; SMILEY 1970; MATO et al. 1972; PRATT and GREENE 1976). These processes have been extensively examined morphologically and recent studies have begun to reveal some of the biochemical regulatory mechanisms controlling this terminal differentiation (see Sect. C).

## C. Cyclic AMP and Palatal Differentiation

CAMP has been implicated as an important modulator of cell differentiation in many developing tissues (ROGAN et al. 1973; CREIGHTON and TREVITHICH 1974; ZALIN and MONTAGUE 1974; ZALIN and LEAVER 1975; MORIYAMA et al. 1976; DESHPANDE and SIDDIQUI 1976; RICKENBERG 1978; NIJJAR 1979; PERRY and OKA 1980). Moreover, it has recently become clearly evident that palatal cAMP levels play a critical role in normal differentiation of the secondary palate. A strong correlation exists between teratogenic agents and mutant genes known to affect palatal de-

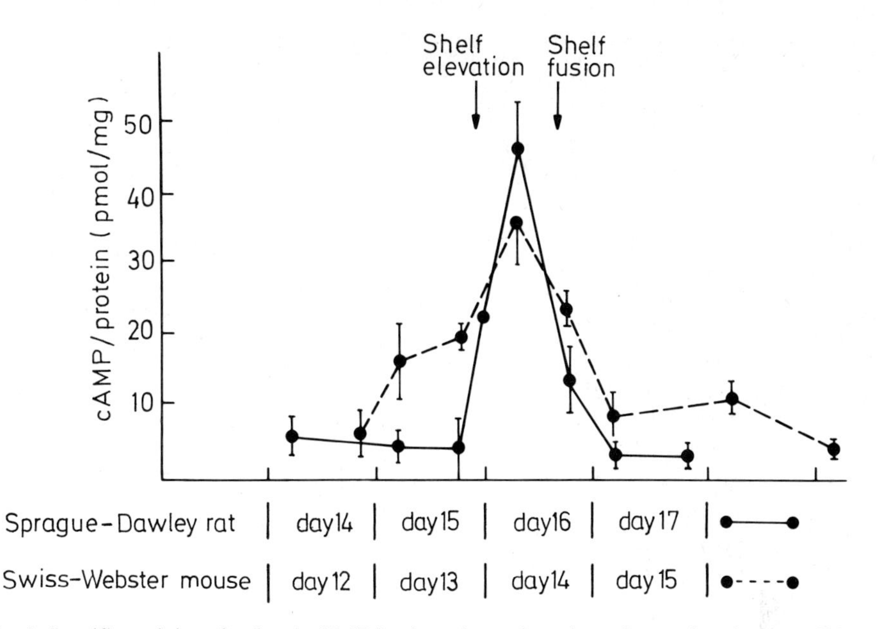


**Fig. 4.** Specific activity of palatal cAMP is plotted as a function of gestational age. *Full line* traces Sprague–Dawley rat palatal cAMP/mg protein. *Broken line* traces Swiss–Webster mouse palatal cAMP/mg protein. GREENE and PRATT (1979b)

velopment adversely and alterations in palatal cAMP levels (ERICKSON et al. 1979; OLSON and MASSARO 1980; PRATT et al. 1980; GREENE et al. 1981).

The initial observation that cAMP levels increase in the secondary palatal shelf just prior to shelf elevation and epithelial differentiation (PRATT and MARTIN 1975), correlates with the gestational period of maximal palatal adenylate cyclase activity (WATERMAN et al. 1976). This increase in palatal cAMP was subsequently shown to be transient (GREENE and PRATT 1979b), with maximal values seen in developing rodent palates corresponding to the gestational period of maximal palatal glycoconjugate synthesis and MEE cell death (Fig. 4). The developing mammalian palate is, however, a heterogeneous tissue, composed of mesenchymal and several types of epithelial cells and it was not determined which population, or populations, of palatal cells were responsible for the measured rise in intracellular cAMP. Recently, using immunohistochemical procedures, we addressed this question and observed a differential localization of cAMP in developing rodent palatal tissue (GREENE et al. 1980). Using specific anti-cAMP antibodies, localization of cAMP was performed utilizing the immunoglobulin–enzyme bridge method of MASON et al. (1969). Staining for cAMP was most intense in palatal epithelium, just prior to and during epithelial adhesion and seam formation with MEE staining most heavily (Fig. 5a, b). CAMP was localized along epithelial and mesenchymal plasma membranes, in addition to intense staining of the midline epithelial cytoplasm.

CAMP immunohistochemical staining intensity can serve as a semiquantitative means to assess cellular cAMP levels (ORTEZ 1978). Studies involving immunohistochemical localization of cyclic nucleotides in a number of mammalian tissues

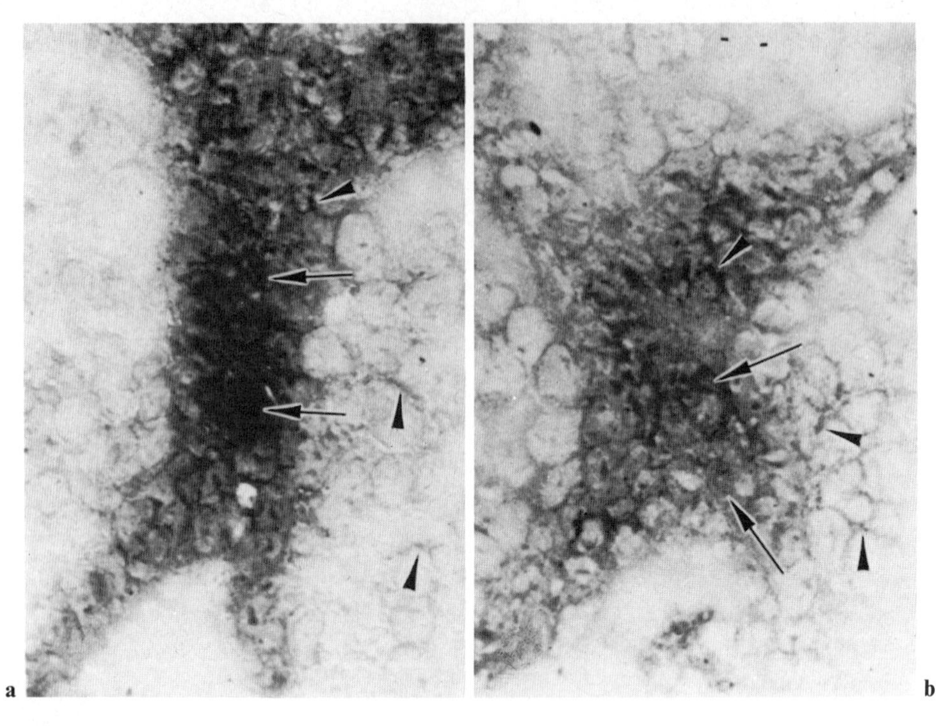

**Fig. 5a, b.** Coronal frozen sections of two apposing rat (**a**) and mouse (**b**) palatal processes immunohistochemically stained for cAMP. Note the intense staining for cAMP in the epithelial cytoplasm (*arrows*) of the intact midline epithelial seam. Note also the distribution of staining along the periphery of epithelial and mesenchymal cells (*arrowheads*). × 125 GREENE et al. (1980)

have repeatedly demonstrated a correlation between intensity of cellular staining for cyclic nucleotides and cellular cAMP content (BLOOM et al. 1973; FALLON et al. 1974; DAVIDOVITCH and SHANFELD 1975; DAVIDOVITCH et al. 1978; DOUSA et al. 1977; STEINER et al. 1978). In the developing secondary palate, increased epithelial staining for cAMP (GREENE et al. 1980) occurred during the developmental period during which palatal cAMP levels transiently elevate (GREENE and PRATT 1979b). Elevated levels of cAMP in the rodent palatal epithelium during epithelial adhesion and cell death suggest a role for this nucleotide in palatal epithelial differentiation. This conclusion is supported by studies which demonstrate that exogenous dibutyryl cAMP, which presumably increases palatal intracellular levels of cAMP, can prevent epidermal growth factor (EGF)-induced inhibition of MEE differentiation (HASSELL 1975; HASSELL and PRATT 1977) and induce precocious MEE differentiation of immature palatal shelves in vitro (PRATT and MARTIN 1975). Thus proper temporal synthesis of palatal cAMP appears to be requisite for normal palatal development.

The precise role which cAMP plays in palatal differentiation is not known. Elevated levels of intracellular cAMP have been correlated, in other systems, with increased cellular adhesiveness (FURMANSKY et al. 1971; NISHIDA et al. 1980) and the

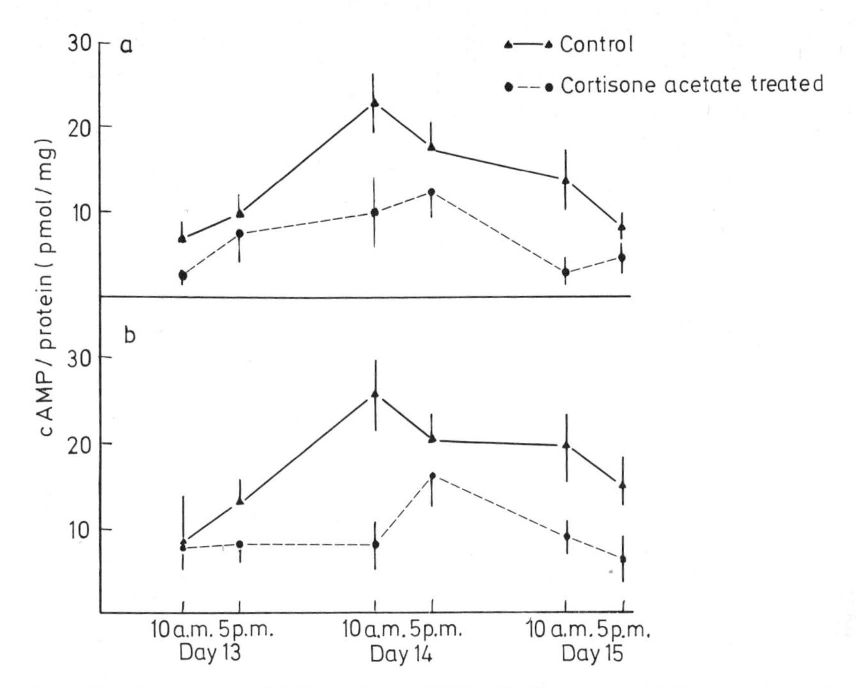


**Fig. 6a, b.** Specific activity of A/Jax (**a**) and C57BL/6J (**b**) palatal cAMP plotted as a function of gestational age. *Full lines* trace control levels of palatal cAMP/mg protein. *Broken lines* trace levels of palatal cAMP/mg protein from fetuses from cortisone-treated dams. GREENE et al. (1981)

induction of autolysis (SHELBURNE et al. 1973; DANIEL et al. 1973; LEMAIRE and COFFINO 1977; STUART and FISHER 1978). Since the transient elevation of palatal cAMP is temporally related to palatal epithelial glycoconjugate synthesis, known to be requisite for palatal epithelial adhesion (GREENE and PRATT 1977) and MEE cell death (PRATT and GREENE 1976; GREENE and PRATT 1979b), and since dibutyryl cAMP can precociously increase glycoconjugate synthesis in immature palatal shelves (PRATT and MARTIN 1975), cAMP may play a key role in regulating the synthesis of glycoconjugates requisite for MEE differentiation.

Many hormones and growth factors, including glucocorticoids (KUEHL et al. 1974; SCHUMACHER et al. 1977; ROSS et al. 1977; GUILLEMANT and GUILLEMANT 1979), which may influence cyclic nucleotide metabolism, appear to be requisite for normal palatal development (see SALOMON and PRATT 1979 for review). The exposure of the embryo to excess glucocorticoids during specific periods of development is known to result in fetal malformations, particularly cleft palate (BAXTER and FRASER 1950; WALKER 1967). Differing susceptibilities to glucocorticoid-induced cleft palate are exhibited by many strains of mice, a partial explanation for which is suggested by differences in levels of orofacial glucocorticoid receptors (see Sect. B.II.2 of Chap. 8). PRATT et al. (1980), however, have reported a correlation between sensitivity to glucocorticoid-induced cleft palate in the brachymorphic mouse and alterations in palatal cAMP levels. Moreover, in recent studies, palatal cAMP was quantitated in developing A/J (steroid-sensitive) and C57BL/6J and 10J (steroid-insensitive) secondary palates after administration of pharmacologic levels of glucocorticoids to pregnant females (ERICKSON et al. 1979; GREENE et al. 1981). A transient rise in palatal cAMP levels was seen in untreated A/J and C57 fetuses, with maximal values occurring during the period of MEE cell differentiation for both strains (Fig. 6). Levels of A/J and C57 palatal cAMP were depressed by maternal administration of teratogenic doses of glucocorticoids (Fig. 6). Immunohistochemical localization of cAMP demonstrated that this decrease in cAMP represented primarily reduced epithelial cAMP (GREENE et al. 1981). These data are further supported by the work of WATERMAN et al. (1977) who demonstrated decreased adenylate cyclase sensitivity in steroid-treated hamster palates. Thus palatal cAMP must be synthesized in proper quantitative levels to facilitate normal palatal development.

Since palatal cAMP levels were equally depressed in a steroid-sensitive (A/J) and a steroid-insensitive (C57 BL/6J) strain (GREENE et al. 1981), differential susceptibility to steroid-induced cleft palate in these two strains does not appear to involve a differential effect on palatal cAMP levels. Three lines of evidence may be interpreted to suggest that excess glucocorticoids may perturb normal development of the secondary palate by affecting palatal medial edge epithelial cAMP levels. After administration of pharmacologic doses of glucocorticoids during midgestation and production of cleft palate (BAXTER and FRASER 1950): (1) medial edge contact, although not extensive, has been shown to occur (GREENE and KOCHHAR 1973; SHAH and TRAVILL 1976; DIEWERT and PRATT 1981); (2) certain phases of medial edge epithelial differentiation are inhibited (HEROLD and FUTRAN 1980; GOLDMAN et al. 1981); and (3) medial edge epithelial palatal cAMP levels are reduced (ERICKSON et al. 1979; GREENE et al. 1981). These data collectively demonstrate that normal development of the mammalian palate is dependent upon proper synthesis, both temporally and quantitatively, of cAMP.

## D. Prostaglandins in the Secondary Palate

Factors controlling cAMP levels during palate morphogenesis are largely unknown, although EGF (NEXØ et al. 1980) and prostaglandins (CHEPENIK and GREENE 1981) have been implicated. Recent studies have suggested that the developing secondary palate is a potential target tissue for the action of EGF–urogastrone (EGF–URO; NEXØ et al. 1980; YONEDA and PRATT 1980). NEXØ et al. (1980) have demonstrated a steady increase in EGF receptor binding in crude membrane fractions from embryos during days 11½–18 of gestation and a more marked increase in membranes from developing maxillae. Moreover, autoradiographic localization of $^{125}$I-labeled EGF–URO binding in the developing secondary palate (NEXØ et al. 1980), as well as studies demonstrating that human palatal mesenchymal cell growth in vitro is dependent on EGF (YONEDA and PRATT 1980), support the contention that palatal mesenchyme and epithelium may serve as target tissues for EGF during development.

Nearly all phases of in vivo palate differentiation occur in vitro (POURTOIS 1966; SMILEY and KOCH 1972; PRATT et al. 1973; GREENE and PRATT 1977). Moreover, since palatal mesenchyme is required to support normal palatal epithelial differentiation (TYLER and KOCH 1977a, b), local mesenchymally derived factors may play a role in modulating palatal cAMP and epithelial and mesenchymal differentiation.

Prostaglandins constitute a diverse family of locally active lipids, many of which are known to be produced by, and stimulate cAMP accumulation in, a wide variety of mammalian cells (SAMMUELSSON et al. 1978). Primary cultures of mouse embryo palate mesenchymal cells were prelabeled with arachidonic acid $^3H$ (C20:4) and stimulated to release compounds which behaved as authentic prostaglandins, identified by thin layer chromatography and radioimmunoassay. Palatal mesenchyme was able to synthesize several compounds which cochromatograph with authentic prostaglandin $E_2$ ($PGE_2$), prostaglandin $F_{2\alpha}$ ($PGF_{2\alpha}$) and 6-keto-$PGF_1$ (the stable breakdown product of prostacyclin; CHEPENIK and GREENE 1981). The prostaglandin-like nature of some of the compounds released by palate mesenchymal cells in vitro was confirmed by radioimmunoassay (ALAM et al. in press), as well as indirectly by the finding that indomethacin, a relatively specific inhibitor of prostaglandin synthesis, inhibited their release (CHEPENIK and GREENE 1981).

Since cAMP is immunohistochemically demonstrable in palatal epithelial and mesenchymal cells (GREENE et al. 1980), these prostaglandins may serve as local modulators of palatal epithelial as well as mesenchymal cAMP formation. To pursue this possibility, responsiveness of fetal mouse palatal mesenchymal cells to prostaglandin $E_2$ ($PGE_2$) and prostacyclin ($PGI_2$) was recently investigated by determining cellular accumulation of cAMP (GREENE et al. 1981). Palatal mesenchymal cells in primary monolayer culture responded to challenge from $PGE_2$ and $PGI_2$ by accumulating cAMP in a dose-dependent relationship (Fig. 7). $PGI_2$ was significantly more effective than $PGE_2$ in stimulating the synthesis and accumulation of cAMP. Physiologic concentrations of $PGI_2$ ($10^{-11}$ *M*) resulted in significant increases in intracellular cAMP (Fig. 7), suggesting that $PGI_2$ may represent the natural ligand. A significant physiologic role for $PGE_2$, the predominant prostaglandin synthesized by these cells (CHEPENIK and GREENE 1981), cannot be ruled out, even though measurable changes in cellular cAMP appear to be minimal in response to low ($10^{-10}$–$10^{-11}$ *M*) doses of $PGE_2$. A shift in the ratio of bound:free cAMP may be sufficient to result in a physiologic response without a detectable change in tissue cAMP levels (DUFAU et al. 1977). Alternatively, palatal epithelium may serve as a target tissue for $PGE_2$ since when organ cultured palates, containing both mesenchyme and epithelium, were acutely challenged with physiologic levels of $PGE_2$, palatal intracellular cAMP levels increased dramatically (R. M. GREENE, unpublished work).

Continuous exposure of palatal mesenchymal cells to $PGE_2$ or 6,9-thia-$PGI_2$, a stable, biologically active analog of $PGI_2$ (NICOLAOU et al. 1977), resulted in accumulation of cAMP for 5 min, after which cells became refractory to further stimulation (Fig. 8). This refractory state was found to be agonist specific. Cells acutely stimulated with $PGE_2$ were refractory to a second exposure of $PGE_2$, but not $PGI_2$ or isoproterenol. When challenged with $PGI_2$, cells became refractory to a second challenge of $PGI_2$, but not $PGE_2$ or isoproterenol (GREENE et al. 1981). This desensitization may serve to modulate the magnitude and duration of response of palatal mesenchymal cells to hormonal stimulation.

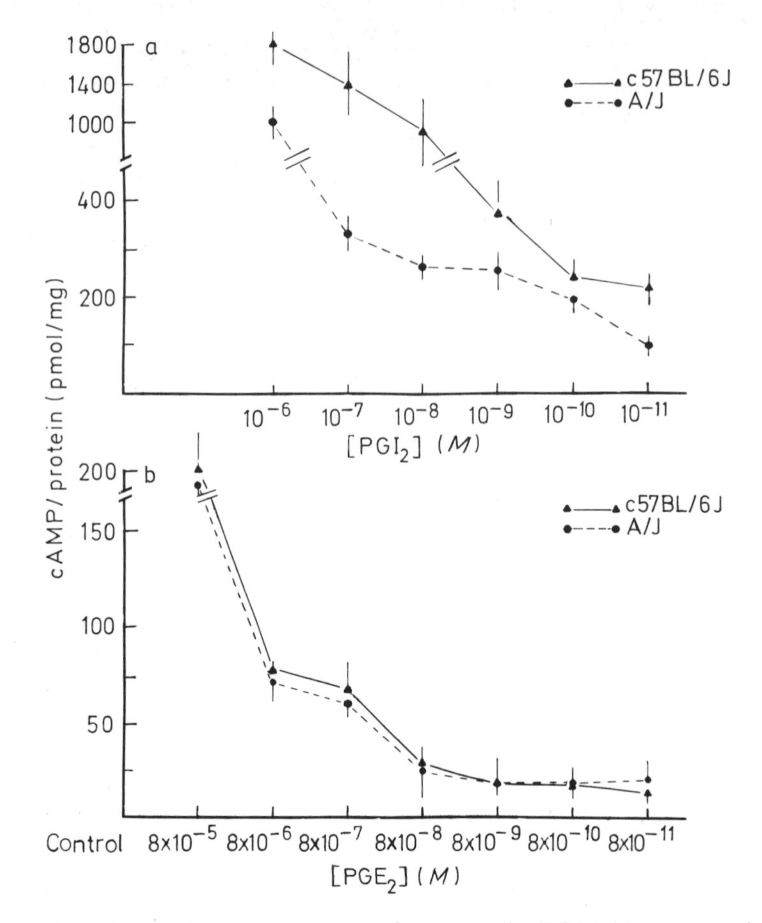


**Fig. 7a, b.** Effect of increasing concentrations of prostacyclin ($PGI_2$) (**a**) or prostaglandin $E_2$ ($PGE_2$) (**b**) on intracellular levels of cAMP in murine palatal mesenchymal cells in monolayer culture. Cells were grown to subconfluency, placed in serum-free media, and stimulation with either $PGI_2$ for 5 min or $PGE_2$ for 15 min. Values represent the mean $\pm$ standard error of quadruplicate determinations

Spontaneous recovery of responsiveness to prostaglandins occurs upon incubation of palatal mesenchymal cells for 6 h in hormone-free medium. Such recovery was inhibited by cycloheximide, colchicine, and cytochalasin B. Thus, maintenance of responsiveness of palatal mesenchymal cells to prostaglandin stimulation may involve transport and insertion of newly synthesized proteins, including prostaglandin receptor proteins, into the plasma membrane.

Palatal mesenchymal, as well as epithelial cAMP, may therefore play a pivitol role in controlling the synthesis of cell products identified with palatal differentiation. Just as epithelial cAMP appears to be critical for synthesis of epithelial glycoconjugates (see Sect. C), mesenchymal cAMP, possibly regulated by palatal prostaglandins, may control synthesis of extracellular matrix components or mesenchymal intracellular contractile elements.

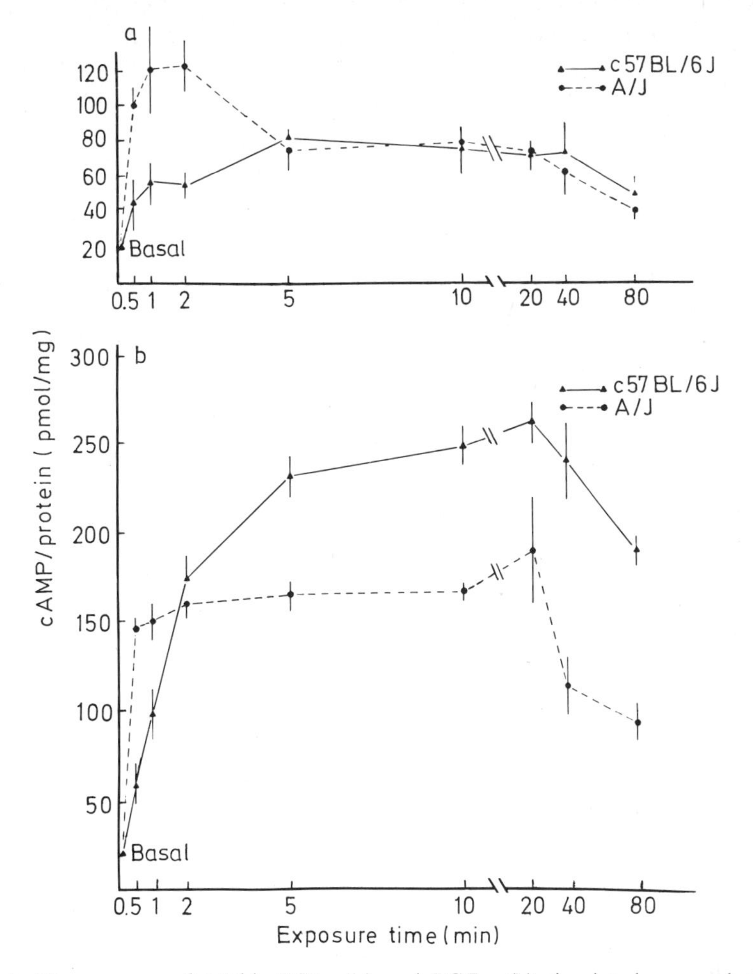


**Fig. 8a, b.** Time course of 6,9thia-$PGI_1$- (**a**) and $PGE_2$- (**b**) stimulated accumulation of cAMP. Cells were grown to subconfluency, placed in serum-free media, and stimulated with 6,9thia-$PGI_2$ ($1 \times 10^{-9}$ *M*) or $PGE_2$ ($8 \times 10^{-6}$ *M*) for from 0.5–80 min. CAMP was extracted at the times indicated after prostaglandin addition. Values represent the mean ± standard error of quadruplicate determinations. Note that accumulation of intracellular cAMP is essentially complete by 5 min, and continuous exposure to either $PGE_2$ or 6,9thia-$PGI_2$ for up to 80 min failed to result in accumulation of any more cAMP than seen with 5 min exposure. Note also that intracellular levels of cAMP declined by 20 min exposure to either prostaglandin. This decline corresponded with a concomitant increase in cAMP in the culture media. Cells failed therefore to maintain extremely high intracellular levels of cAMP by releasing cAMP into the medium

Prostaglandins and glucocorticoids are known to be interrelated in a number of physiologic processes (GRYGLEWSKI et al. 1975; HONG and LEVINE 1976; TAM et al. 1977; FOSTER and PERKINS 1977; PETERS et al. 1977; BRAY and GORDON 1979; RUSSO-MARIE et al. 1979). Moreover, cellular growth and differentiation in the developing secondary palate has been shown to be controlled in part by glucocorticoids (SALOMON and PRATT 1978, 1979; GREENE and SALOMON 1981).

Glucocorticoids more readily induce cleft palate in A/J than in C57Bl/6J strain mouse embryos (WALKER and FRASER 1957) and have also been found to depress mobilization of endogenous arachidonate (C20:4) by cells in vitro (HONG and LEVINE 1976). We labeled palate mesenchymal cells from both strains with $^{14}$C(C20:4) in vitro and then treated with melittin, a putative activator of phospholipase $A_2$, an enzyme thought to regulate release of C20:4 from endogenous phospholipids (SHIER 1979). Melittin stimulated release of radiolabel from cells from both strains in a dose-dependent manner and for any given dose, the relative amount of radioactivity released by C57BL/6J cells was greater than that released by A/J cells (CHEPENIK and GREENE 1981).

Thus, an impaired ability to mobilize endogenous C20:4 (CHEPENIK and GREENE 1981) coupled with a decreased sensitivity to stimulation by prostaglandins (GREENE et al. 1981) would render a prostaglandin-dependent developmental process sensitive to alteration by any agent (i.e., glucocorticoids) or condition which alters arachidonate metabolism. Indeed, TZORTZATOU et al. (1981) have recently suggested that glucocorticoid induction of cleft palate is accompanied by a reduction in available arachidonate in developing fetal maxillae and mandibles.

To define the possible relationships of palatal prostaglandins, glucocorticoids and cAMP to one another, and to palatal development, the effect of dexamethasone on the cAMP response of cultured mouse fetal palatal mesenchymal cells to prostaglandin stimulation was investigated. Preliminary data indicate that preincubation of cells with dexamethasone ($10^{-9}$ *M*), hydrocortisone ($10^{-9}$ *M*), or corticosterone ($10^{-9}$ *M*) results in enhanced responsiveness to $PGE_2$, as determined by accumulation of intracellular cAMP (GREENE and LLOYD 1982). Since glucocorticoids allow many metabolic processes to reach maximal rates (LEFER and SUTFIN 1964; KLETZIEN et al. 1975; HOSHINO et al. 1975; GRANNER et al. 1977), these data suggest that responsiveness of palatal mesenchyme to prostaglandin stimulation may be facilitated, if not maximized, by physiologic levels of glucocorticoid hormones.

## E. Summary

Primary cultures of palatal mesenchymal cells provide a sensitive means to study cellular hormonal control mechanisms in craniofacial development. When combined with organ culture of intact palatal tissue, hormonal control mechanisms, in tissues differing in sensitivity to teratogen-induced craniofacial defects, become especially amenable to study. Although much work remains to be done, the biochemical mechanisms controlling palatal differentiation are now much better understood than a few short years ago. Endogenous palatal glucocorticoids are thought to be facilitory in allowing mesenchymal cells to be maximally responsive to prostaglandin stimulation and, along with EGF, required for proper palatal growth. Palatal mesenchymal cells synthesize several prostaglandin-like compounds which act on palatal mesenchyme, and possibly epithelium, to increase cellular levels of cAMP. This increase in cAMP levels is thought then to modulate differentiation of both palatal epithelial and mesenchymal cells. Continued investigations such as those cited in this chapter, dealing with the underlying biochemical mechanisms controlling normal palatal development are fundamental to an understanding of the etiology of mechanisms of abnormal development. Questions dealing with biochemical mechanisms of action of potential teratogens must be based on a thorough understanding of the normal biochemical events and regulation of these events. Knowledge of mechanisms regulating these events is absolutely essential for understanding how these mechanisms may be perturbed, and thus for understanding the palatal clefts which may result.

*Acknowledgements.* Research support for much of the data presented in this chapter (Sects. C and D) was generously provided by the Department of Anatomy, Jefferson Medical College and in part by PHS grant DE 05550 to the author who is also recipent of NIH Research Career Development Award K04-DE00095. Special thanks are extended to Ms. MARTHA LLOYD for excellent technical assistance provided during the course of many of the studies discussed in this text, and to Mrs. DEBRA LUNDGREN for typing the text.

## References

Alam I, Capitanio A, Smith JB, Chepenik KP, Greene RM (to be published) Radioimmunologic identification of prostaglandins produced by serum stimulated mouse embryo palate mesenchyme cells. Biochim Biophys Acta
Anderson H, Mathiesson ME (1967) Histochemistry of the early development of the human central face and nasal cavity with special reference to the movements and fusion of the palatine processes. Acta Anat (Basel) 68:473–508
Babiarz BS, Allenspach AL, Zimmermann EF (1975) Ultrastructural evidence of contractile systems in mouse palates prior to rotation. Dev Biol 47:32–44
Baxter H, Fraser FC (1950) Production of congenital defects in the offspring of female mice treated with cortisone. McGill Med J 19:245–249
Bloom EE, Wedner HJ, Parker CW (1973) The use of antibodies of study cell structure and metabolism. Pharmacol Rev 25:343–358
Bray MA, Gordon D (1978) Prostaglandin production by macrophages and the effect of anti-inflammatory drugs. Br J Pharmacol 63:635–642
Brinkley LL, Vickerman MM (1978) The mechanical role of the cranial base in palatal shelf movement: an experimental re-examination. J Embryol Exp Morphol 48:93–100
Brinkley LL, Vickerman MM (1979) Elevation of lesioned palatal shelves in vitro. J Embryol Exp Morphol 54:229–240
Brinkley LL, Basehoar G, Avery JK (1978) Effects of craniofacial structures on mouse palatal closure in vitro. J Dent Res 57:402–411
Broaddus PV (1970) Acid hydrolases and their relationship to lysosomes in the mesonephros of the chick embryo. J Exp Zool 75:429–444
Chaudhry AP, Shah RM (1973) Palatogenesis in hamster. II. Ultrastructural observations on the closure of palate. J Morphol 139:329–350
Chepenik KP, Greene RM (1981) Prostaglandin synthesis by primary cultures of mouse embryo palate mesenchyme cells. Biochem Biophys Res Commun 100:951–958
Coleman RD (1965) Development of the rat palate. Anat Rec 151:107–118
Creighton MO, Trevithich JR (1974) Effect of cyclic AMP, caffeine and theophyllone on differentiation of lens epithelial cells. Nature 249:767–768
Daniel V, Litwack G, Tomkins GM (1973) Induction of cytolysis of cultured lymphoma cells by adenosine 3′:5′-cyclic monophosphate and the isolation of resistant variants. Proc Natl Acad Sci USA 70:76–79
Davidovitch Z, Shanfeld JL (1975) Cyclic AMP levels in alveolar bone of orthodontically-treated cats. Arch Oral Biol 20:567–574
Davidovitch Z, Montgomery PC, Yost RW, Shanfeld JL (1978) Immunohistochemical localization of cyclic nucleotides in mineralized tissues: mechanically stressed osteoblasts in vivo. Anat Rec 192:363–374

DeAngelis V, Nalbandian J (1968) Ultrastructure of mouse and rat palatal processes prior to and during secondary palate formation. Arch Oral Biol 13:601–608
DePaola DP, Drummond JF, Lorente C, Zarbo K, Miller SA (1975) Glycoprotein biosynthesis at the time of palate fusion by rabbit palate and maxilla cultured in vitro. J Dent Res 54:1049–1055
Deshpande AK, Siddique MAQ (1976) Differentiation induced by cyclic AMP in undifferentiated cells of early chick embryo in vitro. Nature 263:588–591
Diewert VM (1974) A cephalometric study of orofacial structures during secondary palate closure in the rat. Arch Oral Biol 19:303–315
Diewert V, Pratt RM (1981) Cortisone-induced cleft palate in A/J mice. Failure of palatal shelf contact. Teratology 24:149–162
Dorgan WJ, Schiltz RL (1971) An in vitro study of programmed cell death in rat placental giant cells. J Exp Zool 178:497–512
Dousa TP, Barnes LD, Ong S, Steiner AL (1977) Immunohistochemical localization of 3′:5′-cyclic AMP and 3′:5′-cyclic GMP in rat renal cortex: Effect of parathyroid hormone. Proc Natl Acad Sci USA 74:3569–3573
Dufau ML, Tsuruhara T, Horner KA, Podesta E, Catt KJ (1977) Intermediate role of adenosine 3′:5′-cyclic monophosphate and protein kinase during gonadotropin-induced stenoidogenesis in testicular interstitial cells. Proc Natl Acad Sci USA 74:3419–3423
Erickson RP, Butley MS, Sing CF (1979) H-2 and non H-2 determined strain variation in palatal shelf and tongue adenosine 3′:5′-cyclic morphosphate. J Immunogenet 6:253–262
Fallon EF, Agrawal R, Furth E, Steiner AL, Cowden R (1974) Cyclic quanosine and adenosine 3′,5′-monophosphates in canine thyroid: localization by immunofluorescence. Science 184:1089–1091
Fallon JF, Simandl BK (1978) Evidence of a role for cell death in the disappearance of the embryonic human tail. Am J Anat 152:111–130
Farbman AI (1968) Electron microscopic study of palate fusion in mouse embryos. Dev Biol 18:93–116
Ferguson MWJ (1981) Review: the value of the American alligator (Alligator mississippiensis) as a model for research in craniofacial development. J Craniofacial Genet Dev Biol 1:123–144
Foster SJ, Perkins JP (1977) Glucocorticoids increase the responsiveness of cells in culture to prostaglandin $E_1$. Proc Natl Acad Sci USA 74:4816–4820
Fulton JT (1957) Closure of the human palate in embryo. Am J Obstet Gynecol 74:179–182
Furmansky P, Silverman DS, Lubin M (1971) Expression of differentiated functions in mouse neuroblastoma mediated by dibutyryl-cyclic adenosine monophosphate. Nature 233:413–415
Goldin G, Fabian B (1971) An histochemical investigation of acid phosphatase activity in the pronephros of the developing *Xenopus laevis* tadpole. Acta Embryol Exp (Palermo) 1:31–39
Goldman AS, Herold R, Piddington R (1981) Inhibition of programmed cell death in the fetal palate by cortisol. Proc Soc Exp Biol Med 166:418–424
Granner DK, Lee A, Thompson EB (1977) Interaction of glucocorticoid hormones and cyclic nucleotides in induction of tyrosine aminotransferase in cultured hepatoma cells. J Biol Chem 252:3891–3895
Greene RM, Kochhar DM (1973) Spatial relations in the oral cavity of cortisone-treated mouse fetuses during the time of secondary palate closure. Teratology 8:153–162
Greene RM, Kochhar DM (1974) Surface coat on the epithelium of developing palatine shelves in the mouse as revealed by electron microscopy. J Embryol Exp Morphol 31:683–692
Greene RM, Lloyd M (1982) Glucocorticoids enhance responsiveness of palatal mesenchymal cells to prostaglandins. Teratology 25:46
Greene RM, Lloyd MR, Nicolaou KC (1981) Agonist-specific desensitization of prostaglandin stimulated cyclic AMP accumulation in palatal mesenchymal cell. J Craniofacial Genet Dev Biol 1:261:272

Greene RM, Pratt RM (1976) Developmental aspects of secondary palate formation. J Embryol Exp Morphol 36:225–245
Greene RM, Pratt RM (1977) Inhibition by diazo-oxo-norleucine (DON) of rat palatal glycoprotein synthesis and epithelial cell adhesion in vitro. Exp Cell Res 105:27–37
Greene RM, Pratt RM (1979a) Inhibition of epithelial cell death in vitro in the secondary palate by alteration of lysosome function. J Histochem Cytochem 26:1109–1114
Greene RM, Pratt RM (1979b) Correlation between cyclic AMP levels and cytochemical localization of adenylate cyclase during development of the secondary palate. J Histochem Cytochem 27:924–931
Greene RM, Salomon DM (1981) Glutamine synthetase activity in the developing secondary palate and induction by dexamethasone. Cell Differ 10:193–199
Greene RM, Goldman AS, Lloyd M et al. (1981) Glucocorticoid inhibition of cyclic AMP in the developing secondary palate. J Craniofacial Genet Dev Biol 1:31–44
Greene RM, Shanfeld JL, Davidovitch Z, Pratt RM (1980) Immunohistochemical localization of cyclic AMP in the developing rodent secondary palate. J Embryol Exp Morphol 60:271–281
Gryglewski RJ, Panczenko B, Korbut R, Grodzinska L, Ocetkrewics A (1975) Corticosteroids inhibit prostaglandin release from perfused mesentric blood vessels of rabbit and from perfused lungs of sensitized guinea pigs. Prostaglandins 10:343–355
Guillemant J, Guillemant S (1979) Elevated cyclic GMP concentrations in the rat adrenal cortex after dexamethasone administration. Biochem Biophys Res Commun 88:163–169
Hassell JR (1975) The development of rat palatal shelves in vitro. An ultrastructural analysis of the inhibition of epithelial cell death and palate fusion by the epidermal growth factor. Dev Boil 45:90–102
Hassell JR, Orkin RW (1976) Synthesis and distribution of collagen in the rat palate during shelf elevation. Dev Biol 49:80–88
Hassell JR, Pratt RM (1977) Elevated levels of cAMP alters the effect of epidermal growth factor in vitro on programmed cell death in the secondary palatal epithelium. Exp Cell Res 106:55–62
Hayward F (1969) Ultrastructural changes in the epithelium during fusion of the palatal processes in rats. Arch Oral Biol 14:661–673
Herold RC, Futran N (1980) Effect of cortisol on medial edge epithelium of organ-cultured single palatal shelves from steroid-susceptible mouse strains. Arch Oral Biol 25:423–429
Hong SL, Levine L (1976) Inhibition of arachidonic acid reflease from cells as the biochemical action of anti-inflammatory corticosteroids. Proc Natl Acad Sci USA 73:1730–1734
Hoshino J, Kuhne U, Filjak B, Kroger H (1975) Potentiating effect of a physiological dose of cortisone acetate on the dibutyryl cyclic AMP-mediated induction of tyrosine aminotransferase in rat liver. FEBS Lett 56:62–65
Hudson CD, Shapiro BL (1973) A radioautographic study of DNA synthesis in embryonic rat palatal shelf epithelium with reference to the concept of programmed cell death. Arch Oral Biol 18:77–84
Ilies A (1970) The topography and dynamics of the normal necrotic zones in the human embryo of 11–30 mm CR. IV. The necrotic zones of branchial arches, the extremities, and of the muscular primordia. Histological and histochemical study. Rev Roum Embryol Cytol Ser Embryol 7:117–130
Kletzien RF, Pariza MW, Becker JE, Potter VR (1975) A "permissive" effect of dexamethasone on the glucagon induction of amino acid transport in cultured hepatocytes. Nature 256:46–47
Kochhar DM (1968) Studies of vitamin A-induced teratogenesis: Effects on embryonic mesenchyme and epithelium, and on incorporation of $H^3$-thymidine. Teratology 1:299–310
Krawczyk KWS, Gillon DG (1976) Immunofluorescent detection of actin in non-muscle cells of the developing mouse palatal shelf. Arch Oral Biol 21:503–508
Kuehl FA, Ham EA, Zanetti ME, Sanford CH, Nicol SE, Goldberg ND (1974) Estrogen related increases in uterine guanosine 3′,5′-cyclic monophosphate levels. Proc Natl Acad Sci USA 71:1866–1870

Kuhn EM, Babiarz BS, Lessard JL, Zimmerman EF (1980) Palate morphogenesis. I. Immunological and ultrastructural analysis of mouse palate. Teratology 21:209–223
Larsson KS (1961) Studies on the closure of the secondary palate. III. Autoradiographic and histochemical studies in the normal mouse embryo. Acta Morphol neerl Scand 4:349–367
Lefer AM, Sutfin DC (1964) Cardiovascular effects of catecholamines in experimental adrenal insufficiency. Am J Physiol 206:1151–1155
Lemaire I, Coffino P (1977) Cyclic AMP induced cytolysis in S49 lymphoma cells: selection of an unresponsive "deathless" mutant. Cell 11:149–155
Lessar JL, Wee EL, Zimmerman EF (1974) Presence of contractile proteins in mouse fetal palate prior to shelf elevation. Teratology 9:113–126
Lewis CA, Thibault L, Pratt RM, Brinkley LL (1980) An improved culture system for secondary palate elevation. In Vitro (Rockville) 16:453–460
Mason TE, Phifer RF, Spicer SS, Swallow RD, Dreskin RB (1969) An immunoglobulin-enzyme bridge method for localizing tissue antigens. J Histochem Cytochem 17:563–569
Mato M, Aikawa E, Katahua M (1966) Appearance of various types of lysosomes in the epithelium covering lateral palatine shelves during secondary palate formation. Gunma J Med Sci 15:46–56
Mato M, Aikawa E, Katahua M (1967) Alterations of the fine structure of the epithelium of the lateral palatine shelf during secondary palate formation. Gunma J Med Sci 16:79–99
Mato M, Smiley GR, Dixon AD (1972) Epithelial changes in the presumptive regions of fusion during secondary palate formation. J Dent Res 5:1451–1456
Meller S, Barton LH (1978) Extracellular coat in developing human palatal processes: electron microscopy and ruthenium red binding. Anat Rec 190:223–232
Moriyama Y, Hasegawa S, Murayama K (1976) cAMP and cGMP changes associated with the differentiation of cultured chick embryo muscle cells. Exp Cell Res 101:159–163
Nexø E, Hollenberg MD, Figueroa A, Pratt RM (1980) Detection of epidermal growth factor-urogastrone and its receptor during fetal mouse development. Proc Natl Acad Sci USA 77:2782–2785
Nicolaou KC, Barnette WE, Gasic GP, Magolda RL (1977) 6,9-thia prostacyclin. A stable and biologically potent analogue of prostacyclin ($PGI_2$). J Am Chem Soc 99:7736–7738
Nijjar MS (1979) Role of cyclic AMP and related enzymes in rat lung growth and development. Biochim Biophys Acta 586:464–472
Nishida T, Solish SP, Pomeroy ME, Kobayashi M, Mukai N (1980) Cyclic AMP analog and theophylline increase adhesiveness of retinoblastoma-like tumor cells in culture. J Cell Biol 87:57
Olson FC, Massaro EJ (1980) Developmental pattern of cAMP, adenylcyclase, and cAMP phosphodiesterase in the palate, lung, and liver of the fetal mouse: Alterations resulting from exposure to methylmercury at levels inhibiting palate closure. Teratology 22:155–166
Ortez RA (1978) A semiquantitative method for cyclic nucleotide localization by immunocytochemistry and its application in determining the distribution of cyclic AMP in lungs of normal and pertussis-vaccinated mice following histamine or epinephrine challenge. J Cyclic Nucleotide Res 4:233–244
Perry JW, Oka T (1980) Cyclic AMP as a negative regulator of hormonally induced lactogenesis in mouse mammary gland organ culture. Proc Natl Acad Sci USA 77:2093–2097
Peters HD, Peskar BA, Schönhöfer PS (1977) Glucocorticoids: effects on prostaglandin release, cAMP levels and glycosaminoglycan synthesis in fibroblasts in tissue culture. Naunyn Schmiedebergs Arch Pharmacol 296:131–137
Pourtois M (1966) Onset of acquired potentiality for fusion in the palatal shelves of rats. J Embryol Exp Morphol 16:171–182
Pratt RM, Greene RM (1976) Inhibiton of palatal epithelial cell death by altered protein synthesis. Dev Biol 54:135–145
Pratt RM, King CTG (1972) Inhibition of collagen cross-linking associated with β-aminopropionitrile-induced cleft palate in the rat. Dev Biol 27:322–328

Pratt RM, Hassell JR (1975) Appearance and distribution of carbohydrate rich macromolecules on the epithelial surface of the developing rat palatal shelf. Dev Biol 45:192–198
Pratt RM, Martin GR (1975) Epithelial cell death by altered protein synthesis. Dev Biol 54:135–145
Pratt RM, Goggins JR, Wilk AL, King CTG (1973) Acid mucopolysaccharide synthesis in the secondary palate of the developing rat of the time of rotation and fusion. Dev Biol 32:230–237
Pratt RM, Salomon DR, Diewert VM, Erickson RP, Burns R, Brown KS (1980) Cortisone induced cleft palata in the Brachymorphic mouse. Teratol Carcinog Mutagen 1:15–23
Rickenberg HV (1978) The role of cyclic nucleotides in development. In: Ahmad F (ed) Differentiation and development. Academic Press, New York, pp 149–167
Rogan EG, Schafer MP, Anderson NG, Coggin JH (1973) Cyclic AMP levels in the developing hamster foetus: a correlation with the phasing of foetal antigen in membrane maturation. Differentiation 1:199–204
Ross PS, Manganiello VC, Vaughn M (1977) Regulation of cyclic nucleotide phosphodiesterases in cultured hepatoma cells by dexamethasone and $N^6$,$0^2$-dibutyryl adenosine3′:5′-monophosphate. J Biol Chem 252:1448-1452
Russo-Marie F, Paing M, Duval D (1979) Involvement of glucocorticoid receptors in steroid-induced inhibition of prostaglandin secretion. J Biol Chem 254:8498–8504
Salomon DS, Pratt RM (1978) Inhibition of growth in vitro by glucocorticoids in mouse embryonic facial mesenchyme cells. J Cell Physiol 97:315–328
Salomon DS, Pratt RM (1979) Involvement of glucocorticoids in the development of the secondary palate. Differentiation 13:141–154
Samuelsson B, Goldyne M, Granstrom E, Hamberg M, Hammarstrom S, Malmsten C (1978) Prostaglandins and thromboxanes. Annu Rev Biochem 47:997–1029
Saunders JW (1966) Death in embryonic systems. Science 154:604–612
Schumacher M, Seidel I, Stratling WH (1977) Elevated cyclic GMP concentrations during estrogen induced differentiation of the chick oviduct. Biochem Biophys Res Commun 74:614–620
Shah RM, Chaudhry AP (1974) Light microscopic and histochemical observations on the development of the palate in the golden Syrian hamster. J Anat 117:1–15
Shah RM, Travill AA (1976) Morphogenesis of the secondary palate in normal and hydrocortisone-treated hamsters. Teratology 13:71–84
Shelburne JD, Arstila AU, Trump BF (1973) Studies on cellular autophagocytosis. Cyclic AMP and dibutyryl cAMP stimulated autophagy in rat liver. Am J Pathol 72:521–540
Shier WT (1979) Activation of high levels of endogenous phospholipase $A^2$ in cultured cells. Proc Natl Acad Sci USA 76:195–199
Smiley GR (1970) Fine structure of mouse embryonal palatal epithelium prior to and after midline fusion. Arch Oral Biol 15:287–296
Smiley GR, Koch WE (1972) An in vitro and in vivo study of single palatal processes. Anat Rec 173:405–416
Steiner AL, Koide Y, Earp HS, Bechtel PJ, Beavo JA (1978) Compartmentalization of cyclic nucleotides and cyclic AMP dependent protein kinases in rat liver: immunocytochemical demonstration. In: George WJ, Ignarro LJ (eds) Advances in cyclic nucleotide research, vol 9. Raven Press, New York, pp 691–705
Stuart ES, Fischer MS (1978) In vitro stimulation of tadpole tail regression by cyclic AMP. Biochem Biophys Res Commun 82:621–626
Tam S, Hong SL, Levine L (1977) Relationships among the steroids of anti-inflammatory properties and inhibition of prostaglandin production and arachidonic acid release by transformed mouse fibroblasts. J Pharmacol Exp Ther 203:162–168
Tyler MS, Koch WF (1977a) In vitro development of palatal tissues from embryonic mice. II. Tissue isolation and recombination studies. J Embryol Exp Morphol 38:19–36
Tyler MS, Koch WF (1977b) In vitro development of palatal tissues from embryonic mice. II. Interactions between palatal epithelium and htereotypic oral mesenchyme. J Embryol Exp Morphol 38:37–48

Tyler MS, Pratt RM (1980) Effect of epidermal growth factor on secondary palatal epithelium in vitro: tissue isolation and recombination studies. J Embryol Exp Morphol 58:93–106
Tzortzatou GG, Goldman AS, Boutwell WC (1981) Evidence for a role of arachidonic acid in glucocorticoid-induced cleft palate in rats. Proc Soc Exp Biol Med 166:321–324
Walker BE (1961) The association of mucopolysaccharides with morphogenesis of the palate and other structures in mouse embryos. J Embryol Exp Morphol 9:22–31
Walker BE (1967) Induction of cleft palate in rabbits by several glucocorticoids. Proc Soc Exp Biol Med 125:1281–1284
Walker BE (1969) Correlation of embryonic movement with palate closure in mice. Teratology 2:191–198
Walker BE, Fraser FC (1956) Closure of the secondary palata in three strains of mice. J Embryol Exp Morphol 4:176–189
Walker BE, Fraser FC (1957) The embryology of cortisone-induced cleft palate. J Embryol Exp Morphol 5:201–209
Walker BE, Patterson A (1974) Induction of cleft palate in mice by tranquilizers and barbiturates. Teratology 10:159–163
Walker BW, Quarles J (1976) Palatal development in mouse foetuses after tongue removal. Arch Oral Biol 21:405-412
Waterman RE, Meller SM (1974) Alterations in the epithelial surface of human palatal shelves prior to and during fusion: a scanning electron microscopic study. Anat Rec 180:111–136
Waterman RE, Palmer GC, Palmer SJ, Palmer SM (1976) Catecholamine-sensitive adenylate cyclase in the developing golden hamster palate. Anat Rec 185:125–138
Waterman RE, Palmer GC, Palmer SJ, Palmer SM (1977) In vitro activation of adenylate cyclase by parathyroid hormone and calcitonin during normal and hydrocortisone-induced cleft palate development in the golden hamster. Anat Rec 188:431–444
Wee EL, Zimmerman EF (1980) Palate morphogenesis. II. Contraction of cytoplasmic processes in ATP-induced palate rotation in glycerinated mouse heads. Teratology 21:15–27
Wee EL, Wolfson LG, Zimmerman EF (1976) Palate shelf movement in mouse embryo culture: Evidence for skeletal and smooth muscle contractility. Dev Bol 48:91–103
Wee EL, Babiarz BS, Zimmerman S, Zimmerman EF (1979) Palate morphogenesis. IV. Effects of serotonin and its antagonists on rotation in embryo culture. J Embryol Exp Morphol 53:75–90
Wee EL, Phillips NJ, Babiarz B, Zimmerman EF (1980) Palate morphogenesis. V. Effects of cholinergic agonists and antagonists on rotation in embryo culture. J Embryol Exp Morphol 58:177–193
Wilk AL, King CTG, Pratt RM (1978) Chlorcyclizine induction of cleft palate in the rat: degradation of palatal glycosaminoglycans. Teratology 18:199–210
Yoneda T, Pratt RM (1981) Messenchymal cells from the human embryonic palate are highly responsive to epidermal growth factor. Science 213:563–565
Zalin RJ, Leaver R (1975) The effect of a transient increase in intracellular cAMP upon muscle cell fusion. FEBS Lett 53:33–36
Zalin RJ, Montague W (1974) Changes in adenylate cyclase, cAMP and protein kinase levels in chick myoblasts and their relationship to differentiation. Cell 2:103–108

CHAPTER 7

# Membrane Lipids and Differentiation

K. P. CHEPENIK and S. A. WALDMAN

## A. Introduction

The rationale for studying cell membranes during embryogenesis needs little clarification since, to paraphrase MOSCONA (1974), the notion that such membranes play a most important role in the control of embryonic growth, differentiation, and morphogenesis is generally accepted by development biologists. Recently, KRETSCHMER (1978) pointed specifically to the need for studies of cell membranes in investigations of mechanisms underlying teratogenesis. The rationale for studies of lipid metabolism as related to embryonic cell membranes may not be so obvious without a brief review of the structure of cell membranes in general.

The current concept of cell membranes is that of a fluid mosaic (SINGER and NICOLSON 1972; SINGER 1974, 1977), in which integral, membrane proteins reside in a "two-dimensional bilayer lipid solvent" (SINGER 1977). It is recognized that membrane proteins carry out the chemical processes unique to a particular membrane. However, it is recognized also that the quality and quantity of the lipid matrix may affect (regulate) the activities of many enzymes in the membrane (FOURCANS 1974; TRIGGLE 1970). The "fluid" nature of the cell membrane reflects the fact that the lipid bilayer is in a liquid crystalline state at physiologic temperatures, and that integral proteins (and lipids) may therefore move in the lateral plane of the membrane. The relative degree of "fluidity" of a cell membrane (at a specified temperature) is determined primarily by the acyl composition of the membrane phospholipids (DEMEL et al. 1967; CHAPMAN 1975) and the phospholipid: cholesterol ratio in the membrane (VAN DEENEN et al. 1972; DEMEL and DEKRUYFF 1976). That these characteristics of the cell membrane may change as a function of differentiation is indicated by the general finding that: (1) undifferentiated embryonic cells are more readily agglutinated by some plant lectins than are differentiated ones (MOSCONA 1974; PAULSEN and FINCH 1977; HEWITT and ELMER 1978); and (2) agglutination by plant lectins, in some cases, seems to reflect increased association of binding sites within the cell membrane (HEWITT and ELMER 1978; SACHS 1974).

It should be noted that, in addition to determining membrane fluidity, lipids also may play a role in determining membrane permeability. For example, liposomes prepared with 1,2-diacyl-*sn*-glycero-3-phosphocholine (diacyl-GPC) containing short chain fatty acids are more permeable to glycerol and glucose than those prepared with diacyl-GPC containing long chain fatty acids. An increase in the number of double bonds in the acyl groups of the phospholipids will also affect permeability, as will the amount of cholesterol in the membrane (VAN DEENEN et al. 1972).

## B. Membrane Lipid Composition and Differentiation

The cellular slime mold *Dictyostelium discoideum* has been utilized extensively to study altered membrane lipid composition as a function of differentiation because marked changes occur in its membrane structure and function during its life cycle (ELLINGSON 1974). ELLINGSON (1974) found 1,2-diacyl-*sn*-glycero-3-phosphocholine (diacyl-GPC), -phosphoinositol (diacyl-GPI), and phosphatidic acid increased, whereas monoacyl-*sn*-glycero-3-phosphoethanolamine (lyso-GPE) decreased during development of *D. discoideum*. Since these phospholipids are localized almost exclusively in cellular membranes, one might expect such quantitative changes to be associated with altered membrane function necessary for differentiation. Indeed, WEEKS (1976) was able to inhibit aggregation and differentiation, but not growth, of *D. discoideum* by manipulating the amounts of polyunsaturated fatty acids found in their complex lipids. These studies suggest a correlation between membrane lipid metabolism, composition, and differentiation.

Several investigators have used myoblast fusion, in vitro, as a system with which to study relationships between membrane lipid composition and differentiation of vertebrate cells. It seems that myoblast fusion, in vitro, is an ordered, multistep process, which consists of cell recognition, adhesion, and then membrane fusion (KNUDSEN and HOROWITZ 1977). The fusion event itself appears to be modulated by lipids in that: (1) there is a transient decrease in plasma membrane microviscosity prior to, and during, the process of fusion (PRIVES and SCHNITSKY 1977); and (2) myoblasts grown in media supplemented with fatty acids known to decrease membrane fluidity do not fuse (HOROWITZ et al. 1978, 1979; PRIVES and SCHNITSKY 1977). Furthermore, different membrane lipids may modulate different steps in the fusion process. CORNELL et al. (1980) found that inhibitors of cholesterol synthesis prevent myoblast fusion by inhibiting the cell recognition (aggregation) step in the fusion process. It was suggested that cholesterol availability might modulate assembly of aggregation components into the plasma membrane or maintenance of their activity, since neither the amount of cholesterol nor the cholesterol:phospholipid ratio in the myoblast plasma membrane were altered by inhibiting cholesterol synthesis (CORNELL et al. 1980).

Studies to determine the lipid composition of various organs obtained during embryogenesis in the chicken suggest a correlation between membrane lipid metabolism and differentiation, in vitro. WOOD (1974) reported alterations in the phospholipid composition of brain, heart, and liver obtained from chicken embryos at various stages of differentiation. He found that: (1) the phospholipid composition of each organ was unique to that organ; (2) the acyl composition of the various phospholipid classes was unique to each organ; and (3) there were distinct and unique alterations in the relative amounts of different phospholipids and in their acyl composition as differentiation progressed (WOOD 1974). Though WOOD reported that the acyl composition of chicken embryos phospholipids became more saturated during development, others have found just the opposite to be true (MIYAMOTO et al. 1966; ABAD et al. 1976). The basis for these different findings with the same tissues is not clear. However, increased unsaturation of phospholipid acyl composition would suggest increased membrane fluidity. This is consistent with the findings of KUTCHAI et al. (1976) that the microviscosity of plasma membranes prepared from chicken embryo hearts decreased as development proceeded.

The metabolic basis for the divergent patterns in phospholipid composition of various organs during chicken embryogenesis is not known. That they represent differential expression of enzyme activities would seem obvious. However, which enzymes are expressed, when they are expressed, and what factors modulate their expression are not known.

## C. Lipids as Intracellular Messengers

Lipids may modulate differentiation, not only by their effects on the physical and chemical characteristics of membranes, but also by acting directly as intracellular messengers. Lymphocytes can be stimulated in vivo with the appropriate antigen, and in vitro with mitogens (i.e., phytohemagglutinin, concanavalin A) to undergo blast transformation, a process of differentiation which includes growth, mitosis, and the acquisition of specific functions (LING and KAY 1975; FERBER and RESCH 1977). The mitogenic agent interacts directly with the cell surface and triggers a complex series of biochemical events comprising a membrane-to-nucleus signal sequence resulting in increased DNA synthesis (COFFEY et al. 1981; GREAVES and BAUMINGER 1972). Among the earliest of these events (2–10 min) are cellular accumulations of calcium and calcium-dependent increases in guanylate cyclase activity and intercellular cGMP (COFFEY et al. 1977, 1981; ALLWOOD et al. 1971; WHITNEY and SUTHERLAND 1972; PARKER 1974; HADDEN et al. 1975; HUI and HARMONY 1980; CARPENTIERI et al. 1980). Studies of various enzymes from normal and mitogen-induced lymphocytes revealed that phospholipase A, a calcium-requiring enzyme, is activated early in blast transformation (RESCH et al. 1971; FERBER and RESCH 1977; COFFEY et al. 1981). Agents known to inhibit phospholipase A, such as quinicrine and p-bromophenacyl bromide, also inhibit activation of guanylate cyclase and DNA synthesis in mitogen-stimulated lymphocytes (COFFEY et al. 1981). Also, these activations were inhibited by agents, such as 5,8,11,14-eicosatetraynoic acid and nordihydroguaiaretic acid, which inhibit the oxidative metabolism by lipoxygenase of arachidonate, a product of phospholipase $A_2$ activity, to hydroperoxy and hydroyxy fatty acids (COFFEY et al. 1981). However, activation of guanylate cyclase and DNA synthesis were not inhibited by indomethacin, a relatively specific inhibitor of cycloxygenase which metabolizes arachidonate to prostaglandins (COFFINS et al. 1981). It appears, then, that one of the initial events in blast transformation is a calcium-dependent activation of phospholipase $A_2$ with a concomitant release of membrane-bound arachidonate, which undergoes further oxidation by lipoxygenase to a hydroxy or hydroperoxy fatty acid. This oxidized fatty acid presumably activates guanylate cyclase, and the resulting elevation of cGMP appears to be related to increased DNA synthesis in the nucleus. Thus, membrane-bound lipids and the enzymes metabolizing them play a key role as extracellular messengers in the membrane-to-nucleus signal sequence mediating the differentiation of lymphocytes.

## D. Membrane Lipid Metabolism During Normal and Abnormal Mammalian Embryogenesis

### I. Initial Studies

We have conducted studies of membrane lipid metabolism during normal and abnormal mammalian embryogenesis, in vivo. These studies grew out of our finding that treatment pregnant rats with the teratogen and folic acid antagonist, 9-methylpteroylglutamic acid (9-MePGA) had a differential effect on the rate of synthesis of various subcellular organelles (CHEPENIK and WAITE 1972). We pursued this suggestion by injecting a radiolabeled phospholipid precursor (ethanolamine $^{14}C$) into control and teratogen-treated (9-MePGA) pregnant rats and followed its uptake into different membranous compartments of embryos, placentas, and yolk sacs obtained at various times after the injection (CHEPENIK and WAITE 1973, 1975). We determined the amount of radioactivity incorporated into diacyl-GPC, 1,2-diacyl-*sn*-glycero-3-phosphoethanolamine (diacyl-GPE), and monoacylphosphatidylethanolamine (monoacyl-GPE) extracted from subsellular fractions rich in either mitochondria, lysosomes, microsomes, or soluble components (cytosol). Those phospholipids were studied because: (a) ethanolamine is utilized in the synthesis of diacyl-GPE, the second most common phospholipid in cell membranes (generally speaking); (b) diacyl-GPE may be sequentially methylated (BREMER 1969) to form diacyl-GPC, the most common phospholipid found in cell membranes; and (c) monoacyl-GPE is a degradation product of diacyl-GPE. The amount of radioactivity found in diacyl-GPE declined and the amount in diacyl-GPC increased in a reciprocal fashion when these phospholipids were examined at various times after injection of the radiolabel (Figs. 1, 2). This was true for all tissues (embryos, placentas, and yolk sacs), and was interpreted to mean that the embryo, placenta, and yolk sac might be capable of synthesizing dicacyl-GPE de novo and then methylating it to form diacyl-GPC.

Following injection of ethanolamine $^{14}C$, the amount of radioactivity found in diacyl-GPC was equal to that found in diacyl-GPE, first in the yolk sac and maternal liver, then in the placenta, and then in the embryo (Table 1). These data were interpreted to mean that the yolk sac tended to take up phospholipids as it found them in serum lipoproteins (since serum lipoproteins almost entirely originate in the liver), that the placenta may synthesize diacyl-GPE as a precursor to diacyl-GPC as well as take diacyl-GPC up from the maternal serum, and that the embryo might either synthesize diacyl-GPE and then diacyl-GPC, or take these compounds up from the placenta. Furthermore, the teratogen treatment altered the rate of incorporation of radiolabel into phospholipids from subcellular fractions of embryos and placentas (Figs. 1, 2), indicting an alteration in the rate of synthesis or turnover of subcellular membranes in those tissues. The teratogen-induced alteration in rates of accumulation of radiolabeled diacyl-GPE and diacyl-GPC was reflected in: (1) a shortening of the time after injection of ethanolamine $^{14}C$ that the amount of radioactivity in diacyl-GPC equaled the amount in diacyl-GPC in embryos and placentas (Table 1); and (2) an alteration in the temporal sequence of accumulation of radioactivity in one cellular fraction of the embryo compared with another (Table 2).

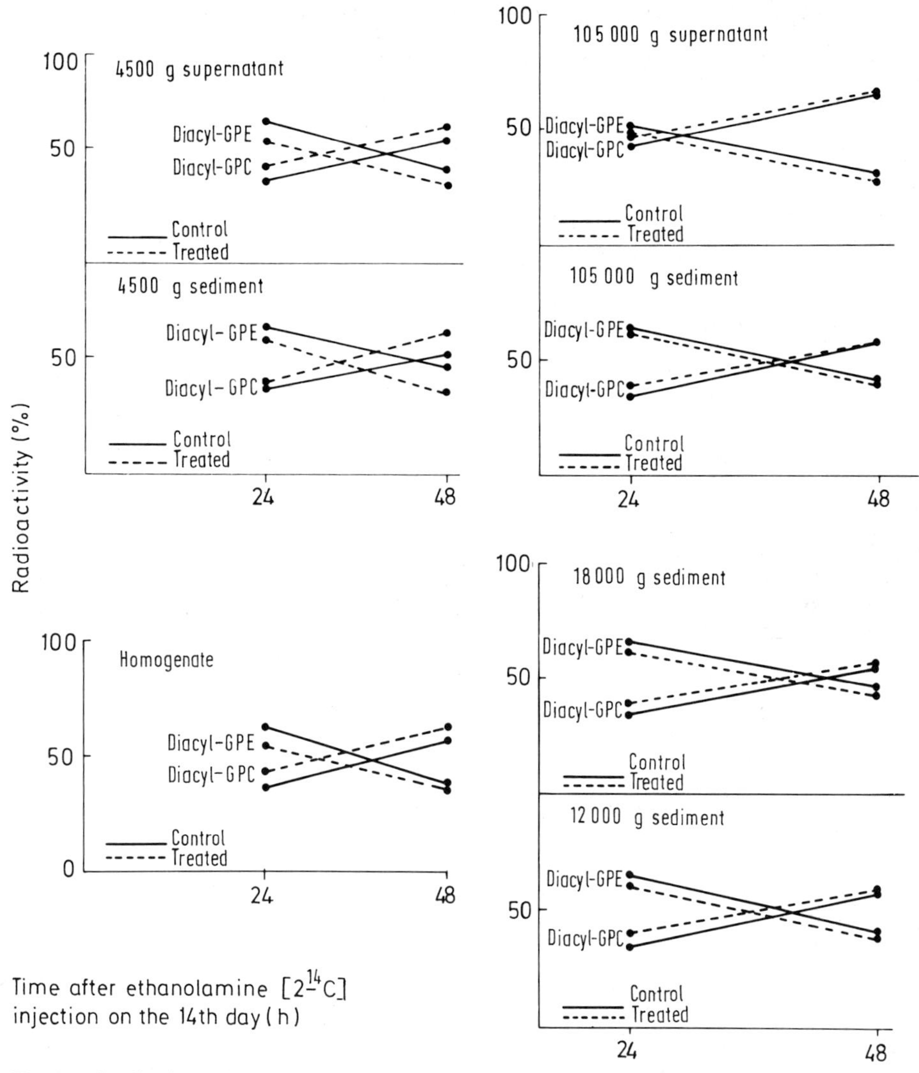


**Fig. 1.** Distribution of radioactivity as diacyl-GPC or diacyl-GPE in various fractions of control and treated embryos. Pregnant rats were fed a synthetic, teratogenic diet containing the folate antagonist 9-MePGA from the 11th to 14th days of gestation. Ethanolamine [2-$^{14}$C] was injected into the maternal circulation on the 14th day and tissues collected at various times thereafter for analysis as described in CHEPENIK and WAITE (1973)

These data were interpreted to mean the teratogen (9-MePGA) had altered the ability of the embryo to synthesize diacyl-GPC from diacyl-GPE, and that the embryo had been shifted to a greater dependence on phospholipid metabolism in the placenta. It seemed that in turn placental phospholipid uptake had been altered. We speculated that the folic acid antagonist may have produced the observed effects on diacyl-GPC synthesis: (a) by altering some transmethylation reactions necessary for the synthesis of *S*-adenosylmethionine (SAM), the key compound in the

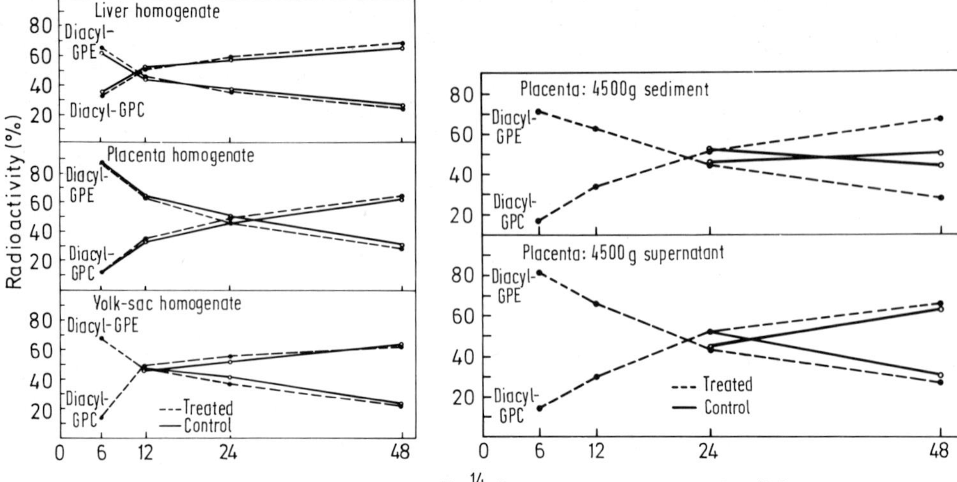


**Fig. 2.** Distribution of radioactivity as diacyl-GPC or diacyl-GPE in homogenates of maternal liver, yolk sac, and placenta, and two subcellular fractions. Pregnant rats were fed a synthetic, teratogenic diet containing the folate antagonist 9-MePGA from the 11th to 14th days of gestation. Ethanolamine [2-$^{14}$C] was injected into the maternal circulation on the 14th day and tissues collected at various times thereafter for analysis as described in CHEPENIK and WAITE (1975)

**Table 1.** Time after ethanolamine [2-$^{14}$C] injection on the 14th day of gestation that diacyl-GPC:diacyl-GPE = 1:1 in homogenates of control and treated[a] embryos, placentas, yolk sacs, and maternal liver[b]

| Tissue | Time (h) | |
|---|---|---|
| | Control | Treated |
| Liver | 10.1 | 11.4 |
| Yolksac | 12.7 | 11.2 |
| Placenta | 27.2 | 22.3 |
| Embryo | 38.6 | 31.3 |

[a] Pregnant rats were fed a synthetic, teratogenic diet containing the folate antagonist 9-MePGA from the 11th to 14th days of gestation

[b] The data were obtained by constructing a perpendicular line between the abcissa and the points of intercept of the diacyl-GPC and diacyl-GPE lines in Fig. 1 and 2

methylation of diacyl-GPE to diacyl-GPC; or (b) by directly affecting the activation of methionine (to yield SAM) by decreasing the amount of ATP in the embryo (CHEPENIK et al. 1970). In any event, these experiments resulted in data which documented (for the first time, as far as we know) that a maternal teratogenic treatment could alter the rate of accumulation of basic components of cellular mem-

**Table 2.** Time after ethanolamine [2-$^{14}$C] injection on the 14th day that diacyl-GPC:diacyl-GPE=1:1 in various fractions of control and treated embryos[a, b]

| Fraction[c] (control) | Time (h) | Fraction[c] (treated) | Time (h) |
|---|---|---|---|
| Cytosol | 28.6 | Cytosol | 25 |
| Microsomes | 38.2 | Mitochondria | 34.2 |
| Lysosomes | 41.6 | Microsomes | 36.2 |
| Mitochondria | 43.2 | Lysosomes | 37.4 |

[a] Pregnant rats were fed a synthetic, teratogenic diet containing the folate antagonist 9-MePGA from the 11th to 14th days of gestation

[b] The data were obtained by constructing a perpendicular line between the abcissa and the points of intercept of the diacyl-GPC and diacyl-GPE lines in Figs. 1 and 2

[c] Subcellular fractions were prepared from homogenates and characterized for "marker" enzymes as described in CHEPENIK and WAITE (1973)

branes in selected membranous compartments of the embryo and its hemochorial placenta. The data led us to think about factors which regulate the synthesis and composition of cellular membranes during normal development, and the possibility that one basic mechanism underlying abnormal embryogenesis could be an alteration in the chemistry and function of selected cellular membranes.

## II. Role of the Placenta

On reviewing the literature, it became apparent that the metabolic pathways available for synthesis, degradation, or transformation of phospholipids had not been determined in early mammalian embryos and placentas. Furthermore, there seemed to be discrepancies in some of the in vivo studies of placental and fetal phospholipid metabolism. In an elegant series of experiments BIEZENSKI (1968, 1969) and BIEZENSKI et al. (1971) have shown clearly that the rabbit placenta at term does not transfer phospholipids intact from the maternal to the fetal circulation. Rather, it seems the rabbit placenta hydrolyzes the maternal blood phospholipids and presents the products of hydrolysis as well as newly synthesized phospholipids to the fetus. POPJAK (1954) reported also that neither the rat nor the rabbit placenta transferred intact phospholipids from the maternal to fetal circulation. Both POPJAK and BIEZINSKI were able to find radiolabeled inorganic phosphorus in the rabbit (and rat) fetal liver following injection of $^{32}$P-labeled phospholipids into the maternal circulation.

In contrast, EISENBERG et al. (1967) reported that no measurable amount of radioactivity was found in the rat fetus following injection of lysolecithin $^{32}$P into the maternal circulation. Therefore, these investigators agree that: (1) the placenta does not transfer intact phospholipids from the maternal circulation to the fetal circulation; (2) the fetus (liver and carcass) is capable of phospholipid synthesis; and (3) the fatty acid portion of maternal blood phospholipids may be utilized by the fetus for synthesis of its phospholipids (BIEZENSKI et al. 1971; EISENBERG et al.

1967). There is disagreement concerning the products of phospholipid hydrolysis that are presented to the fetus in that POPJAK (1954) and BIEZENSKI (1968) found inorganic phosphorous derived from maternal phospholipids in fetal phospholipids; EISENBERG and coinvestigators (1967) did not. Only BIEZENSKI addressed the question of whether or not the placenta secreted intact phospholipids into the fetal circulation. He found that it did. Our finding that a teratogen-induced shift towards increased uptake of diacyl-GPC by the embryo was accompanied by a similar shift in the placenta supports the idea the placenta secretes intact phospholipids into the circulation of the embryo.

## III. Experimental Approaches

Information regarding factors which regulate the ability of the mammalian embryo and its placenta to synthesize, degrade, and transform phospholipids is critical to our understanding the qualitative and quantitative nature of cell membrane formation during normal embryogenesis and the mechanisms by which an agent might affect such membrane characteristics. Since phospholipid metabolism is so complex, one must use a number of experimental approaches in pursuit of such information, as follows:

1. In vitro characterization of key enzymes involved in phospholipid synthesis, degradation, and transformation. Such studies define the metabolic capabilities of the tissue and the subcellular localization of those capabilities.
2. In vivo studies in which carefully selected, radiolabeled phospholipid precursors are injected, either singly or in combination, into the pregnant animal and their rates of distribution into specific phospholipids of the maternal blood, placenta, and embryo are determined. These studies aim to characterize the phospholipid metabolic pathways operative in vivo, and give some indication of possible relationships between the quality and quantity of phospholipids synthesized by the placenta or taken up by it from the maternal blood and the phospholipids found in the embryo.
3. In vitro studies in which selected structures of the embryo, its yolk sac, and placental slices are incubated separately with selected radiolabeled phospholipid precursors and their rates of distribution into various lipids are determined. These studies aim to characterize the phospholipid metabolic pathways operative in tissues of the embryo or its placentas in the absence of influences by other sources (i.e., maternal blood).
4. Careful characterization of classes and molecular species of phospholipids present in embryos, selected tissues and cells of embryos, subcellular fractions of the embryos, and their associated placentas. In part, such studies aim to characterize the relative utilization of various phospholipid metabolic pathways by normal and abnormal embryos and their placentas. That is, the metabolic pathway by which phospholipids are produced determines to a great extent their fatty acid composition (in rat liver LYMAN et al. 1973, 1975; REITZ and LANDS 1968; HILL et al. 1968). Therefore, the detection of a change in the acyl composition of phospholipids in the embryo or embryonic cells during sequential stages of development or in response to a teratogenic treatment might be suggestive as to which metabolic pathway is the dominant one in vivo. Such studies also aim to detect subtle changes

in the chemical composition of cellular membranes of the embryo as a function of normal or abnormal differentiation, and provide data which may be used in the construction of model membranes with which the physical characteristics of cellular membranes may be determined. This approach has been used most elegantly by WAITE and his group in relating alterations in lipid metabolism and composition to alterations in the physical characteristics of cellular membranes from tumors (MORTON et al. 1976; WAITE et al. 1977).

5. Sampling of umbilical vein blood during the period of organogenesis and determination of the quality and quantity of phospholipids present therein as a function of normal and abnormal differentiation. By using carefully selected radiolabeled precursors and sampling umbilical vein blood at short intervals after their injection into the maternal blood, it should be possible to determine with precision the quality and quantity of lipids (or anything else, for that matter) transferred to the embryonic circulation, and detect any alteration in placental function during gestation or in response to a teratogenic treatment. In part, such studies should define possible relationships between embryonic metabolism and placental function.

## IV. Results

In the following paragraphs are presented some of the kinds of data obtained with some of these approaches, their interpretation, and where applicable, alterations detected in response to a maternal teratogen treatment.

### 1. In Vitro Enzyme Studies

So far, the presence of the do novo phospholipid synthetic pathway (CHEPENIK et al. 1977) and the reacylating pathway (CHEPENIK et al. 1976; EAST et al. 1978) in the rat embryo and its associated placentas has been demonstrated. The ability of the hemochorial placenta to deacylate phospholipids has been demonstrated (EAST et al. 1975). In all cases, the specific enzymes studied (cholinephosphotransferase, EC 2.7.8.2; Lysolecithin acyltransferase, EC 2.3.1.23; and phospholipases A, EC 3.1.1.4 and EC 3.1.1.32) were quite similar in their subcellular localization, cofactor requirements, and pH optima to those described for adult tissues. Most importantly, these studies document the ability of the embryo and its placentas to synthesize and transform phospholipids. By comparing the activities of an enzyme in one tissue to its activity in another, some insight into the relative importance of the metabolic pathway represented by that enzyme might be obtained. For example, it was found that cholinephosphotransferase activity was higher in the placenta than in embryo (CHEPENIK et al. 1977). This was somewhat surprising since the embryo has a higher mitotic rate than placenta, and hence might the expected to synthesize membranes (and membrane precursors) faster than placenta. One interpretation, then, of the difference in cholinephosphotransferase activities between placenta and embryo is that phospholipid destined for membrane biogenesis in the embryo might be synthesized by a metabolic pathway other than the de novo pathway, or arise outside the embryo. Another possibility is that phospholipid turnover is greater in placenta than embryo, thus requiring greater synthetic ability on the part of placenta.

## 2. In Vivo Metabolic Studies

By using carefully selected radiolabeled precursors, it is possible to obtain some insight into metabolic pathways operative in vivo. The difficulty with this approach in studying something as complex as phospholipid metabolism during mammalian embryogenesis is that the precursor might be utilized by a number of different tissues (i.e., placenta, embryo, maternal liver). For example, when ethanolamine $^{14}C$ was injected into pregnant rats, the radiolabel appeared first in diacyl-GPE and then in diacyl-GPC of the embryo, placenta, yolk sac, and maternal liver (CHEPENIK and WAITE 1973, 1975). One interpretation of these data is that all of these structures have the ability to methylate diacyl-GPE to diacyl-GPC via phosphatidylethanolamine methyltransferase (EC 2.1.1.7, BREMER 1969).

Another interpretation is that placenta, embryo, and yolk sac take up diacyl-GPC containing the radiolabel from the blood, since liver, the source of almost all blood-borne lipoproteins, is known to be able to synthesize diacyl-GPC from diacyl-GPE (VAN GOLDE and VAN DEN BERG 1977). In order to distinguish between these possibilities, a mixture of ethanolamine $^{3}H$ and glycerol $^{14}C$ (5 μCi [$^{3}H$]/μCi [$^{14}C$]) was injected into the circulation of a pregnant rat on either the 14th or 16th days of gestation, and the isotopic ratio in diacyl-GPC obtained from embryos, placentas, yolk sacs, maternal liver, and blood, 2 h and 4 h after injection was determined (Table 3). The great reduction in the ratio of [$^{3}H$]:[$^{14}C$] in diacyl-GPC of the embryo compared with placenta (or blood) suggests the embryo takes up little phospholipid from the placenta. That any $^{3}H$ should appear in diacyl-GPC of the embryo suggests some ability to methylate diacyl-GPE to diacyl-GPC, though at a seemingly low rate. This interpretation is supported further by our finding some radiolabel in diacyl-GPC when minced embryos are incubated with ethanolamine $^{14}C$ in defined media (K. P. CHEPENIK, unpublished work 1973).

**Table 3.** Ratio of [$^{3}H$]:[$^{14}C$] in diacyl-GPC and diacyl-GPE extracted[a] from maternal liver, plasma, embryos, and their placentas following maternal injection of ethanolamine $^{3}H$ and glycerol $^{14}C$ [b]

| | Liver | Plasma[c] | Placenta | Yolk sac | Embryo |
|---|---|---|---|---|---|
| 14th day of gestation[d] | | | | | |
| Diacyl-GPC | 86 | 46 | 8 | 9.4 | 0.11 |
| Diacyl-GPE | 286 | | 224 | 111 | 8.2 |
| 16th day of gestation[d] | | | | | |
| Diacyl-GPC | 59 | 44 | 8 | 2 | 0.3 |
| Diacyl-GPE | 305 | | 194 | 37 | 15.3 |

[a] Diacyl-GPC and diacyl-GPE were separated by thin layer chromatography of $CHCl_3$ extracts of liver, placentas, embryos, and maternal plasma as described in CHEPENIK and WAITE (1973)

[b] Ethanolamine [1-$^{3}H$] and glycerol [1-$^{14}C$] were injected into the maternal circulation in a ratio of 5 μCi [$^{3}H$]/μCi [$^{14}C$] at the beginning of the 14th or 16th day of gestation

[c] Maternal plasma was obtained by centrifugation of whole blood, collected in syringes which contained heparin

[d] Tissues were collected 4 h after injection of radioisotopes on the designated days of gestation

### 3. In Vitro Metabolic Studies

Incubation of selected structures or cells of the embryo with carefully chosen radio-labeled precursors permits the mapping of lipid metabolic pathways operative in those structures as they undergo normal and abnormal differentiation. In preliminary experiments, embryonic forelimbs, hindlimbs, livers, yolk sacs, and placentas were obtained from normal and teratogen-treated (9-MePGA) mothers on the 14th or 15th days of gestation. This teratogenic treatment is known to produce a high incidence of skeletal malformations in the neonate (CHEPENIK et al. 1970). The various structures were incubated in defined media containing palmitate $^{14}C$ for up to 1 h, and the rate of incorporation of radiolabel into various lipids was determined by qualitative and quantitative analysis of lipids extracted from those tissues. It was found (CHEPENIK et al. 1978) that:

1. The rate of incorporation of radiolabel into phosphatidylcholine was linear as a function of time or amount of tissue. Most importantly, there was no lag in the uptake of radiolabel.
2. When the fatty acid methyl esters of diacyl-GPC or diacyl-GPE extracted from the various structures were subjected to $AgNO_3$ chromatography, about 10% of the total radioactivity could be recovered as monoenoic species.
3. Embryonic tissues and yolk sacs synthesized fatty alcohols and other neutral lipids at a greater rate than did placenta or maternal liver (Table 4).
4. Forelimbs and hindlimbs from treated embryos incorporated radiolabel into diacyl-GPC at a faster rate than did controls on the 15th day (Table 5); no such differences were seen on the 14th day or in the other tissues studied.

These data are interpreted to mean that:

1. Neither substrate concentration, diffusion, nor uncharacterized enzyme inhibitors were limiting in the rate of conversion of substrate to product. If any of

**Table 4.** Incorporation of palmitate [1-$^{14}C$] into neutral lipids[a, b]. Incorporation (nmol $g^{-1} \times h^{-1}$)

| Structure | Fatty alcohols | Neutral lipids (triglyceride, cholesterol esters, wax esters, fatty acid methyl esters) |
|---|---|---|
| Embryo[c] | | |
| Forelimb | 60 | 120 |
| Hindlimb | 74 | 130 |
| Liver | 70 | 193 |
| Yolk sac | 52 | 193 |
| Placenta (slices) | 11 | 80 |
| Maternal liver (slices) | 19 | 30 |

[a] The various structures were incubated for 60 min in Krebs-Ringer phosphate buffer containing 75 nmol palmitate [1-$^{14}C$] (4.22 μCi)
[b] Lipids were extracted into $CHCl_3$. Neutral lipids were separated by thin layer chromatography in hexane:diethyl ether:acetic acid (50:50:1 v/v), and their radioactivity determined by scintillation spectrometry
[c] Structures obtained on the 15th day of gestation

**Table 5.** Incorporation of palmitate [1-$^{14}$C] into phospholipids by embryonic tissues and their placentas[a]. Incorporation (nmol $g^{-1} \times h^{-1}$)

| | | Diacyl-GPC | | Diacyl-GPE | |
|---|---|---|---|---|---|
| | | Day 14 | Day 15 | Day 14 | Day 15 |
| Embryo[b, c] | | | | | |
| Forelimb | C | 116±34 | 58±12 | 24±12 | 15±41 |
| | T | 128±15 | 107±35 ($P<0.05$) | 37±10 | 20± 8 |
| Hindlimb | C | | 56±14 | | 12± 4 |
| | T | | 156±87 ($0.05<P<0.10$) | | 35±17 ($0.02<P<0.05$) |
| Liver | C | | 127±34 | | 37±17 |
| | T | | 151±64 | | 28±16 |
| Yolk sac[d] | C | | 123 | | 38 |
| | T | | 100 | | 26 |
| Placenta[d] | C | | 34 | | 9 |
| | T | | 40 | | 6 |
| Maternal liver[d] | C | | 18 | | 7 |
| | T | | 19 | | 5 |

[a] The designated tissues were obtained from pregnant rats killed on the 14th or 15th day of gestation. The tissues were dissected in Krebs-Ringer phosphate buffer and placed in tared vials containing 1 ml Krebs-Ringer phosphate buffer; 5 μl ethanol containing 75 nmol of palmitate [1-$^{14}$C] (56 μCi/μmol) was added. The vials were incubated for 60 min at 37 °C. The reaction was terminated by the addition of $CHCl_3$, and the lipids were extracted. The various lipids were separated by thin layer chromatography, identified by staining with 2,7-dichlorofluorescein. Their radioactivities were determined by scintillation spectroscopy

[b] C=controls; pregnant rats were fed a synthetic diet containing folic acid from the 11th to the 15th day of gestation. T=treated; pregnant rats were fed a synthetic diet lacking in folic acid and containing the teratogen and folic acid antagonist 9-MePGA from the 11th to the 14th day of gestation; they were fed the folic acid supplemented diet from the 14th to the 15th day of gestation. This treatment is known to produce a high incidence (94%) of skeletal malformations in the neonate

[c] Values represent the means of at least three separate determinations ± the standard deviation

[d] Values are from one determination only

these phenomena were operative, there would not have been linearity in amount of product produced as a function of amount of tissue present in the media, nor would the line describing product formation as a function of time extrapolate through the zero time, zero product point.

2. The embryonic tissues are able to desaturate fatty acids (at least palmitate); whether they are able to desaturate and elongate essential fatty acids is yet to be determined.

3. The embryonic tissues and yolk sac very rapidly reduce fatty acids to fatty alcohols, compared with placentas or liver. This is in keeping with our finding a high content of plasmalogen in embryos (CHEPENIK et al. 1980), and a rapid rate of incorporation of hexadecanol [1-$^{14}$C] into plasmalogen by yolk sac (K. P. CHEPENIK et al., unpublished work 1978). Fatty alcohols are the precursors to the alkyl- and alk-1-enyl groups found in ether glycerides (SNYDER 1972).

4. The teratogen may have selectively affected phospholipid metabolism in the structure which developes abnormally (limb). Another interpretation is that the altered phospholipid metabolism in teratogen-treated forelimbs on the 15th, but not 14th, day may simply reflect a developmental delay. That is, inspection of histologic preparations of 9-MePGA-treated and control embryos revealed that by the 14th day, mesenchymal condensation had not occurred in the treated embryos to the same degree as controls, nor had chondrogenesis progressed to the same degree in the treated embryos as it had in the controls by the 15th day. The conclusion that the phospholipid data reflect a developmental delay may be a bit premature, however. That is, folic acid antagonists are known to inhibit cell replication (MUELLER et al. 1962), and hence might be expected to alter the rate of membrane biogenesis. However, the rate of synthesis of a membrane precursor (diacyl-GPC) was not different between teratogen-treated limbs and controls at a time when the treated embryos were still exposed to the 9-MePGA (14th day). It may be then, that either the cells of the embryo have excaped from the inhibitory effects of the teratogen by the 14th day, or that the rate of incorporation of palmitate $^{14}C$ is a measure of both synthesis of phospholipid as well as turnover of the acyl group on the phospholipid. Further experimentation should discriminate between these possibilities. In any event, it should be clear that this approach can yield information about metabolism as it takes place in relatively discrete structures of the embryo, and can detect alterations associated with altered development.

## 4. Acyl Composition of Embryo and Placental Phospholipids

As noted earlier in this chapter, the acyl composition of membrane phospholipids influences certain physical characteristics of the membrane. Furthermore, the synthetic pathway by which phospholipids are produced determines to a great extent their fatty acid composition (in rat liver) (LYMAN et al. 1973, 1975; REITZ and LANDS 1968; HILL et al. 1968). Therefore, the detection of a change in the fatty acid composition of phospholipids in the embryo during sequential stages of development, or in response to a teratogen treatment, might be suggestive as to which metabolic pathway is the predominant one in vivo. For these reasons, studies to determine the acyl composition of phospholipids isolated from normal and teratogen-treated rat embryos and their associated placentas were initiated. Preliminary studies revealed that diacyl-GPC isolated from the embryo was enriched in saturated and monoenoic species, and deficient in polyenoic species when compared with that of placenta or maternal plasma (Table 6). This relative increase in saturation in diacyl-GPC is reflected in a lower double bond index (percentage of the acyl moieties C 16:1, C 18:1, C 18:2, C 20:4, C 22:5, C 22:6, multiplied by the number of double bonds of the acid) for the embryo (78) when compared with that of the placenta (138), or maternal plasma (153). Diacyl-GPE isolated from rat embryos also had a lower double bond index (206) than that of placenta (236) or maternal plasma (248) (Table 7), though the differences among the tissues was not as dramatic as that found for diacyl-GPC. Whether the relatively high content of saturated fatty acids in phospholipids of the embryo reflects: (1) the inability of the embryo to elongate and unsaturate essential fatty acids or to incorporate polyenoic fatty acids via the acylation pathway; or (2) a failure of transfer of polyenoic fatty

**Table 6.** Fatty acid composition (wt. %) of diacyl-GPC[a, b] isolated from maternal plasma, placentas, and embryos[c] of rats

| Acyl moiety[d] | Plasma[e] | Placenta | Embryo |
|---|---|---|---|
| C14:0 | | 1.0 | 2.7 |
| C16:0 | 12.1 | 26.8 | 42.9 |
| C16:1 | | 2.9 | 8.2 |
| C18:0 | 29.2 | 19.7 | 8.0 |
| C18:1 | 4.2 | 10.2 | 22.5 |
| C18:2 | 16.4 | 16.6 | 4.2 |
| C22:0/20:3 | 3.4 | | |
| C20:4/22:1 | 24.6 | 22.9 | 9.7 |
| C22:4/24:1 | | | |
| C22:5 | 1.3 | | |
| C22:6 | 1.9 | | |

[a] Values are the means of gas-liquid chromatographic analysis of at least two separate preparations of fatty acyl methyl esters
[b] In some cases the percentages may not add to 100% since compounds constituting less than 1% of the total are not included
[c] All samples obtained on the 14th day of gestation
[d] Acyl moieties designated by number of carbon atoms: followed by number of double bonds in that compound
[e] Plasma obtained by centrifugation of maternal blood collected in syringes which contained heparin

acids to the embryo by placenta, are areas currently under investigation. It has been found that membrane preparations from rat embryos have high lysophospholipase activities (WALDMAN et al., to be published). These enzymes degrade the lysophospholipid substrate utilized in the synthesis of phospholipids containing polyunsaturated fatty acids.

## V. Vitamin A and Glucocorticoids

A number of agents known to alter differentiation in vivo and in vitro have recently been identified as having an effect on membrane lipid metabolism. Specifically, vitamin A alters chondrogenesis in vivo (KOCHHAR 1977) and in vitro (KOCHHAR 1977; LEWIS et al. 1978). It has also been found to enhance the deacylation of phospholipids, in vitro, with a concomitant increase in prostaglandin synthesis (LEVINE and OHUCHI 1978). Also, vitamin A was reported recently to have an enzyme-mediated effect on membrane microviscosity (MEEKS et al. 1981). Hydrocortisone is known to produce cleft palate (BLAUSTEIN et al. 1971) and cartilage defects (JURAND 1968) in the newborn mouse. This drug, and its more potent analog dexamethasone, have been reported to depress prostaglandin synthesis by altering the activity of phospholipase A (HONG and LEVINE 1976; HIRATA et al. 1980), a key enzyme in controlling release of free fatty acids from phospholipids. From the previous discussion, one might expect any agent which alters membrane lipid metab-

**Table 7.** Fatty acid composition (wt. %) of ethanolamine phospholipids isolated from maternal plasma, placentas, and embryos of rats[a, b, c]

| Alipatic[d, e] moiety | Plasma[f] | Placenta | Embryo |
|---|---|---|---|
| C14:0 | 2.4 | 4.0 | |
| C16:0 DMA | | | 6.1 |
| C16:0 | 7.2 | 7.2 | 8.1 |
| C16:1 | 1.8 | | 1.9 |
| C18:0 DMA | | | 4.1 |
| C18:0 | 16.7 | 26.4 | 15.4 |
| C18:1 DMA | | | 4.4 |
| C18:1 | 8.6 | 7.4 | 13.4 |
| C18:2 | 6.9 | 6.6 | 1.9 |
| C18:3/20:1 | | | |
| C22:0/20:3 | 4.6 | | |
| C20:4/22:1 | 33.1 | 30.3 | 24.0 |
| C24:0/22:3 | | | |
| C22:4/24:1 | 8.3 | 10.4 | 8.8 |
| C22:5 | 2.9 | 2.6 | 3.6 |
| C22:6 | 7.3 | 6.6 | 5.7 |
| Other[g] | | | 2.7 |

[a] Values are the means of gas chromatographic analysis of two separate preparations of fatty acyl methyl esters
[b] Tissues obtained on the 14th day of gestation
[c] In some cases the percentages may not add up to 100% since compounds constituting less than 1% of the total are not included
[d] DMA indicates alk-1-enyl groups analyzed as dimethylacetals of fatty aldehydes; all other numbers represent acyl moieties
[e] Aliphatic moieties designated by number of carbon atoms: followed by number of double bonds in that compound
[f] Plasma obtained by centrifugation of maternal blood, collected in syringes which contained heparin
[g] Unidentified components having retention times longer than that of 22:6

olism to alter differentiation per se. Furthermore, the recent findings that mouse embryo palate mesenchyme cells (CHEPENIK and GREENE 1981) and chick embryo limb bud mesenchyme cells (CHEPENIK et al. 1981) are able to synthesize prostaglandins suggest another mechanism by which vitamin A or hydrocortisone could alter differentiation.

## E. Conclusion

In summary, the foregoing has demonstrated that across taxonomic groups, in a variety of systems, in vivo and in vitro, the lipid composition of cellular membranes changes with differentiation. Some evidence has been presented that agents which alter differentiation so as to result in birth defects have an effect on membrane lipid metabolism, suggesting an area for mechanistic studies in teratology. It should be remembered that, although membrane modification may be a primary mechanism involved in normal and abnormal differentiation, the physical and chemical properties of membranes are not under direct control of the genome. However, the enzymes responsible for such modifications are genetically controlled. Since differentiation is a process of selective gene expression, it is reasonable to suggest that membrane modifications are secondary to differential expression of the genes controlling enzymes of lipid metabolism. Hence an area for future research is the correlation of developmental alterations in lipid metabolism with modifications of membrane lipid composition, and their role in normal and abnormal differentiation.

*Acknowledgments.* Original data reported herein was obtained under the auspices of either National Institutes of Health grant HD-04269, HD-08433, or a grant from the Dean's Overage Research Program of Thomas Jefferson University Medical College. We thank Mrs. DEBRA LUNDGREN for her diligence in typing this manuscript.

## References

Abad C, Bosch MA, Municio AM, Ribera A (1976) Age differences in the positional distribution of phosphoglycerides and molecular species of choline phosphoglycerides during development of the chick embryo liver. Biochim Biophys Acta 431:62–74

Allwood G, Asherson GL, Davey MJ, Goodford PJ (1971) The early uptake of radioactive calcium by human lymphocytes treated with phytohemagglutimin. Immunology 21:509–516

Biezenski JJ (1968) Origin of fetal plasma phospholipids. Excerpta Med Int Congr Ser 183:221–239

Biezenski JJ (1969) Role of placenta in fetal lipid metabolism. I. Injection of phospholipids double labeled with $^{14}$C-glycerol and 32P into pregnant rabbits. Am J Obstet Gynecol 104:1177–1189

Biezenski JJ, Carrozza J, Li J (1971) Role of placenta in fetal lipid metabolism. III. Formation of rabbit plasma phospholipids. Biochim Biophys Acta 239:92–97

Blaustein FM, Feller R, Rosenzweig F (1971) Effect of ACTH and adrenal hormones on cleft palate frequency in CD-1 mice. J Dent Res 50:609–612

Bremer J (1969) Phosphatidylethanolamine: Adenosylmethiomine methyltransferase(s) from animal liver. In: Lowenstein JM (ed) Methods in enzymology, vol 14. Academic Press, New York, p 125

Carpentieri U, Minguell JJ, Haggard ME (1980) Variation of activity of protein kinases in unstimulated and phytohemagglutimin – stimulated normal and leukemic human lymphocytes. Cancer Res 40:2714–2718

Chapman D (1975) Lipid dynamics in cell membranes. In: Weissman G, Claiborn R (eds) Cell membranes: biochemistry, cell biology, and pathology. H.P. Publishing, New York, p 130

Chepenik KP, Greene RM (1981) Prostaglandin synthesis by primary cultures of mouse embryo palate mesenchyme cells. Biochem Biophys Res Commun 100:951–958

Chepenik KP, Waite BM (1972) Effects of transitory maternal pteroylglutamic acid (PGA) deficiency on respiratory control ratios, phosphorylative capacity, and cytochrome oxidase activities of mitochondria from developing rat embryos. Teratology 5:191–198

Chepenik KP, Waite BM (1973) Incorporation of a phospholipid precursor into the subcellular organelles of teratogen-treated rat embryos. Teratology 8:175–189

Chepenik KP, Waite BM (1975) Incorporation of a phospholipid precursor into the subcellular organelles of placentas and yolk-sacs associated with teratogen-treated embryos. Teratology 11:247–256

Chepenik KP, Johnson EM, Kaplan S (1970) Effects of transistory maternal pteroylglutamic acid (PGA) deficiency on levels of adenosine phosphates in developing rat embryos. Teratology 3:229–236
Chepenik KP, East JM, Waite BM, Nelowet VA (1976) Phospholipid transformation during mammalian embryogenesis. Teratology 13:19A
Chepenik KP, Borst DE, Waite BM (1977) Cholinephosphotransferase activities in early rat embryos and their associated placentas. Dev Biol 60:463–472
Chepenik KP, Malone B, Blank M, Borst DE, Snyder F (1978) Lipid metabolism during abnormal limb morphogenesis. Teratology 17:32A
Chepenik KP, Blank M, Snyder F, Waite BM (1980) On the presence of plasmalogens in developing rat embryos. Int J Biochem 11:605–607
Chepenik KP, Waite BM, Parker C (1980) Arachidonate metabolism during chondrogenesis, in vitro. J Cell Biol 87:21 a
Coffey RG, Hadden EM, Hadden JW (1977) Evidence for cyclic AMP and calcium mediation of lymphocyte activation by mitogens. J Immunol 119:1387–1394
Coffey RG, Hadden EM, Hadden JW (1981) Phytohemagglutimin stimulation of guanylate cyclase in human lymphocytes. J Biol Chem 256:4418–4424
Cornell RB, Nissley SM, Horowitz AF (1980) Cholesterol availability modulates myoblast fusion. J Cell Biol 86:820–824
Demel RA, DeKruyff (1976) The function of sterols in membranes. Biochim Biophys Acta 475:109–132
Demel RA, Van Deenen LLM, Pethica BA (1967) Monolayer interactions of phospholipids and cholesterol. Biochim Biophys Acta 135:11–19
East JM, Chepenik KP, Waite BM (1975) Phospholipase(s) A activities in rat placentas of 14 days gestation. Biochim Biophys Acta 388:106–112
East JM, Chepenik KP, Waite BM (1978) Deacylation-reacylation of phospholipids by rat embryos and their associated placentas. I. Placental acyltransferases. Biol Neonate 35:213–220
Eisenberg S, Stein Y, Stein O (1967) The role of placenta in lysolecithin metabolism in rats and mice. Biochim Biophys Acta 137:115–120
Ellingson JS (1974) Changes in the phospholipid composition in the differentiating slime mold, *Dictyostelium discoideum*. Biochim Biophys Acta 337:60–67
Ferber E, Resch K (1977) Structure and physiologic role of lipids in the lymphocyte membrane. In: Marchalonis JJ (ed) The lymphocyte. Structure and function. M. Dekker, New York, Basel, p 593
Fourcans B (1974) Role of phospholipids in transport and enzymic reactions. Adv Lipid Res 12:147–226
Greaves MF, Bauminger S (1972) Activation of T and B lymphocytes by insoluble phytomitogens. Nat New Biol 235:67–70
Hadden JW, Johnson EM, Hadden EM, Coffey RG, Johnson LD (1975) Cyclic GMP and lymphocyte stimulation. In: Rosenthal AS (ed) Immune recognition. Academic Press, New York, p 359
Hewitt AT, Elmer WA (1978) Developmental modulation of lectin-binding sites on the surface membranes of normal and Brachypod mouse limb mesenchymal cells. Differentiation 10:31–38
Hill EE, Husbands DE, Lands WEM (1968) The selective incorporation of $^{14}C$-glycerol into different species of phosphatidic acid, phosphatidylethanolamine, and phosphatidylcholine. J Biol Chem 243:4440–4451
Hirata F, Schiffmann E, Venkatasubramanian K, Salomon D, Axelrod J (1980) A phospholipase $A_2$ inhibitory protein in rabbit neutrophils induced by glucocorticoids. Proc Natl Acad Sci USA 77:2533–2536
Hong S, Levine L (1976) Inhibition of arachidonic acid release from cells as the biochemical action of anti-inflammatory corticosteroids. Proc Natl Acad Sci USA 73:1730–1734
Horowitz AF, Wight A, Ludwig P, Cornell R (1978) Interrelated lipid alterations and their influence on the proliferation and fusion of cultured myogenic cells. J Cell Biol 77:334–357

Horowitz AF, Wight A, Knudsen K (1979) A role for lipid in myoblast fusion. Biochem Biophys Res Commun 86:514–521
Hui DY, Harmony JAK (1980) Inhibition by low density lipoproteins of mitogen-stimulated cyclic nucleotide production by lymphocytes. J Biol Chem 255:1413–1419
Johnson EM (1965) Electrophoretic analysis of abnormal development. Proc Soc Exp Biol Med 118:9–11
Jurand A (1968) The effect of hydrocortisone acetate on the development of mouse embryos. J Embryol exp Morph 20:355–366
Knudsen KA, Horowitz A (1977) Tandem events in myoblast fusion. Dev Biol 58:328–338
Kochhar DM (1977) Cellular basis of congenital limb deformity induced in mice by vitamin A. Birth defects. Orig Article Ser XIII:111–154
Kretchmer N (1978) Perspectives in teratologic research. Teratology 17:203–211
Kutchai H, Barenholz Y, Ross TF, Wermer DE (1976) Developmental changes in plasma membrane fluidity in chick embryo heart. Biochim Biophys Acta 436:101–112
Levine L, Ohuchi K (1978) Retinoids as well as tumor promoters enhance deacylation of cellular lipids and prostaglandin production in MDCK cells. Nature 276:274–275
Lewis CA, Pratt RM, Pennypacker JP, Hassel JR (1978) Inhibition of limb chondrogenesis in vitro by vitamin A: alterations in cell surface characteristics. Dev Biol 64:31–47
Ling NR, Kay JE (1975) Lymphocyte stimulation. Revised edition. North Holland, Amsterdam
Lyman RL, Sheehan G, Tinnoco J (1973) Phosphatidylethanolamine metabolism in rats fed a low methionine, choline-deficient diet. Lipids 8:71–79
Lyman RL, Giotas C, Medwadowski B, Miljanick P (1975) Effect of low methionine, choline deficient diets upon major unsaturated phosphatidylcholine fractions of rat liver and plasma. Lipids 10:157–167
Meeks RG, Zaharevitz D, Chen RF (1981) Membrane effects of retinoids: Possible correlation with toxicity. Arch Biochem Biophys 207:141–147
Miyamoto K, Stephanides LM, Bernsohn J (1966) Fatty acids of glycerophosphatides in developing chick embryonic brain and liver. J Lipid Res 7:664–670
Morton R, Cunningham C, Jester R, Waite M, Miller N, Morris HP (1976) Alteration of mitochondrial function and lipid composition in Morris 7777 hepatoma. Cancer Res 36:3246–3254
Moscona AA (1974) Surface specification of embryonic cells: Lectin receptors, cell recognition, and specific cell ligands. In: Moscona AA (ed) The cell surface in development. Wiley & Sons, New York, p 67
Mueller GC, Kajiwara K, Stubblefield E, Rueckert R (1962) Molecular events in the reproduction of animal cells. I. The effect of puromycin on the duplication of DNA. Cancer Res 22:1084–1090
Parker CW (1974) Correlation between mitogenicity and stimulation of calcium uptake in human lymphocytes. Biochem Biophys Res Co 61:1180–1186
Paulsen DF, Finch RA (1977) Age and region-dependent concanavalin A reactivity of chick wing-bud mesoderm cells. Nature 268:639–641
Popjak G (1954) The origin of fetal lipids. Cold Spring Harbor Symp Quant Biol 19:200–208
Prives J, Shinitzky M (1977) Increased membrane fluidity precedes fusion of muscle cells. Nature 268:761–763
Reitz RC, Lands WEM (1968) Effects of ethylenic bond position upon acyltransferase activity with isomeric cis, cis-octadecadienoyl coenzyme A thiol esters. J Biol Chem 243:2241–2246
Resch K, Ferber E, Odenthal J, Fischer H (1971) Early changes in the phospholipid metabolism of lymphocytes following stimulation with phytohemagglutimin and with lysolecithin. Eur J Immunol 1:162–165
Sachs L (1974) Lectins as probes for changes in membrane dynamics in malignancy and cell differentiation. In: Miscona AA (ed) The cell surface in development. Wiley & Sons, New York, p 127
Singer SJ (1974) The molecular organization of membranes. Annu Rev Biochem 43:805–833
Singer SJ (1977) The proteins of membranes. J Colloid Interface Sci 58:452–458

Singer SJ, Nicolson GL (1972) The fluid mosaic model of the structure of cell membranes. Science 175:720–731
Snyder F (1972) The enzymic pathways of ether-linked lipids and their precursors. In: Snyder F (ed) Ether lipids: Chemistry and biology. Academic Press, New York, p 121
Triggle DJ (1970) Some aspects of the role of lipids in lipid-protein interactions and cell membrane structure and function. Recent Prog Surf Sci 3:273–290
Van Deenen LLM, DeGier J, Demel RA (1972) Relations between lipid composition and permeability of membranes. In: Ganguly J, Smellie RMS (eds) Current trends in the biochemistry of lipids. Proceedings of the international symposium of lipids 3–4 December 1971. Biochem Soc Symp No 5. Academic Press, New York, p 377
Van Golde LMG, Van den Berg SG (1977) Liver. In: Snyder F (ed) Lipid metabolism in mammals, vol 1. Plenum Press, New York, p 35
Waite M, Parce B, Morton R, Cunningham C, Morris HP (1977) The deacylation and reacylation of phosphoglyceride in microsomes of Morris hepatoma 7777 and host rat liver. Cancer Res 37:2092–2098
Waldman SA, Chepenik KP, Waite BM (to be published) Acyl composition and metabolism in plasma membranes isolated from rat embryos. Arch Biochem Biophys
Weeks G (1976) The manipulation of the fatty acid composition of *Dictyostelium discoideum* and its effect on cell differentiation. Biochim Biophys Acta 450:21–32
Whitney RB, Sutherland RM (1972) Requirement for calcium ions in lymphocyte transformation stimulated by phytohemagglutimin. J Cell Physiol 80:329–338
Wood R (1974) Embryonic vs tumor lipids. II. Changes in phospholipids of developing chick brain, heart, and liver. Lipids 9:429-439

CHAPTER 8

# Hormone Receptors and Malformations

D. S. SALOMON

## A. Introduction

Differentiation may be considered as an orderly progression of various morphological, cellular, and biochemical events which occur temporally and spatially during development in specific cell types. During embryogenesis, an array of cellular interactions are proceeding along genetically and epigenetically defined pathways. These interactions can be direct cell–cell or tissue–tissue interactions such as occur between the epithelium and adjacent mesenchyme in the developing pancreas, thyroid, salivary glands, lung, intestine, kidney, mammary gland, and secondary palate (SALOMON and PRATT 1979; KRATOCHWIL 1972; SAXÉN 1972; LE DOUARIN 1970), as mediated by the extracellular matrix (GROBSTEIN 1975). Alternatively, indirect interactions perform equally important roles during development. These interactions occur between adjacent or distant cell types and are mediated by extracellular or intracellular chemical messengers (hormones, growth factors, and cyclic nucleotides). Hormones are compounds which are specific products of one or more groups of cells (endocrine tissue) that are transported in the vascular system to other groups of cells (target tissue) which are capable of responding in a specific physiologic and biochemical manner. Cells of one tissue may also produce growth factors locally which affect an adjacent, but different, cell type (paracrine) without entering the vascular system. There is also evidence for autocrine growth regulation in which a cell which is producing a growth factor can also respond to that same growth factor (SPORN and TODARO 1980). Paracrine or autocrine regulation of growth and/or differentiation could play an important role during development under circumstances where one cell type is locally influencing the differentiation of a second cell type (SALOMON et al. 1981; SAXÉN 1972).

In a variety of fetal tissues, specific hormones either individually or in concert are necessary for both triggering and/or maintaining the differentiation and maturation of specific embryonic cells (SALOMON and PRATT 1979, RUTTER et al. 1973). In contrast, in the adult organism, hormones are necessary for the control of normal homeostasis. In other words, in providing the organism with adaptive signals emanating from environmental changes which are capable of being transduced into appropriate physiologic responses. The nature and duration of the physiologic or developmental response are determined by several factors such as: (1) the chemical nature of the homone or hormones; (2) type of target tissue or tissues; (3) the physiologic or developmental state of the organism with respect to the receptivity of the target tissue for the hormone; (4) the concentration of hormone at the target tissue; and (5) adaptive responses to the hormone (feedback mechanisms).

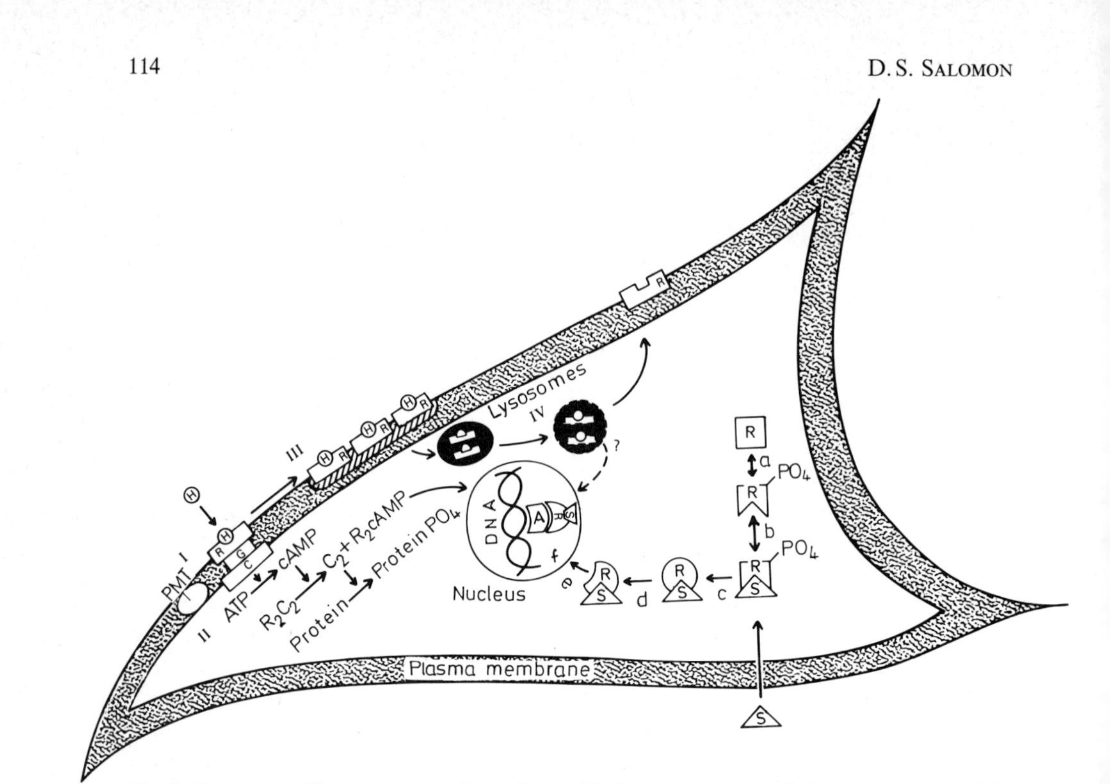


**Fig. 1.** Receptor–effector systems for polypeptide hormones, growth factors, and steroids. Steroid hormones (*S*) freely diffuse across the plasma membrane and bind to specific high affintiy cytoplasmic, soluble, receptor proteins (*b*) with may exist (*a*) in an unactivated, nonphosphorylated state, incapable of binding the steroid but, upon phosphorylation, may be capable of binding the steroid (activation). Upon steroid binding, the steroid–receptor complex undergoes "transformation" (conformational change) (*c, d*), a metabolically dependent process allowing translocation (*e*) and binding of the complex to specific nuclear acceptor proteins (*A*) in chromatin (*f*), resulting in the modulation of specific mRNA molecules. In contrast, polypeptide hormones and growth factors (*H*) bind to cell surface glycoprotein receptors (*I*). For those hormones which function through the adenylate cyclase–protein kinase system (*II*), the hormone–receptor complex is coupled to and activates the adenylate cyclase catalytic unit through the G regulatory protein. Transient elevation in cyclic AMP (cAMP) leads to the activation of protein kinase ($R_2C_2$) by causing a dissociation of the catalytic and regulatory subunits. During this process, cAMP is bound to the receptor (*R*) subunit. The catalytic unit (*C*) can then phosphorylate specific proteins, with this latter event or possibly translocation of the $R_2$–cAMP complex to the nucleus leading to a specific set (or sets) of physiologic responses. For other hormones or growth factors which do not act via this system (e.g., insulin and EGF), there is a clustering (*III*) of the ligand–receptor complex in clathrin-coated pits, followed by internalization of the complex (*IV*) and subsequent lysosomal-mediated degradation. Clustering of the receptor–ligand complex, as well as coupling through the G binding protein, may be influenced by local changes in membrane fluidity, as affected by methylation of phospholipids by phosphomethyltranferases (PMT) in the membrane

Hormones and growth factors reside in four major chemical classes of compounds: (1) peptides and polypeptides; (2) catecholamines; (3) steroids (and sterols and retinoids); and (4) iodothyronines. For all hormones and growth factors, response in a target tissue is dictated by the presence of specific receptors for the particular ligand (KAHN 1976; O'MALLEY and SCHRADER 1976). A receptor is a class of proteins or glycoproteins which interacts in a specific noncovalent manner with the ligand (hormone or growth factor) with high affinity, low capacity, and reversibility. Upon ligand recognition and binding to the receptor, a specific program of biochemical changes ensues within the target cell that results in a particular set of physiologic or developmental responses (transduction). Receptors may be particulate (membrane bound) or soluble components of the target cell (Fig. 1).

Polypeptide hormones, peptide growth factors, and catecholamines interact at the cell membrane with receptors that are integral components of the membrane structure (KAHN 1976; CATT et al. 1979). For several of these systems, there is a rapid coupling of the receptor to and activation of the adenylate cyclase system with the generation of intracellular cyclic AMP (cAMP) and the subsequent activation of cAMP-dependent enzymes (e.g., protein kinases). For other ligands such as insulin, growth hormone, prolactin, epidermal growth factor (EGF), and the somatomedins, the nature of the intracellular signal is unknown (ROTH et al. 1979; CARPENTER and COHEN 1979). In contrast, the plasma carrier protein for cholesterol, low density lipoprotein (LDL), interacts with a specific receptor and is subsequently transported into the target cell for the delivery of cholesterol (GOLDSTEIN et al. 1979). A large body of evidence exists suggesting that, following binding of the ligand to surface receptors, there is also a rapid clustering of the ligand–receptor complexes to clathrin-coated pits on the membrane, with the subsequent endocytosis or internalization of these complexes (GOLDSTEIN et al. 1979). The result is degradation of the ligand and/or receptor and a reduction in the level of receptors on the target cell surface (GOLDSTEIN et al. 1979; CATT et al. 1979). The significance of these latter events as to the production of biologic responses is unknown. However, they may serve to desensitize the target cell to further challenge and response to the hormone or growth factor.

Steroids, retinoids and sterols (vitamin D) enter target cells via passive diffusion, and interact with specific, soluble intracellular receptor proteins in the cytoplasmic (cytosol) cell fraction (Fig. 1); (O'MALLEY et al. 1976; MUNCK and LEUNG 1977; SANI et al. 1978). Following binding to the receptor, at least in the case of steroid hormones, the hormone–receptor complex undergoes a temperature-dependent, conformational change (transformation), allowing the complex to translocate to the nucleus. Unbound cytosol receptor also may exist in various phosphorylated states which determines its ability to bind the steroid (activation). This process may be controlled by various soluble activators or inhibitors (GOIDL et al. 1977; PRATT 1978; SATO et al. 1980). After nuclear transfer, the transformed, activated hormone–receptor complex interacts with specific acceptor sites which are components of the acidic nuclear proteins (O'MALLEY et al. 1976; O'MALLEY and SCHRADER 1976). This interaction (or interactions) results in alterations in transcriptional processes. These molecular events are then ultimately expressed as specific cellular responses.

During the last several years, a large body of evidence has accumulated illustrating that receptors for various hormones and carrier proteins are involved in the etiology of specific disease states (LIPPMAN 1976; ROTH et al. 1979; POLLET and LEVEY 1980). Receptor defects in target tissues, including an absence or reduction in receptors, decreased or increased binding to receptors, and the presence of antibodies to receptors, have been implicated in such diverse pathologic states as leukemia, breast cancer, familial hypercholesterolemia, obesity, diabetes, Graves' disease, acromegaly, Addison's disease, and myasthenia gravis. It is the purpose of this chapter to review some of the possible roles of receptor alterations in the etiology of certain congential malformations. Evidence will be presented to illustrate that disorders in receptor design and/or function as well as postreceptor (effector) alterations may be involved in specific genetic abnormalities which result from insensitivity, enhanced sensitivity, or response defects in target tissues for a particular hormone or growth factor.

## B. Steroids

### I. Androgens

#### 1. Testicular Feminization

Genetic sex is determined at fertilization. A variety of genetic sexual anomalies or intersex syndromes such as Turner's or Klinefelter's syndromes have been described that result in sexual abnormalities due to meiotic dysjunctions. Gonadal or primary sex is determined later in development by the genetic sex of the organism. Differentiation of the indifferent gonads begins following migration of the germ cells from the embryonic yolk sac to the gonadal ridge (JOST et al. 1973; WILSON 1978). In the male, H–Y antigens determine germ cell development into sperm (OHNO 1976). In the absence of H–Y antigens, ovarian development results in the embryo. Establishment of mammalian secondary (phenotypic) sexual characteristics begins during midgestation (days 12–14) in the rodent, and in the latter part of the first trimester in humans. Internal secondary sex organs arise from the wolffian and müllerian ducts which are derivatives of the mesonephric kidney. During midgestation, these embryonic ducts traverse a period during which their development can be irreversibly altered by the presence or absence of androgens, but not estrogens (JOST et al. 1973). In the female embryo, the wolffian ducts regress while the müllerian ducts differentiate into the oviducts and uterus, while in the male, the müllerian ducts regress and the wolffian ducts give rise to the epididymis, vas deferens, and seminal vesicle.

Retention and differentiation of the müllerian ducts with concomitant regression of the wolffian ducts in female embryos are processes which require neither fetal ovaries nor testes (JOST 1972; JOST et al. 1973). In contrast, differentiation of the wolffian ducts into appropriate male accessory sex organs requires the presence of exogenous androgens or steroidogenically competent fetal testes. Female secondary sexual organogenesis therefore results in the absence of an androgenic environment, the absence or presence of ovaries being unimportant. Male accessory sex organ development, however, must be imposed by androgens against a basic female body trend (JOST et al. 1973; WILSON 1978). Development of the wolffian ducts requires the presence of testosterone or dihydrotestosterone (DHT) at a specific time in development when the tissue is receptive to the hormone. Whether specific androgen receptors are expressed in the tissue at this time is not known owing to the size and amount of embryonic tissue available for biochemical analysis. However, specific uptake of $^3H$ testosterone has been demonstrated in the wolffian ducts in male, but not female, embryos at this time (WILSON and SIITERI 1973).

There are several genetic mutations which result in abnormal development of the secondary sex organs (GOLDSTEIN and WILSON 1975). Of these, male pseudohermaphroditism, type 2, in humans and testicular feminization (Tfm) in mice and humans have been extensively studied at the biochemical and molecular levels (DUNN et al. 1973; ATTARDI and OHNO 1974; GOLDSTEIN and WILSON 1975). Type 2 pseudohermaphroditism is an autosomal recessive defect in which derivatives of the urogenital sinus differentiate in genotypic males into female (clitoris and vagina), rather than male (penis and scrotum) structures. This occurs owing to an inability of the urogenital sinus to convert testosterone to DHT, as a result of a deficiency in the level of the 5α-reductase enzyme which converts testosterone to DHT (GOLDSTEIN and WILSON 1975). Tfm is inherited as an X-linked recessive trait (LYON and HAWKES 1970). Affected individuals are genotypically male (X/Y) with cryptorchid (intraabdominal), steroidogenically competent testes that exhibit external phenotypic female body traits (WILSON 1978). Wolffian and müllerian duct internal accessory sex organs fail to develop in such individuals. The failure of the embryonic wolffian ducts to differentiate into male organs is due to the nonresponsiveness of the target tissue (end organ insensitivity) to endogenous or even exogenous androgens.

In fact, all androgen target organs, including nonsecondary sex organ derivatives such as kidney, submaxillary gland, brain, and the male mammary buds, fail to respond to androgen action (GOLDSTEIN WILSON 1975; ATTARDI 1976). Since individuals expressing complete penetrance of the defect, Tfm hemizygotes (Tfm/Y♀), lack any male secondary sex organs, study of the defect has been conducted on tissues such as kidney, brain, skin fibroblasts, and submaxillary glands in which specific biochemical responses are normally induced in response to androgens (Table 1). The molecular cause or causes of Tfm mutation have been most studied in tissues from mice, although recent data suggest that one or more similar lesions may be expressed in human tissue (MEYER et al. 1975; AMRHEIN et al. 1976; VERHOEVEN and WILSON 1979). In humans, Tfm occurs at a frequency ranging from 1 in 20,000 to 1 in 64,000 male newborns, and is the most common form of familial male pseudohermaphroditism.

**Table 1.** Androgen-induced responses in nonsecondary sex organ target tissues

| Tissue | Response |
|---|---|
| Kidney | Alcohol dehydrogenase<br>β-Glucuronidase<br>Arginase |
| Submaxillary gland | α-Amylase<br>Proteases (A and D)<br>Epidermal growth factor<br>Nerve growth factor |
| Male embryonic mammary buds | Mammary epithelial regression via mammary mesenchyme |
| Brain (hypothalamic-preotic) | Male behavioral and neuroendocrinologic patterns |

The primary molecular defect in tissues that express the Tfm mutation, as observed in Tfm/Y♀ hemizygous mice, is end organ insensitivity to the androgen-inducible phenotypes in all target tissues (ATTARDI 1976). Heterozygotes, Tfm/+, exhibit intermediate inductive responses to androgens (TETTENBORN et al. 1974) as a consequence of random X inactivation in cells constituting the target tissue. Although synthesis of testosterone and DHT is reduced in the testes and other organs in adult Tfm/Y mice compared with wild-type, normal males (X/Y), 6–8-week-old Tfm/Y mice synthesize approximately equal amounts of these androgens as X/Y mice (GOLDSTEIN and WILSON 1972). This result suggested that reduced plasma levels of androgens in Tfm/Y adult mice was a secondary effect due to a failure of response in androgen target tissues (BARDIN et al. 1973), thereby promoting through a feedback mechanism a decrease in androgen biosynthesis. In kidney and preputial glands from Tfm/Y mice, testosterone and DHT fail to concentrate, either in the cytosol or nucleus (GOLDSTEIN and WILSON 1975; ATTARDI 1976). Further investigations subsequently revealed that Tfm/Y kidney and preputial gland cytosol lacks, or is markedly depleted in the 8 *S* form of the cytoplasmic androgen receptor (BARDIN et al. 1973; GOLDSTEIN and WILSON 1975). This absence or reduction in demonstrable cytosol receptor correlated with a reduction in the specific translocation of testosterone or DHT in isolated kidney nuclei from Tfm/Y mice (GEHRING et al. 1971). A deficiency in the 8 *S* form of the androgen receptor was also noted in Tfm/Y submaxillary gland cytosol (DUNN et al. 1973).

From these studies, it was concluded that end organ insensitivity was a consequence of the inability of cells expressing the Tfm mutation to affect a receptor-mediated transfer of androgens to nuclear sites for promotion of biologic response. Either a complete absence of, or structural alteration to, the cytoplasmic receptor would account for the defect (ATTARDI and OHNO 1974; GEHRING and TOMKINS 1974). A structural alteration in the receptor at the steroid binding site could reduce its ability to bind to the steroid. Alternatively, modification of a site (or sites) on the receptor, which associates with specific acceptor sites in the nucleus in the 20%–30% of the remaining and detectable cytosol receptors present in the Tfm/Y target cells, could also account for androgen nonresponsiveness (ATTARDI 1976). In fact, it has recently been demonstrated that the Tfm mutation does not produce merely a reduction in the level of wild-type cytosol receptor, but that the residual remaining receptor population in cells expressing the mutation are also altered receptors in that they exhibit different elution profiles following DNA–cellulose chromatography (WIELAND and FOX 1979). Therefore, both quantitative and/or qualitative differences in specific subsets of cytoplasmic forms of the androgen receptor could account for the degrees of penetrance of the Tfm syndrome (i.e., "complete" or "partial" forms).

The Tfm syndrome in humans has a strong analogy to the malformation in mice with respect to both symptoms and molecular defects in the androgen receptors (WILSON 1978). Dermal fibroblasts from normal males or females possess approximately 1,200–19,000 androgen receptor sites for each cell (MEYER et al. 1975). Cells from six of ten Tfm patients had reduced or undetectable androgen binding in intact cells. The remaining four individuals exhibited normal cytoplasmic and nuclear binding for the hormone. All ten Tfm patients by pedigree were found to have an X-linked association with the syndrome. The four Tfm individuals that possessed normal androgen binding and translocation may express the mutation, as in the case of mice, owing to alterations in the region of the androgen receptor that interacts with nuclear acceptor sites, or alterations in other accessory proteins that mediate androgen-dependent transcription (AMRHEIN et al. 1976).

## II. Glucocorticoids

### 1. Cystic Fibrosis

Cystic fibrosis (CF) is an autosomal recessive disease occurring once in every 1,600–2,500 births (BRESLOW et al. 1978b). Affected individuals have pulmonary and gastrointestinal problems. The biochemical defect or defects associated with this birth defect have not yet been identified. EPSTEIN et al. (1977) have demonstrated that fibroblasts obtained from CF individuals are more resistant to the cytotoxicity of dexamethasone, a synthetic glucocorticoid, than are normal cells. Cytotoxicity was evaluated by colony formation after 14–21 days in the absence or presence of the steroid or other drugs. Ouabain, a drug which inhibits membrane-bound $Na^+,K^+$-ATPase, also showed a similar correlation for cytotoxicity between fibroblasts from CF and normal individuals. EPSTEIN et al. (1977) suggested that resistance to both ouabain and dexamethasone cytotoxicity was due to a common mechanism related to the sterol nucleus. Subsequently, BRESLOW et al. (1978a) demonstrated that CF fibroblasts exhibited cross-resistance for cytotoxicity to dexamethasone and the sex steroids, 17$\beta$-estradiol, DHT, and progesterone. The variation in resistance to dexamethasone cytotoxicity in CF and normal fibroblasts was not due to differences in the level or affinity of cytoplasmic receptors for glucocorticoids. They suggested that quantitative differences in the level of glucocorticoid receptors between CF and normal fibroblasts could not account for the diminished cytotoxicity of the glucocorticoids in CF cells. Nevertheless, alterations in receptor nuclear translocation, association with chromosomal acceptor sites, or responses distal to the receptor could have accounted for the differences between CF and normal fibroblasts (SIBLEY and YAMAMOTO 1979). However, no demonstrable receptors for estrogens were found in either male or female fibroblasts obtained from either CF or normal individuals. Since 17-$\beta$-estradiol as well as DHT and progesterone were equally as effective as dexamethasone in producing cytotoxicity in normal, but not CF cells, an alternate mechanism (or mechanisms) other than through a receptor pathway for cell killing was suggested as being operative. Further evidence arguing against a receptor-mediated cytotoxicity in this system was provided following analysis of androgen receptors in fibroblasts from Tfm patients and the cytotoxicity to DHT in these cells versus normal cells (BRESLOW et al. 1979). Tfm fibroblasts lacked any measurable specific binding for DHT, in contrast to cells obtained from normal individuals. However, both Tfm and normal fibroblasts were equally sensitive to the cell killing induced by DHT.

The mechanism (or mechanisms) by which steroids induce cell killing in this system still remains obscure. Until this question is resolved, attempts to address the differences in sensitivity to steroid-induced cytotoxicity in fibroblasts obtained from CF and normal individuals can only be speculative. However, this qualification does not distract from the usefulness of these observations as potential criteria for prenatal diagnosis of CF. In fact, it was found that cells obtained after amniocentesis from a woman at high risk of producing a CF child exhibited marked resistance to dexamethasone, whereas amniocentesic cells from other individuals with no familial history of CF were sensitive to the steroid (BRESLOW et al. 1978 b).

## 2. Cleft Palate

Glucocorticoids administered in pharmacologic doses to a variety of animals during midpregnancy inhibit closure of the secondary palate and cause specific limb malformations (WALKER 1967; SHAH and KILISTOFF 1976; SALOMON and PRATT 1979). In nonhuman primates, glucocorticoids can function as teratogens when administered in excessive doses. In bonnet and rhesus monkeys, atrophy of thymus and lymphoid tissues, skeletal defects, and cleft palate (CP) have been observed following administration of pharmacologic doses of triamcinolone acetonide (HENDRICKX et al. 1975). Women treated with glucocorticoids to support pregnancy in the presence of infertility problems give birth to infants with markedly low birth weight (REINISCH et al. 1978). However, evidence to suggest that glucocorticoids are teratogenic in humans with respect to CP production is not definitive.

Different strains of mice exhibit various degrees of susceptibility to glucocorticoid-induced CP (BAXTER and FRASER 1950; KALTER 1954; SALOMON and PRATT 1979). For example, all of the offspring of A/J mice treated with glucocorticoids between days 11 and 14 of gestation have CP, whereas C57BL/6J (C57) mice treated with the same dose of the steroid over this period produce 20%–25% offspring with CP. A number of factors could contribute to glucocorticoid-induced CP, and have been proposed to explain the response differences of various strains of mice to the teratogenic effect of glucocorticoids (Table 2; GREENE and KOCHHAR 1975; SALOMON and PRATT 1979). The synthesis and metabolism of glucocorticoids differ among adult mice of various strains (BADR and SPICKETT 1965). However, during midgestation, at least in A/J and C57 mice, no significant differences were found in the concentration of maternal or fetal corticosterone, the major naturally occurring glucocorticoid in rodents (SALOMON et als. 1979).

Glucocorticoids can traverse the rodent placenta (ZARROW et al. 1970). Furthermore, although maternal metabolism of exogenously administered glucocorticoids is higher in more sensitive strains (ZIMMERMAN and BOWEN 1972 a), a large fraction of the steroid reaches the fetus unmetabolized. In fact, the active terato-

**Table 2.** Possible factors involved in the control of glucocorticoid-induced cleft palate

I. Maternal modulation – genetic differences in the maternal rate of metabolism of endogenous or exogenously administered steroid
   1. Faster in more resistant strains
II. Formation of one or more teratogenic metabolites by the mother or fetus from the administered steroid
   1. Increased in the more sensitive strains
III. Variable distribution of the steroid at different stages in development in embryonic, extraembryonic, or maternal tissues
IV. Variable biologic sensitivity of embryonic target organ (or organs) toward the steroid at different developmental stages

**Table 3.** Glucocorticoid receptors in rodent embryonic maxillary processes and forepaws

| Tissue | Sites/cell | $K_d(M)$ |
|---|---|---|
| Maxillary Processes | | |
| A/J | 16,300 | $1.7 \times 10^{-8}$ |
| C57BL/6J | 7,200 | $7.9 \times 10^{-9}$ |
| Sprague-Dawley rat | 10,372 | $9.6 \times 10^{-9}$ |
| Forepaws | | |
| A/J | 3,798 | $7.9 \times 10^{-9}$ |
| C57BL/6J | 6,150 | $2.9 \times 10^{-8}$ |
| Sprague-Dawley rat | 13,025 | $1.2 \times 10^{-8}$ |

genic agent represents unmetabolized glucocorticoid (ZIMMERMAN and BOWEN 1972b). A direct metabolic effect of glucocorticoids on the embryo has been suggested as one of the determining factors controlling glucocorticoid teratogenicity (SALOMON and PRATT 1979). Protein and RNA synthesis are inhibited in the embryo following glucocorticoid administration to the mother (ZIMMERMAN et al. 1970). Moreover, the total amount of radioactive glucocorticoid administered to the mother and associated with palatal and other fetal tissues, correlates with the degree of inhibition of RNA and protein synthesis and the teratogenic susceptibility in various strains of mice.

Mouse and rat embryonic facial (maxillary) mesenchhyme cells possess high affinity, specific receptor proteins for glucocorticoids (Table 3; SALOMON and PRATT 1976, 1979). Moreover, A/J facial mesenchyme cells contain 2–3 times more cytoplasmic receptors than C57 cells, which correlates with the higher sensitivity of A/J mice than C57 mice to steroid-induced CP. The correlative strain difference in embryonic glucocorticoid receptor levels are generally restricted to areas of the orofacial region since the concentration of receptors in the embryonic forepaws of A/J and C57 mice fail to show a correlation with teratogenic susceptibility. The difference in glucocorticoid receptor levels between A/J and C57 maxillary mesenchyme cells is reflected in the magnitude of inhibition of growth and DNA synthesis produced in these cells by glucocorticoids (SALOMON and PRATT 1978). A/J cells are more sensitive to glucocorticoids than C57 cells with respect to inhibition of growth and DNA synthesis as well as to the induction of glutamine synthetase (GREENE and SALOMON 1981).

Owing to their size and the limited amount of palatal tissue available for biochemical analysis, glucocorticoid receptors prepared from whole midgestation fetuses have been characterized with respect to their physiochemical properties compared with those of receptors in maternal liver (SALOMON et al. 1978). The embryonic cytosol receptors in both A/J and C57 mice are heat-labile, sulfhydryl-dependent proteins which bind with high affinity either dexamethasone or triamcinolone acetonide. The embryonic receptors exhibit sedimentation properties (7–9 *S*) and elution profiles from DE-52 ion-exchange columns that are similar to adult, maternal hepatic receptors. Furthermore, these binding proteins can be biochemically distinguished from plasma transcortin, a serum glucocorticoid transport protein.

**Table 4.** Maxillary cytoplasmic glucocorticoid receptors and cleft palate frequency

| Strain | Sites/cell | Cleft palate (%) |
|---|---|---|
| SWR/FR | 83,960 | 100 |
| SWR/NIH | 61,500 | 100 |
| DBA/1J | 29,216 | 94 |
| A/J | 16,300 | 100 |
| CBA/J | 10,764 | 12 |
| C5BL/6J | 7,073 | 25 |

**Table 5.** Frequency of glucocorticoid-induced cleft palate and H-2 haplotypes

| Strain | Cleft palate (%) | H-2 haplotypes |
|---|---|---|
| A/J | 100 | H-$2^a$ |
| B.10A | 81 | H-$2^a$ |
| SWR/J | 100 | H-$2^q$ |
| DBA/1J | 94 | H-$2^q$ |
| C57BL/6J | 25 | H-$2^b$ |
| C57BL/10 ScSn | 21 | H-$2^b$ |
| A.By | 85 | H-$2^b$ |
| CBA/J | 12 | H-$2^k$ |
| C3H/HeJ | 63 | H-$2^k$ |
| bm/bm | 100 | H-$2^b$ |

The correlation of glucocorticoid receptor levels in embryonic maxillary tissue and strain susceptibility to steroid-induced CP is not limited to A/J and C57 mice. In other strains, the levels of cytoplasmic glucocorticoid receptors in maxillary mesenchyme cytosols are also correlated with the sensitivity of these animals to glucocorticoid-induced CP (Table 4). GOLDMAN et al. (1977) have confirmed and extended these observations. Furthermore, they demonstrated that the concentration of receptors was higher, both in fetal and maternal secondary palates, in animals possessing the H-$2^a$ haplotype than those having the H-$2^b$ haplotype, an association which also correlates with glucocorticoid-induced CP susceptibility (Table 5; BONNER and SLAVKIN 1975; TYAN and MILLER 1978).

Whereas an association between receptor levels and H-2 haplotypes was found in both fetal and maternal palatal tissues, no correlation was observed in adult mouse liver from H-2 congenic strains (BUTLEY et al. 1978) although intrastrain differences in receptor concentration were noted in these studies. Furthermore, PRATT et al. (1980) were also unable to demonstrate a clear association with steroid resistance and possession of the H-$2^b$ haplotype. Specifically, C57 mice and bm/bm mice possess the same haplotype, H-$2^b$. However, they differ at a single locus which is not associated with the H-2 complex. Homozygous brachymorph (bm/bm) mice are as sensitive to glucocorticoid-induced CP as A/J mice. However, the level of

**Table 6.** Glucocorticoid receptor defects in S49 mouse lymphoma cells

| Designation | Phenotype |
|---|---|
| $r^-$ | Absence of cytosol receptor or defect in steroid binding site |
| $nt^-$ | Deficiency in nuclear translocation |
| $nt^i$ | Enhanced nuclear translocation – alteration in binding to acceptor sites in nucleus |
| $d^-$ | Deathless defect distal to receptor or lesions in nonreceptor, transformation, or activation components |

glucocorticoid receptors in embryonic facial mesenchyme cells in bm/bm mice were similar to the concentration of receptors in the parental, wild-type, resistant C57 strain. Therefore, one or more genes other than those associated with the H-2 locus also probably contribute to genetic differences between these strains with respect to steroid-induced CP susceptibility (BIDDLE and FRASER 1977; SALOMON and PRATT 1979). Furthermore, differences other than quantitative variations in the level of steroid receptors must also be involved in controlling the genetic response frequency differences. Alterations or lesions distal to the level of the receptor may function to regulate the magnitude of the response produced by the steroid.

GOLDMAN et al. (1978) have subsequently extended their studies and have presented evidence for the presence of glucocorticoid receptors in cultured mesenchyme cells obtained from fused human fetal palates. PRATT and SALOMON (1980) have also characterized glucocorticoid receptors in cultured dermal fibroblasts obtained from skin biopsies of normal individuals and women or offspring of women who have a history of children with cleft lip and/or CP. In these studies, an inverse correlation was noted between the level of glucocorticoid receptors in the fibroblasts and the pedigree. Cells obtained from offspring of women with a history of orofacial malformations had fewer receptors and were less responsive to glucocorticoid-induced growth inhibition or inhibition of colony formation than cells from individuals without a history of CP. YONEDA et al. (1981) have extended these observations to a larger sampling of individuals with histories of cleft lip and/or cleft palate. They found a decrease in the number of glucocorticoid receptors in skin biopsies from individuals with cleft lip and/or palate, and suggested that this observation might serve as a valuable diagnostic criterion for screening individuals who might be at risk of producing offspring with cleft lip and/or palate.

The data at hand, therefore, argue against simplistic explanations for ascribing any one particular defect in the etiology of steroid-induced CP. Certainly, altered levels of glucocorticoid receptor proteins may be one factor serving to predispose certain strains of mice or humans to either steroid-induced or spontaneous CP. Nevertheless, other differences, either distal to the receptor or involving metabolism or distribution of glucocorticoids in the maternal or fetal compartments, are also likely to contribute to the etiology of CP. Furthermore, the interactions of glucocorticoids with other hormones or growth factors such as epidermal growth factor (EGF), which is known to play a role in normal palatogenesis (SALOMON and PRATT 1979), should be considered in attempting to decipher the molecular defects in CP production.

It should also be stressed that a spectrum of pathologic and genetic variations in sensitivity to glucocorticoids have been described in mice and humans (HARRIS and BAXTER 1979). Some of these disorders can be traced to quantitative differences in the level of glucocorticoid receptors. However, more subtle defects in steroid receptor design and function occur which are related to genetic variations in glucocorticoid sensitivity. For example, mouse S49 lymphoma cells are normally killed by glucocorticoids. Mutant cell lines have been selected for steroid resistance, and exhibit various receptor abnormalities (SIBLEY and YAMAMOTO 1979). These variant clones differ in their phenotypes (Table 6) by possessing specific lesions at various points in the steroid receptor pathway which all confer resistance. Description of this system merely serves to illustrate the complexity, even at the level of the receptor, of attempting to define CP susceptibility solely on the basis of quantitative variations in steroid receptor levels.

# C. Cholesterol

## I. Low Density Lipoprotein

### 1. Familial Hypercholesterolemia

Cholesterol is delivered to and acquired by animal cells through a plasma binding protein, low density lipoprotein (LDL). Cells possess specific membrane-bound receptors for LDL which are located in clathrin-coated pits (GOLDSTEIN et al. 1979). Following binding to the receptor, LDL and associated cholesterol, as well as the receptor, are internalized and delivered to lysosomes. In the lysosomes, the cholesteryl ester components of LDL are hydrolyzed to unesterified cholesterol, and the receptor and protein portions of LDL are degraded. Recycling of the receptor requires de novo protein synthesis and occurs within 6–10 h, whereas internalization or endocytosis of the LDL–receptor complex occurs within 10 min after ligand binding (BROWN et al. 1975; GOLDSTEIN et al. 1979).

Several structural mutations have been described for the LDL receptor which are responsible for the genetic disease, familial hypercholesterolemia (FH) (Table 7). FH is an autosomal dominant disorder, characterized by an elevation

**Table 7.** Low density lipoprotein receptor defects in familial hypercholesterolemia

| Designation | Phenotype |
|---|---|
| $R^{b^0}$ | Absence of LDL cell surface receptor |
| $R^{b^-}$ | Defect in receptor binding site for LDL |
| $R^{b^+, i^0}$ | Absence of internalization of LDL receptor |

in the plasma levels of LDL with the subsequent accumulation of cholesterol in body tissues which leads to the formation of xanthomas and atherosclerosis (BROWN et al. 1975; POLLET and LEVEY 1980). Intracellular cholesterol concentrations are regulated by the rate-limiting enzyme in cholesterol biosynthesis, 3-hydroxy-3-methylgluturyl coenzyme A reductase (HMG CoA reductase). In FH patients, there is an overproduction of endogenous cholesterol owing to the failure of LDL to suppress HMG CoA reductase activity (BROWN et al. 1975). In these circumstances, LDL fails to enter the cell because of mutations in the LDL receptor system, resulting in an overproduction of peripheral cholesterol and elevated plasma levels of cholesterol.

The LDL receptor defects have been studied in cultured dermal fibroblasts from skin biopsies and peripheral lymphocytes obtained from FH patients and normal individuals. Originally, two mutant alleles associated with LDL receptor structure were characterized (GOLDSTEIN et al. 1979). The receptor-negative ($R^{b^0}$) phenotype was found to bind less than 1% of the LDL compared with normal, wild-type (+/+) cells. Heterozygous individuals for this allele (+/$R^{b^0}$) possess an LDL receptor which binds approximately 50% of the wild-type amount of LDL. Cells from FH subjects who are homozygous for the the receptor-negative allele ($R^{b^0}/R^{b^0}$) were found to show no high affinity binding of LDL. In both $R^{b^0}$ heterozygotic and homozygotic individuals, the plasma levels of LDL are 2- to 6-fold above normal. Subsequently, GOLDSTEIN et al. (1979) identified a second class of mutant alleles that expresses a phenotype in which the LDL receptor exhibits a defect (or defects) in binding for LDL (receptor-defective, $R^{b^-}$). The receptor for LDL in cells from FH individuals expressing this mutation in the homozygous state ($R^{b^-}/R^{b^-}$) binds less than 10% of the wild-type amount of LDL. Cells from both $R^{b^-}$ heterozygotes and homozygotes exhibit a reduction in the internalization and subsequent degradation of the LDL–receptor complex in proportion to the reduced level of binding of LDL to these cells.

Recently, GOLDSTEIN et al. (1977) have described a third mutation, involving the LDL receptor, which is distinct from the $R^{b^0}$ and $R^{b^-}$ defects. The mutation involves a defect in the internalization of the LDL–receptor complex. Fibroblasts from a patient exhibiting this lesion were able to bind normal amounts of LDL at the cell surface, but subsequent to binding failed to internalize the bound LDL. The pedigree revealed that this patient inherited paternally the $R^{b^+,i^0}$ phenotype and maternally the $R^{b^0}$ phenotype. Both parents were heterozygotes, with the father being +/$R^{b^+,i^0}$ and the mother +/$R^{b^0}$. This patient represents a compound heterozygote whose cells possess two different alleles for the LDL receptor and is therefore $R^{b^0}/R^{b^+,i^0}$. Further investigation revealed that fibroblasts possessed a normal number of clathrin-coated pits, to which the LDL–receptor complex normally associated at 37 °C. However, the LDL receptors from the patient's cells were not located in these pits, but were scattered randomly over the plasma membrane (ANDERSON et al. 1977). From these studies, it was concluded that the LDL receptor consists of at least two distinct binding sites. One site binds the ligand, LDL, since the $R^{b^0}$ mutant allele disrupts this function. The second site controlled by the $R^{b^+,i^0}$ allele is necessary for receptor incorporation of, or coupling to, the clathrin-coated pits in the membrane so as to facilitate internalization of the LDL–receptor complex. The recognition site on the receptor which is necessary for internalization probably is involved in binding the receptor to clathrin in the coated pits. These conclusions were reached since the $R^{b^0}$ and $R^{b^+,i^0}$ mutations were found to be noncomplementing with respect to receptor function.

# D. Thyroid Hormones

## I. Triiodothyronine

### 1. Familial Thyroid Hormone Resistance

Receptors for thyroid hormones are soluble, nuclear binding proteins which have been identified in liver, kidney, and lymphocytes (SAMUELS and TSAI 1973; OPPENHEIMER et al. 1976). Familial end organ resistance to thyroid hormones (FTHR) was first reported by REFETOFF et al. (1972). Children exhibiting this syndrome were characterized by high circulating levels of L-thyroxine ($T_4$) and L-triiodothyronine ($T_3$), goiter, deaf mutism, and epiphyseal defects. The syndrome appears to be inherited in certain cases as an autosomal dominant or codominant trait. Various tissues such as the pituitary, in which thyroid-stimulating hormone (TSH) is normally suppressed by high $T_3$ or $T_4$ levels, were not affected by these hormones in FTHR individuals. Specifically, TSH suppression was not markedly affected after exogenous $T_3$ or $T_4$ administration (POLLET and LEVEY 1980). However, labeled $T_3$ and $T_4$ were able to penetrate such tissues as liver. Furthermore, conversion of $T_4$ to $T_3$ occurred normally in peripheral tissues of FTRH patients.

BERNAL et al. (1978) considered the possibility that an alteration in the interaction of thyroid hormones at the cellular receptor might partially account for the peripheral end organ resistance to these hormones. They characterized $T_3$ nuclear binding sites in peripheral lymphocytes, and cultured biopsied dermal fibroblasts obtained from normal and FTHR subjects. In lymphocytes from an FTHR individual, the affinity of nuclear binding for $T_3$ was ten-fold less than the affinity measured in normal lymphocytes. For fibroblasts, high and low affinity nuclear binding components, or negative cooperativity, were demonstrated in FTHR cultured cells. In contrast, normal fibroblasts exhibited only the high affinity binding component, or lacked cooperativity for $T_3$ binding. BERNAL et al. (1978) suggested that the presence of a low affinity binding site for $T_3$, or the enhanced sensitivity to $T_3$ owing to negative cooperativity of a single class of binding sites, could lead to $T_3$ resistance as a result of hypersensitivity at the target organ for the hormone. There is also evidence to suggest that postreceptor alterations may contribute to thyroid hormone resistance (VERHOEVEN and WILSON 1979). In ob/ob mice, thyroxine fails to increase the level of $Na^+,K^+$-ATPase activity in hepatocytes. In these animals, other thyroid hormone parameters were apparently normal (YORK et al. 1978).

# E. Polypeptide Hormones

## I. Growth Hormone

### 1. Levi-Lorain Dwarfism and Snell Dwarf

The peripheral effects of growth hormone on target tissues are mediated by somatomedins, a class of insulin-related growth factors produced in the liver (VAN WYK and UNDERWOOD 1975; DAUGHADAY et al. 1975). These growth factors are low molecular weight polypeptides (6,000–10,000 datons). A variety of biologic responses in vivo and in vitro have been described in different cell types following somatomedin administration or changes in somatomedin plasma levels (VAN WYK et al. 1978).

One congenital form of resistance to growth hormone (GH) is the Levi-Lorain dwarf in humans (POLLET and LEVEY 1980). This type of dwarfism is an autosomal recessive mutation in which affected individuals exhibit craniofacial disproportions, truncal obesity, and various dermatologic syndromes. Plasma GH levels are elevated in these individuals. However, stimulation or suppression of GH secretion is normal. Serum somatomedin levels are generally suppressed and are not elevated in response to exogenous GH therapy. Since somatomedin levels are not elevated, and since GH does not produce an increase in endogenous somatomedins in these patients, the defect appears to be at the level of the GH receptor in responsive target tissues such as liver. However, no conclusive evidence for this has been presented to date. Nevertheless, in the mouse, there is an autosomal recessive mutation, Snell dwarf mouse, which in the homozygous state (dw/dw) resembles certain aspects of the human Levi-Lorain dwarf syndrome.

In contrast to the human Levi-Lorain dwarf, the mouse Snell dwarf has low plasma levels of GH as well as TSH and prolactin (Prl). These animals are stunted, infertile, and immunologically incompetent. In dw/dw animals, there is an absence of somatotropic and lactotropic cells in the anterior pituitary. Owing to an absence or reduction in circulating levels of GH and Prl, receptors for these hormones might be modified. KNAZEK et al. (1977) have demonstrated a reduction in the number of GH receptors in livers from dw/dw mice compared with their normal littermates. In contrast, no Prl binding could be observed in dw/dw livers, while normal littermates exhibited appreciable activity. However, Prl binding sites were induced or exposed in dw/dw mice following ectopic pituitary transplantation or GH administration. In a subsequent study, KNAZEK et al. (1978) demonstrated that either GH or Prl were equally effective in causing the appearance of Prl receptors following in vivo administration. Pretreatment of dw/dw mice with cycloheximide did not prevent the GH-induced appearance of Prl receptors. Likewise, GH administration failed to cause an increase in GH receptors in dw/dw mice. The authors suggested that these results indicated the presence of cryptic or nonfunctional Prl receptors in the dw/dw mouse that could be exposed following GH treatment. The Levi-Lorain dwarf may exhibit a similar masking of GH receptors in target tissues such as the liver.

## II. Parathyroid Hormone

### 1. Pseudohypoparathyroidism

Parathyroid hormone (PTH) regulates calcium and phosphorus metabolism. Pseudohypoparathyroidism (PsHP) is an X-linked or autosomal dominant disorder described by Albright as one of the first congential hormone resistance syndromes (also referred to as the Albright–McCune–Sternberg syndrome or osteitis fibrosa disseminata). It is characterized by hypoparathyroidism with elevated serum levels of PTH, hypocalcemia, and hyperphosphatemia. PsHP is often associated with Albright's hereditary osteodystrophy in which individuals exhibit short stature, obesity, brachydactyly, short metacarpals and metatarsals, and soft tissue calcifi-

**Table 8.** Components of the receptor–effector adenylate cyclase system

| Designation | Function |
|---|---|
| R | Hormone receptor |
| G | Guanine nucleotide binding protein |
| NAD glycohydrolase | ADP ribosylation |
| PMT (I, II) | Phospholipid methyltransferases I and II |
| C | Catalytic unit |

cations (WHITE and MARX 1978; POLLET and LEVEY 1980). CHASE et al. (1969) demonstrated that PsHP individuals fail to respond to exogenous PTH administration, as measured by elevations in urinary cyclic AMP levels. These results suggested that the primary defect in PsHP was in the PTH–receptor–adenylate cyclase system (Table 8). Subsequently, DREZNER and BURCH (1978) found a normal PTH receptor in renal cortical plasma membranes obtained from a PsHP patient. However, generation of cyclic AMP from ATP in response to PTH was depressed if GTP was omitted from the reaction when compared with adenylate cyclase activity in normal renal cortical plasma membranes. The Michaelis constant $K_m$ of adenylate cyclase for the substrate ATP was sifnificantly higher in PsHP plasma membrane fractions than the $K_m$ in membranes from control subjects. However, after addition of GTP the apparent $K_m$ was lowered to control levels. The authors suggested that the defect in the hormone–receptor–effector adenylate cyclase system was due to an abnormal nucleotide regulatory site promoting a partial uncoupling of the receptor and adenylate cyclase units.

Adenylate cyclase consists of a catalytic unit and a guanine nucleotide regulatory protein (G unit; Table 8). The catalytic unit is located on the inner surface of the plasma membrane while the receptor component is situated on the external side (KASLOW et al. 1979). The G unit functions as a transducer to couple the catalytic unit to the receptor, thereby mediating the enzymatic activation of adenylate cyclase by hormones, guanine nucleotides, fluoride, and cholera toxin. The activity of the G unit, with respect to its coupling function for the receptor and cyclase units, can be modified by ADP ribosylation through an NAD glycohydrolase. In this reaction, ADP ribose is transferred from NAD to an arginine residue on the G unit. Likewise, there are two phospholipid methyltransferases (PMT I and II) located within the plasma membrane which may serve to facilitate the juxtaposition of the receptor and G units by increasing membrane fluidity (HIRATA and AXELROD 1980). Defects at any one of these postreceptor sites could have accounted for the data presented by DREZNER and BURCH (1978) with regard to PTH insensitivity in target cells from PsHP patients.

LEVINE et al. (1980) demonstrated a reduction in the amount of G unit protein in erythrocyte membranes from PsHP individuals. Erythrocyte membranes were utilized because they lack a $\beta$-andrenergic and catalytic unit. Reconstitution experiments were performed with membranes from the G unit-deficient S49. Mouse lymphoma adenylate cyclase-deficient ($Cyc^-$) mutants. Although no alteration in the affinity of the G units for GTP from PsHP membranes was observed, there was a 50% reduction in the amount of G unit activity compared with normal individuals. The authors suggested that since the G unit is common to other hormones which function through the adenylate cyclase system, alteration in the G unit in PsHP may be reflected in resistance to other hormones. In fact, TSH and gonadotropin insensitivity have been reported in patients with PsHP.

## F. Conclusion

It was the goal of this chapter to provide a broad overview of some of the more frequent and pathogenically defined congential syndromes associated with resistance or enhanced sensitivity to various classes of hormones. Both metabolic and/or anatomic malformations are associated with several of these conditions. The pathophysiology of these syndromes can in many instances be traced to primary defects in the receptor, in which there is an absence of or elevated receptors or defect in the hormone recognition and binding site (e.g., Tfm, Snell dwarf, FH, CP, and FTHR). Alternatively, subtle quantitative and/or qualitative alterations in postreceptor, effector, or transducing components may be involved in the etiology of some of these defects. For steroid hormones, transformation and activation components are necessary for normal biologic functioning of the receptor. Likewise, the presence of nuclear acceptor sites associated with chromatin are obligatory components in the pathway for recognition of the steroid–receptor complex before a biologic response can be produced in target cells. Certain subclasses of the Tfm mutation in specific tissues in mice and humans may be due to alterations or defects in receptor transformation, activation, or nuclear translocation. Moreover, modification of nuclear acceptor sites could contribute to a change in hormone sensitivity in target cells (e.g., S49 mouse lymphoma glucocorticoid-resistant variants). For example, the incomplete association of glucocorticoid-induced CP susceptibility in mice with H-2 haplotype (congenic) may also indicate that one or more non-H-2 associated genes may be important in regulating postreceptor components for these hormones.

For ligands which interact with specific membrane-bound receptors, the data also indicate that lesions in any of the steps distal to the receptor (effector components) may be modified, and thereby contribute to the pathogenesis of hormone-resistant syndromes. Hormones which function through the adenylate cyclase–protein kinase system may be particularly sensitive to genetic mutations owing to the complexity of this pathway. Receptor coupling and activation of adenylate cyclase through the G binding protein (e.g., PsHP) and the subsequent steps leading to activation of cAMP-dependent protein kinases are potential targets for genetic lesions. In fact, in S49 mouse lymphoma cells, specific mutants have been isolated which are resistant to the cytolytic effects of hormones which function through the adenylate cyclase–protein kinase system (Table 9). An absence or reduction in the G binding protein or catalytic unit are examples of proximal defects leading to hormone resistance. Likewise, distal structural or regulatory mutations in the protein kinase molecule (catalytic or regulatory subunits) have also been identified and shown to be involved in resistance to cytolysis by hormones or exogenous cyclic AMP (INSEL et al. 1975; SCHLEIFER et al. 1980). The LDL receptor–

**Table 9.** Adenylate cyclase–protein kinase defects in S49 mouse lymphoma cells

| Designation | Phenotype |
|---|---|
| I Cyclase mutants | |
| Cyc$^-$ | Deficiency in G binding protein |
| UNC | Uncoupled receptor and catalytic units, alteration in G binding protein |
| II Kinase mutants | |
| Kin A | $K_m$ mutants, alteration in regulatory (R) subunit |
| Kin B | $V_{max}$ mutants, deficiency in protein kinase |
| Kin C | PK$^-$ mutants, lack protein kinase |

effector mutations further illustrate that the processing mechanism (or mechanisms) for the ligand–receptor complex may also be prone to genetic variation. For example, the LDL receptor phenotype, $R^{b^+, i^0}$, exhibits a defect in the clustering and subsequent internalization of the LDL–receptor complex, although a normal receptor for LDL is present on the target cell.

From this discourse it is apparent that several of these congenital syndromes can consist of a mixture of heterogeneous defects, resulting from quantitative and/or qualitative alterations in any of a number of steps in the hormone–receptor–effector pathway. This wide range in genetic–pathogenic heterogeneity may contribute to the degree of penetrance of a particular syndrome and may also explain the association of certain functional metabolic disturbances with specific anatomic malformations (POLLET and LEVEY 1980). It must also be stressed that intertissue differences may exist with respect to hormone sensitivity, and these might fluctuate as a function of the developmental state of the tissue (HARRIS and BAXTER 1979). Therefore, one organ or set of organs may be more prone to genetic or environmental insult at a specific time in development than other target organs. Likewise, other hormones or growth factors may synergistically or antagonistically influence the degree of sensitivity in a target tissue to a particular hormone.

Investigations concerned with definition of the molecular mechanisms of various hormones and growth factors should provide information regarding the etiology of these various genetic diseases and malformations. Furthermore, the use of animal mutants (e.g., Tfm/Y, dw/dw, ob/ob, and bm/bm mice), which resemble certain human genetic diseases related to hormone dysfunction, will provide suitable model systems in which to conduct these studies.

## References

Amrhein JA, Meyer WJ, Jones HW, Migeon CJ (1976) Androgen insensitivity in man: evidence for genetic heterogeneity. Proc Natl Acad Sci USA 73:891–894

Anderson RGW, Goldstein JL, Brown MS (1977) A mutation that impairs the ability of lipoprotein receptors to localize in coated pits on the cell surface of human fibroblasts. Nature 270:695–699

Attardi B (1976) Genetic analysis of steroid hormone action. Trends Biochem Sci Nov:241–244

Attardi B, Ohno S (1974) Cytosol androgen receptor from kidney of normal and testicular feminized (Tfm) mice. Cell 2:205–212

Badr FM, Spickett SG (1965) Genetic variation in the biosynthesis of corticosteroids in *Mus musculus*. Nature 205:1088–1090

Bardin WC, Bullock LP, Sherins RJ, Mowszowicz I, Blackburn WR (1973) II. Androgen metabolism and mechanism of action in male pseudohermaphroditism: a study of testicular feminization. Recent Prog Horm Res 29:65–108

Baxter H, Fraser FC (1950) Production of congenital defects in the offspring of female mice treated with cortisone. McGill Med J 19:245–249

Bernal J, Refetoff S, Degroot LJ (1978) Abnormalities of triiodothyronine binding to lymphocyte and fibroblast nuclei from a patient with peripheral tissue resistance to thyroid hormone action. J Clin Endocrinol Metab 47:1266–1272

Biddle FG, Fraser FC (1977) Cortisone-induced cleft palate in the mouse: a search for the genetic control of the embryonic response trait. Genetics 85:289–302

Bonner JJ, Slavkin HC (1975) Cleft palate susceptibility linked to histocompatibility-2 (H-2) in the mouse. Immunogenetics 2:213–218

Breslow JL, Epstein J, Fontaine JH (1978a) Dexamethasone-resistant cystic fibrosis fibroblasts show cross-resistance to sex steroids. Cell 13:663–669

Breslow JL, Epstein J, Fontaine JH, Forbes GB (1978b) Enhanced dexamethasone resistance in cystic fibrosis cells: potential use for heterozygote detection and prenatal diagnosis. Science 201:180–182

Breslow JL, Epstein J, Forbes GB, Fontaine JH (1979) Steroid hormone toxicity in human fibroblasts does not correlate with high afifnity receptor content. J Cell Physiol 99:343–348

Brown MS, Brannan PG, Bohmfalk HA et al. (1975) Use of mutant fibroblasts in the analysis of the regulation of cholesterol metabolism in human cells. J Cell Physiol 85:425–436

Butley MS, Erickson RP, Pratt WB (1978) Hepatic glucocorticoid receptors and the H-2 locus. Nature 275:136–138

Carpenter G, Cohen S (1979) Epidermal growth factor. Annu Rev Biochem 48:193–216

Catt KJ, Harwood JP, Aguilera G, Dufau ML (1979) Hormonal regulation of peptide receptors and target cell responses. Nature 280:109–116

Chase LR, Melson GL, Aurbach GD (1969) Pseudohypoparathyroidism: defective excretion of 3′,5′-AMP in response to parathyroid hormone. J Clin Invest 48:1832–1844

Daughaday WH, Herington AC, Phillips LS (1975) The regulation of growth by endocrines. Recent Prog Horm Res 31:211–244

Drezner MK, Burch WM (1978) Altered activity of the nucleotide regulatory site in parathyroid hormone-sensitive adenylate cyclase from the renal cortex of a patient with pseudohypoparathyroidism. J Clin Invest 62:1222–1227

Dunn JF, Goldstein JL, Wilson JD (1973) Development of increased cytoplasmic binding of androgen in the submandibular gland of the mouse with testicular feminization. J Biol Chem 248:7819–7825

Epstein J, Breslow JL, Davidson RL (1977) Increased dexamethasone resistance of cystic fibrosis fibroblasts. Proc Natl Acad Sci USA 74:5642–5646

Gehring U, Tomkins GM (1974) Characterization of a hormone receptor defect in the androgen-insensitivity mutant. Cell 3:59–64

Gehring U, Tomkins GM, Ohno S (1971) Effect of the androgen-insensitivity mutation on a cytoplasmic receptor for dihydrotestosterone. Nature New Biol 232:106–107

Goidl JA, Cake MH, Dolan KP, Parchman G, Litwack G (1977) Activation of the rat liver glucocorticoid-receptor complex. Biochemistry 16:2125–2130

Goldman AS, Katsumata M, Yaffe SJ, Gusser DL (1977) Palatal cytosol cortisol-binding protein associated with cleft palate susceptibility and H-2 geneotype. Nature 265:643–645

Goldman AS, Shapiro BH, Katsumata M (1978) Human fetal palatal corticoid receptors and teratogens for cleft palate. Nature 272:464–466

Goldstein JL, Wilson JD (1972) Studies on the pathogenesis of pseudohermaphroditism in the mouse with testicular feminization. J Clin Invest 51:1647–1658

Goldstein JL, Wilson JD (1975) Genetic and hormonal control of male sexual differentiation. J Cell Physiol 85:365–378
Goldstein JL, Brown MS, Stone NJ (1977) Genetics of the LDL receptor: evidence that the mutations affecting binding and internalization are allelic. Cell 12:629–643
Goldstein JL, Anderson RGW, Brown MJ (1979) Coatal pits, coated vessels and receptor-mediated endocytosis. Nature 279:679–685
Greene RM, Kochar DM (1975) Some aspects of corticosteroid-induced cleft palate: a review. Teratology 11:47–55
Greene RM, Salomon DS (1981) Glutamine synthetase activity in the developing rodent secondary palate and induction by dexamethasone. Differentiation 10:193–201
Grobstein C (1975) Developmental role of intercellular matrix: retrospective and prospective. In: Slavkin HC, Grenlich RC (eds) Ectracellular matrix influences gene expression. Academic Press, New York, p 9
Harris AW, Baxter JD (1979) Variations in cellular sensitivity to glucocorticoids: observations and mechanisms. In: Baxter JD, Rousseau GG (eds) Glucocorticoid hormone action. Monogr Endocrinol 12:423
Hendrickx AG, Sawyer RH, Terrell TG, Osburn BI, Hendrickson RV, Steffek AJ (1975) Teratogenic effects of triamcinolone on the skeletal and lymphoid systems in nonhuman primates. Fed Proc 34:1661–1665
Hirata F, Axelrod J (1980) Phospholipid methylation and biological signal transmission. Science 209:1082–1092
Insel PA, Bourne HR, Coffino P, Tomkins GM (1975) Cyclic AMP-dependent protein kinase: pivotal role in regulation of enzyme induction and growth. Science 190:896–898
Jost A (1972) A new look at the mechanism controlling sex differentiation in mammals. Johns Hopkins Med J 130:38–53
Jost A, Vigier B, Prepin J, Perchellet JP (1973) Studies on sex differentiation in mammals. Recent Prog Horm Res 29:1–38
Kahn RC (1976) Membrane receptors for hormones and neurotransmitters. J Cell Biol 70:261–286
Kalter H (1954) Inheritance of susceptibility to the teratogenic action of cortisone in mice. Genetics 39:185–196
Kaslow HR, Farfel Z, Johnson GL, Bourne HR (1979) Adenylate cyclase assembled in vitro: cholera toxin substrates determine different patterns of regulation by isoproterenol and guanosine 5′-triphosphate. Mol Pharmacol 15:472–483
Knazek RA, Liu SC, Gullino PM (1977) Induction of lactogenic binding sites in the liver of the Snell dwarf mouse. Endocrinology 101:50–58
Knazek RA, Liu SC, Graeter RL et al. (1978) Growth hormone causes rapid induction of lactogenic receptor activity in the Snell dwarf mouse liver. Endocrinology 103:1590–1596
Kratochwil K (1972) Tissue interaction during embryonic development: general properties. In: Tarin G (ed) Tissue interactions in carcinogenesis. Academic Press, New York, p 1
Le Douarin N (1970) Induction of determination and induction of differentiation during development of the liver and certain organs of endomesodermal origin. In: Wolf E (ed) Tissue interactions during organogenesis. Gordon and Breach, New York, p 37
Levine MA, Downs RW, Singer M, Marx SJ, Aurbach GD, Spiegel AM (1980) Deficient activity of guanine nucleotide regulatory protein in erythrocytes from patients with pseudohypoparathyroidism. Biochem Biophys Res Commun 94:1319–1324
Lippman M (1976) Steroid hormone receptors in human malignancy. Life Sci 18:143–152
Lyon MF, Hawkes SG (1970) X-linked gene for testicular feminization in the mouse. Nature 227:1217–1219
Meyer WJ, Migeon BR, Migeon CJ (1975) Locus on human X chromosome for diyhdrotestosterone receptor and androgen insensitivity. Proc Natl Acad Sci USA 72:1469–1472
Munck A, Leung K (1977) Glucocorticoid receptors and mechanisms of action. In: Pasqualini JR (ed) Receptors and mechanisms of action of steroid hormones, vol 8, Modern pharmacology-toxicology. M Dekker, New York Basel, p 311
Ohno S (1976) Major regulatory genes for mammalian sexual development. Cell 7:15–21
O'Malley BW, Schrader WT (1976) The receptors of steroid hormones. Sci Am Feb:32–44

O'Malley BW, Schwartz RJ, Schrader WT (1976) A review of regulation of gene expression by steroid hormone receptors. J Steroid Biochem 7:1151–1159
Oppenheimer JH, Koerner D, Schwartz HL, Surks HI (1972) Specific nuclear triiodothyronine binding sites in rat liver and kidney. J Clin Endocrinol Metab 35:330–333
Pollet RJ, Levey GS (1980) Principles of membrane receptor physiology and their application to clinical medicine. Ann Int Med 92:663–680
Pratt RM, Salomon DS (1980) Glucocorticoid receptors and cleft palate in mice and man. In: Melnick M, Bixlee D, Shields ED (eds) Progress in clinical and biological research. Etiology of cleft lip and palate. Alan R Liss, New York. 46:149–169
Pratt RM, Salomon DS, Diewert VM, Erickson RP, Burns R, Brown KS (1980) Cortisone-induced cleft palate in the brachmorphic mouse. Teratogenesis, Carcinogenesis and Mutagenesis 1:15–23
Pratt WB (1978) The mechanism of glucocorticoid effects in fibroblasts. J Invest Dermatol 71:24–35
Refetoff S, Degroot LJ, Bernard B, DeWind LT (1972) Studies of a sibship with apparent hereditary resistance to the intracellular action of thyroid hormone. Metabolism 21:723–756
Reinisch JM, Simon NG, Karow WG, Gandelman R (1978) Prenatal exposure to prednisone in humans and animals retards intrauterine growth. Science 202:436–438
Roth JB, Lesniak MA, Bar RJ et al. (1979) An introduction to receptors and receptor disorders. Proc Soc Exp Biol Med 162:3–12
Rutter WJ, Pictet RN, Morris RW (1973) Toward molecular mechanisms of developmental processes. Annu Rev Biochem 42:601–646
Salomon DS, Pratt RM (1976) Glucocorticoid receptors in murine embryonic facial mesenchyme cells. Nature 264:174–177
Salomon DS, Pratt RM (1978) Inhibition of growth in vitro by glucocorticoids in mouse embryonic facial mesenchyme cell. J Cell Physiol 97:315–328
Salomon DS, Pratt RM (1979) Involvement of glucocorticoids in the development of the secondary palate. Differentiation 13:141–154
Salomon DS, Zubairi Y, Thompson EB (1978) Ontogeny and biochemical properties of glucocorticoid receptors in mid-gestation mouse embryos. J Steroid Biochem 9:95–107
Salomon DS, Gift VD, Pratt RM (1979) Corticosterone levels during midgestation in the maternal plasma and fetus of cleft-palate-sensitive and -resistant mice. Endocrinology 103:154–156
Salomon DS, Liotta LA, Kidwell WR (1981) Differential growth factor responsiveness of rat mammary epithelium plated on different collagen substrata in serum-free medium. Proc Natl Acad Sci USA 78:382–386
Samuels HH, Tsai JS (1973) Thyroid hormone action in cell culture: demonstration of nuclear receptors in intact cells and isolated nuclei. Proc Natl Acad Sci USA 70:3488–3492
Sani BP, Titus BC, Banerjee CK (1978) Determination of binding affinities of retinoids to retinoic acid-binding protein and serum albumin. Biochem J 171:711–717
Sato B, Keizo N, Nishizawa Y, Nakao K, Matsumoto K, Yamamura Y (1980) Mechanism of activation of steroid receptors: involvement of low molecular weight inhibitor in activation of androgen, glucocorticoid and estrogen receptor systems. Endocrinology 106:1142–1148
Saxén L (1972) Interactive mechanisms in morphogenesis. In: Tarin D (ed) Tissue interactions in carcinogenesis. Academic Press, New York, p 49
Schleifer LS, Garrison JC, Sternweis PC, Northup JK, Gilman AG (1980) The regulatory component of adenylate cyclase from uncoupled S49 lymphoma cells differs in charge from the wild type protein. J Biol Chem 255:2641–2644
Shah RM, Kilistoff A (1976) Cleft palate induction in hamster fetuses by glucocorticoid hormones and their synthetic analogues. J Embryol Exp Morphol 36:101–108
Sibley CH, Yamamoto KR (1979) Mouse lymphoma cells: mechanism of resistance to glucocorticoids. In: Baxter JD, Rousseau GG (eds) Glucocorticoid hormone action. Monogr Endocrinol 12:357
Sporn MB, Todaro GJ (1980) Autocrine secretion and malignant transformation of cells. N Engl J Med 303:878–881

Tettenborn U, Dofuku R, Ohno S (1974) Noninducible phenotype exhibited by a proportion of female mice heterozygous for the X-linked testicular feminization mutation. Nature New Biol 234:37–40
Tyan ML, Miller KK (1978) Genetic and environmental factors in cortisone induced cleft palate. Proc Soc Exp Biol Med 158:618–621
Van Wyk JJ, Underwood LE (1975) Relation between growth hormone and somatomedin. Annu Rev Med 26:427–441
Van Wyk JJ, Furlanetto RW, Plet AS, D'Ercole J, Underwood LE (1978) The somatomedin group of peptide growth factors. In: Sanford KK (ed) Third decennial review conference: cell, tissue and organ culture-gene expression and regulation in cultured cells. Natl Cancer Inst Monogr 48:141
Verhoeven GF, Wilson JD (1979) The syndromes of primary hormone resistance. Metabolism 28:253–289
Walker BE (1967) Induction of cleft palate in rabbits by several glucocorticoids. Proc Soc Exp Med 125:1281–1284
White BJ, Marx SJ (1978) Dermatoglyphic and radiographic findings in a mother and daughter with pseudohypoparathyroidism. Clin Genet 13:359–368
Wieland SJ, Fox TO (1979) Putative androgen receptors distinguished in wild-type and testicular feminized (Tfm) mice. Cell 17:781–787
Wilson JD (1978) Sexual differentiation. Annu Rev Physiol 40:279–306
Wilson JD, Siiteri PK (1973) Developmental pattern of testosterone synthesis in the fetal gonad of the rabbit. Endocrinology 92:1182–1191
Yoneda T, Goldman AS, Van Dyke DC, Wilson LS, Pratt RM (1981) Decreased number of glucocorticoid receptors in dermal fibroblasts from individuals with facial clefting: a preliminary report. J Craniofacial Gen and Develop Biol 1:229–234
York DA, Bray GY, Yukimura Y (1978) An enzymatic defect in the obese (ob/ob) mouse: loss of thyroid-induced sodium- and potassium-dependent adenosine triphosphatase. Proc Natl Acad Sci USA 75:477–481
Zarrow MX, Philpott JE, Denenberg VH (1970) Passage of $^{14}$C-4-corticosterone from the rat mother to the fetus and neonate. Nature 226:1058–1059
Zimmerman EF, Bowen D (1972a) Distribution and metabolism of triamcinolone acetonide in mice sensitive to its teratogenic effects. Teratology 5:57–70
Zimmerman EF, Bowen D (1972b) Distribution and metabolism of triamcinolone acetonide in inbred mice with different cleft palate sensitivities. Teratology 5:335–344
Zimmerman EF, Andrew F, Kalter H (1970) Glucocorticoid inhibition of RNA synthesis responsible for cleft palate in mice: a model. Proc Natl Acad Sci USA 67:779–785

CHAPTER 9

# Mutagens as Teratogens: A Correlative Approach

C. A. SCHREINER and H. E. HOLDEN, JR.

## A. Introduction

The recent development and application of short-term tests for the detection of mutagenic activity has generated several efforts to determine th extent of the interrelationship of genotoxicity with other pathologic end points. The most enthusiastic of these efforts has been directed toward the correlation of mutagenic and carcinogenic activities (MCCANN et al. 1975). Several major studies have shown that this correlation is in the range of about 67% (KAWACHI et al. 1980) to about 90% (MCCANN et al. 1975). This correlation has permitted the use of short-term assay results to predict the probability of carcinogenic hazard or safety of a variety of test substances. Other pathologic end points, such as teratology, have not given such clear-cut correlation with genetic toxicity (KALTER 1971). The most significant correlation should include a representative sampling from most classes of existing compounds, weighted according to the importance of that class in exposure to the population. However, the scientific impetus to evaluate all aspects of toxicity for chemicals with known biologic activity has resulted in a disproportionate number of cancer chemotherapeutic agents and alkylating agents among those compounds tested to date for teratology and genetic toxicology. Although this condition may have a marked influence on the degree of correlation, the comparative process must begin.

Attempts to explore the correlation between mutagenic and teratogenic activity have been generally frustrated and diffused by such factors as inadequately standardized protocols and test models and ambiguous criteria for positive results. Furthermore, such physiologic factors as the placental barrier, the transport of active metabolites produced in the maternal liver to the fetus, and development stage at time of exposure are expected to diminish the concurrence of mutagenicity and teratogenicity data. Also adding to the complexity of this correlation is the diversity of genetic end points which are measured in the broad scope of genetic toxicology. These span the range from alteration of a single base-pair to gross disruption of chromosome structure and number.

In general, point mutations tend to be somewhat insidious, with phenotypic expression only after a considerable latent period. In a fetus, the presence of such a mutation would not be expected to result in a frank teratogenic event. However, the correlation of point mutation induction with reproductive problems induced by carcinogens that cross the placenta should be recognized. The use of in vitro microbial point mutation assays as predictors of potential carcinogenic activity has been widely explored in recent years. DIPAOLO and KOTIN (1966) showed that the

**Table 1.** Literature survey of compounds studied for both teratology and in vivo cytogenetic effects

| Compound | Teratology | | | | | | In vivo cytogenetics | | | |
|---|---|---|---|---|---|---|---|---|---|---|
| | Mouse | Rat | Hamster | Rabbit | Primate | Human | Teratogenic? | Somatic | Germ cell | Mutagenic? |
| Acetylsalicylic acid | + [1] | + [2] | | | | − [3] | Yes | − [4] | | No |
| Actinomycin D | | + [5] | | + [6] | | | Yes | + [7] | + [8] | Yes |
| Adriamycin | − [9] | + [10] | | − [10] | | | Yes | + [11] | | Yes |
| Aldrin | + [12] | | + [12] | | | | Yes | + [13] | − [8] | Yes |
| Aminopterin | | + [14] | | | | Inc. [15] | Yes | | − [8] | No |
| 1-β-Arabinofuranosylcytosine | | + [16] | | + [17] | | | Yes | + [11] | | Yes |
| Azacytidine | + [18] | + [19] | | | | | Yes | | − [8] | No |
| Azathioprine | − [20] | − [20] | | + [20] | | | Yes | + [21] | | Yes |
| Benomyl | | − [22] | | | | | No | + [23] | | Yes |
| Benzene | + [24] | − [25] | | | | | Yes | + [26] | − [27] | Yes |
| Benzo[a]pyrene | − [28] | − [29] | | | | | No | + [30] | + [30] | Yes |
| 5-Bromodeoxyuridine | + [31] | + [32] | + [33] | − [34] | | | Yes | | − [8] | No |
| Busulfan | | + [35] | | | | | Yes | + [36] | + [8] | Yes |
| Butylated hydroxytoluene | − [37] | − [37] | | | | | No | | − [8] | No |
| Cadmium | | + [38] | + [39] | | | − [40] | Yes | | + [41] | Yes |
| Caffeine | +/− [42] | +/− [42] | | +/− [42] | | +/− [42] | Inc. | − [21] | − [43] | No |
| Captan | | − [44] | − [44] | − [45] | − [46] | | No | − [47] | − [47] | No |
| Carbaryl | | − [48] | − [49] | − [49] | | | No | − [50] | − [8] | No |
| Carbofuran | | − [51] | | − [51] | | | No | − [50] | | No |
| Chlorambucil | | + [32] | | | | | Yes | + [52] | | Yes |
| Chloramphenicol | − [53] | − [53] | | − [53] | − [54] | | No | − [55] | − [8] | No |
| Chlorpromazine | | − [56] | | | | − [56] | No | | − [8] | No |
| Cyclamate | − [57] | − [58] | | − [58] | | | No | Inc. [59] | Inc. [59] | Inc. |
| Cyclohexylamine | − [60] | | | | | | No | + [61] | − [59] | Yes |
| Cyclophosphamide | + [62] | + [63] | | + [64] | + [65] | | Yes | + [66] | + [8] | Yes |
| Daunomycin | | + [10] | | | | | Yes | + [67] | | Yes |
| DDT | − [68] | − [69] | | − [70] | | | No | | − [8] | No |
| 2,4-Dichlorophenoxyacetic acid | | + [71] | | | | | Yes | + [22] | − [8] | Yes |
| Dichlorvos | | − [73] | | − [73] | | | No | − [74] | − [74] | No |
| Dieldrin | − [75] | | | | | | No | | − [8] | No |

| | | | | | | | | | | |
|---|---|---|---|---|---|---|---|---|---|---|
| Diethylnitrosamine | | –[76] | | | | | No | –[77] | | No |
| Diethylstilbesterol | | | | | | ±[78] | Yes | –[79] | | No |
| Dimethoate | –[86] | | | | | | No | –[50] | | No |
| Dimethylbenzanthracene | +[80] | +[81] | | | | | Yes | +[82] | | Yes |
| Dimethylsulfoxide | –[83] | –[84] | +[85] | | | | Yes | | –[8] | No |
| 2,4-Dinitrophenol | –[87] | –[88] | | | | | No | +[89] | | Yes |
| Diphenylhydantoin | +[90] | | | | | +[91] | Yes | –[92] | –[8] | No |
| Diquat | | +[93] | | | | | Yes | | –[94] | No |
| Ergotamine | –[95] | –[95] | | –[95] | | | No | –[96] | | No |
| Ethanol | +[97] | –[98] | | | | Inc.[42] | Inc. | –[99] | | No |
| *N*,*N*-Ethylene thiourea | | +[100] | | +[100] | | | Yes | +[50] | –[101] | Inc. |
| Ethylnitrosourea | | +[102] | | | | | Yes | +[103] | | Yes |
| 5-Fluorouracil | +[104] | +[32] | | | | | Yes | +[11] | | Yes |
| Formaldehyde | | –[105] | | | | | No | | –[8] | No |
| Griseofulvin | | +[106] | | | | | Yes | | –[8] | No |
| Hycanthone | +[107] | | | | | | Yes | +[108] | –[109] | Yes |
| Hydroxyurea | | +[110] | | | | | Yes | | –[8] | No |
| *N*-Hydroxyurethane | | +[110] | | | | | Yes | +[77] | | Yes |
| Ifosfamide | +[111] | | | | | | Yes | +[77] | | Yes |
| Imipramine | –[112] | –[112] | | –[112] | –[113] | –[114] | No | –[115] | | No |
| 5-Iododeoxyuridine | +[116] | +[116] | | +[117] | | | Yes | | –[8] | No |
| Lead | +[118] | +[118] | +[118] | | | | Yes | –[119] | | No |
| Meprobamate | | –[120] | | | Inc.[121,122] | | Inc. | Inc. | –[8] | No |
| 6-Mercaptopurine | +[16] | +[16] | | +[16] | | | Yes | +[123] | +[124] | Yes |
| Metepa | | +[125] | | | | | Yes | +[126] | +[127] | Yes |
| Methotrexate | +[128] | | | –[129] | | | Yes | +[130] | –[130] | Yes |
| Methyl carbamate | | –[131] | | | | | No | | –[8] | No |
| Methylcholanthrene | Inc.[42] | | | | | | Inc. | +[132] | –[133] | Yes |
| Methylmethanesulfonate | +[134] | | | | | | Yes | +[135] | +[136] | Yes |
| *N*-Methyl-*N*-nitro-*N*-nitrosoguanidine | +[137] | | | | | | Yes | –[138] | +[139] | Yes |
| *N*-Methyl-*N*-nitrosourea | | +[140] | | | | | Yes | | +[139] | Yes |
| Mitomycin C | +[141] | –[16] | | | | | Yes | +[142] | +[8] | Yes |
| Nicotine | +[143] | | | | | | Yes | +[144] | | Yes |
| Nitrilotriacetic acid | –[145] | –[146] | | –[146] | | | No | | –[8] | No |
| Ozone | +[147] | –[148] | | | | | Yes | –[149] | | No |
| Paraquat | | +[150] | | | | | Yes | | –[94] | No |

**Table 1** (continued)

| Compound | Teratology | | | | | | In vivo cytogenetics | | | |
|---|---|---|---|---|---|---|---|---|---|---|
| | Mouse | Rat | Hamster | Rabbit | Primate | Human | Teratogenic? | Somatic | Germ cell | Mutagenic? |
| Patulin | −[151] | | | | | | No | | −[151] | No |
| Phenylbutazone | | −[152] | | −[152] | | | No | −[55] | | No |
| 1-Phenyl-3,3-dimethyltriazene | | +[76] | | | | | Yes | +[153] | | Yes |
| Procarbazine | | +[154] | | | | | Yes | +[77] | | Yes |
| Quinacrine | | −[155] | | | | | No | +/−[156] | | Inc. |
| Reserpine | | +[157] | | −[157] | | | Yes | | −[8] | No |
| Styrene | | −[158] | | −[158] | | | No | +[159] | | Yes |
| Thalidomide | −[42] | −[42] | | +[42] | +[42] | +[42] | Yes | | −[8] | No |
| Theophylline | | | | | | −[160] | No | | −[8] | Yes |
| Thio-TEPA | +[161] | +[162] | | | | | Yes | +[11] | +[8] | Yes |
| Tolbutamide | +[163] | +[164] | | −[165] | | −[165] | Yes | | −[8] | No |
| Toxaphene | | −[166] | | | | | No | | −[8] | No |
| Triacetyl-6-azauridine | | | | | Inc.[167] | | Inc. | | −[8] | No |
| 2,4,5-Trichlorophenoxyacetic acid | +[168] | −[169] | | −[169] | | −[170] | Yes | +[171] | | Yes |
| Triethylene melamine (TEM) | +[172] | +[16] | | | | | Yes | +[173] | +[174] | Yes |
| Triethylene phosphoramide (TEPA) | | +[175] | | | | | Yes | +[176] | +[177] | Yes |
| Uracil mustard | | +[16] | | | | | Yes | | −[8] | No |
| Urethane | +[178] | +[179] | | | | | Yes | +[17] | −[8] | Yes |
| Vinblastine sulfate | | +[42] | +[42] | +[42] | +[42] | | Yes | | −[8] | No |
| Vincristine | | +[42] | +[42] | +[42] | +[42] | | Yes | +[11] | | Yes |

Inc. = inconclusive

[1] LARSSON and ERIKKSON 1966; [2] WARKANY and TAKACS 1959; [3] TURNER and COLLINS 1975; [4] FRANK et al. 1978; [5] WILSON 1966; [6] TUCHMANN-DUPLESSIS and MERCIER-PAROT 1960; [7] ARRIGHI and HSU 1965; [8] EPSTEIN et al. 1972; [9] OHGURO et al. 1973; [10] THOMPSON et al. 1978; [11] MAIER and SCHMID 1976; [12] OTTOLENGHI et al. 1974; [13] GEORGIAN 1975; [14] BARANOV 1966; [15] THIERSCH 1952; [16] CHAUBE and MURPHY 1968; [17] OHKUMA et al. 1973; [18] SCHMAHL 1978; [19] TAKEUCHI and MURAKAMI 1978; [20] TUCHMANN-DUPLESSIS and MERCIER-PAROT 1968; [21] TSUCHIMOTO and MATTER 1977; [22] SHERMAN et al. 1975; [23] SEILER 1976; [24] WATANABE and YOSHIDA 1970; [25] GREEN et al. 1978; [26] PHILIP and JENSEN 1970; [27] LYON 1976; [28] MACKENZIE et al. 1979; [29] RIGDON and RENNELS 1964; [30] BASLER and ROHBORN 1976; [31] DIPAOLO 1964; [32] CHAUBE and MURPHY 1968; [33] RUFFOLO and FERM 1965; [34] ADAMS et al. 1961; [35] MURPHY et al. 1958; [36] LEONARD and LEONARD 1978; [37] CLEGG 1965; [38] BARR 1973; [39] FERM and CARPENTER 1967a; [40] THUERAUT et al. 1975; [41] SHIMADA et al. 1976; [42] SHEPARD 1980; [43] AESCHBACHER et al. 1978;

[44] Kennedy et al. 1968; [45] Fabro et al. 1966; [46] Vondruska et al. 1971; [47] Tezuka et al. 1978; [48] Weil et al. 1973; [49] Robens 1969; [50] Seiler 1977; [51] McCarthy et al. 1971; [52] Lawler and Lele 1972; [53] Fritz and Hess 1971a; [54] Courtney and Valerio 1968; [55] Jensen 1972; [56] Kalter 1968; [57] Kroes et al. 1977; [58] Vogin and Oser 1969; [59] Machemer and Lorke 1976; [60] Becker and Gibson 1970; [61] Legator et al. 1969; [62] Gibson and Becker 1968; [63] Chaube et al. 1967; [64] Fritz and Hess 1971b; [65] Wilk et al. 1978; [66] Goetz et al. 1975; [67] Jensen and Philip 1971; [68] Ware and Good 1967; [69] Ottoboni 1969; [70] Hart et al. 1971; [71] Schwetz et al. 1971; [72] Pilinskaya 1974; [73] Thorpe et al. 1972; [74] Dean and Thorpe 1972; [75] Dix et al. 1977; [76] Druckrey 1973a; [77] Wild 1978; [78] McLachlan and Dixon 1977; [79] Bishun et al. 1977; [80] Lambert and Nebert 1977; [81] Currie et al. 1970; [82] Rees et al. 1970; [83] Caujolie et al. 1967; [84] Thiersch 1971; [85] Ferm 1966; [86] Budreau and Singh 1973; [87] Gibson 1973; [88] Goldman and Yakova 1964; [89] Mitra and Manna 1971; [90] Harbinson and Becker 1969; [91] Monson et al. 1973; [92] Alving et al. 1976; [93] Khera et al. 1970; [94] Anderson et al. 1976; [95] Grauwiler and Schon 1973; [96] Matter 1976; [97] Chernoff 1977; [98] Sandor and Amels 1971; [99] Chaubey et al. 1977; [100] Ruddick and Khera 1975; [101] Schupback and Hummler 1977; [102] Druckrey et al. 1966; [103] Soukoup and Au 1975; [104] Dagg 1960; [105] Puskine et al. 1968; [106] Klein and Beall 1972; [107] Moore 1972; [108] Holden et al. 1975; [109] Green et al. 1973; [110] Chaube and Murphy 1966; [111] Bus and Gibson 1973; [112] Harper et al. 1965; [113] Hendrickx 1975; [114] Banister et al. 1972; [115] Bishun et al. 1974; [116] Percy 1975; [117] Itoi et al. 1975; [118] Ferm and Carpenter 1967b; [119] Schmid and Bauchinger 1973; [120] Brar 1969; [121] Hartz et al. 1975; [122] Milkovich and Vandenberg 1974; [123] Holden et al. 1973; [124] Generoso et al. 1975; [125] Gaines and Kimbrough 1966; [126] Richardson 1974; [127] Epstein 1969; [128] Skalko and Gold 1974; [129] Adams et al. 1961; [130] Melnyk et al. 1971; [131] Yashuda 1972; [132] Sugiyama 1973; [133] Muller et al. 1978; [134] Beliles et al. 1973; [135] Brewen et al. 1970; [136] Parlington and Bateman 1964; [137] Inouye and Murakami 1978; [138] Matter and Grauwiler 1974; [139] Parkin et al. 1973; [140] Napalko and Alexandrov 1968; [141] Tanimura 1968a; [142] Michelmann et al. 1977; [143] Nishimura and Nakai 1958; [144] Bishun et al. 1972; [145] Tjalve 1972; [146] Nolen et al. 1971; [147] Veninga 1967; [148] Kavlock et al. 1979; [149] McKenzie et al. 1977; [150] Khera et al. 1970; [151] Reddy et al. 1978; [152] Scharadien et al. 1969; [153] Newton et al. 1977; [154] Tuchmann-Duplessis and Mercier-Parot 1967; [155] Rothschild and Levy 1950; [156] Jenssen et al. 1974; [157] Kalter 1968; [158] Murray et al. 1978; [159] Meretoja et al. 1977; [160] Heinonen et al. 1977; [161] Tanimura 1968b; [162] Murphy et al. 1958; [163] Smithberg and Runner 1963; [164] Tuchmann-Duplessis and Mercier-Parot 1959; [165] Lazarus and Volk 1963; [166] Kennedy et al. 1973; [167] van Wagener et al. 1970; [168] Roll 1971; [169] Emmerson et al. 1971; [170] Nelson et al. 1979; [171] Majumdar and Hall 1973; [172] Kageyama and Nishimura 1961; [173] Schmid et al. 1971; [174] Hastings et al. 1976; [175] Thiersch 1957b; [176] Adler et al. 1971; [177] Epstein et al. 1971; [178] Sinclair 1950; [179] Takaori et al. 1966

majority of carcinogens exert teratogenic effects, although carcinogens make up only a small fraction of total teratogenic agents. Chromosomal mutations in a developing fetus would be expected to have a more severe and immediate effect because of the multiplicity of genetic systems involved. Clearly, the nature of an induced genetic lesion should be considered in determining the extent of correlation with teratogenic activity.

In this chapter, attention is directed first to those agents which have been studied for teratogenic effects and genetic activity at the chromosomal level and second, to those for which carcinogenic, teratogenic, and point mutational data are available. An empirical approach to study the mutagenic and teratogenic activities of a large number to chemicals would undoubtedly be most satisfactory. This would permit standardization of protocols, test models, and judgment of results. However, the nature of both teratogenic and mutagenic studies precludes the development of an adequate data base with sufficient numbers of chemicals in diverse chemical classes. An alternative approach, and the one taken here, is to examine the available literature in both areas and determine, retrospectively, the extent of correlation. In the first compilation, the mutagenicity is limited to in vivo cytogenetic effects. In the second, only in vitro cytogenic results are considered. Third, the correlation between teratology and spindle disruption is examined. And finally, the relationship of point mutations, carcinogenesis, and teratogenesis is addressed.

Teratology data is limited to structural malformations induced in five commonly used mammalian models or in humans. The principle sources of this information are SHEPARD (1980) and WEINSTEIN (1976). The decision whether a compound is positive or negative in a particular animal model is, where possible, the decision of the originating authors. In those cases where diverse opinions were expressed in more than one paper, using the same species, the results are identified as "+/−". The ultimate label of "teratogen" is based on the spectrum of results in the individual models. A compound positive in any species is judged "teratogenic", even though it is recognized that results from some models may be more significant than others in terms of predicting human health hazard.

## B. In Vivo Cytogenetics Versus Teratology

Because teratogenicity is, by nature, an in vivo process, it might be expected that results of in vivo cytogenetic studies would be most pertinent in developing a correlation. Ideally, this survey should be limited to studies of the effects of substances on the chromosomes of the developing fetus in utero. Clearly, such studies are extremely rare. Much more common are studies measuring the cytogenetic effects of substances on mammalian somatic or germ cells in vivo or somatic cells in vitro. These models have the capability of detecting induced changes in chromosome structure (i.e., clastogenicity) or chromosome number (i.e., disruption of normal anaphase disjunction).

Table 1 is a compilation of compounds for which in vivo cytogenetic results and teratology data are available. Cytogenetic results are listed as: (1) somatic effects in metaphase analyses or micronucleus tests; or (2) germ cell results from cytologic studies on gonadal tissue, dominant lethal assays, or heritable translocation tests.

**Table 2.** Teratology versus in vivo cytogenetics

| | |
|---|---|
| A. Positive teratology, positive cytogenetics | 34 |
| B. Negative teratology, negative cytogenetics | 19 |
| C. Positive teratology, negative cytogenetics | 19 |
| D. Negative teratology, positive cytogenetics | 6 |
| E. Inconclusive teratology or cytogenetics | 8 |
| F. Total compounds surveyed | 86 |
| Total correlation $[(A+B)/F \times 100]$ | 62% |

The methods employed in these assays are described in BRUSICK (1980). Mutagenic activity in either somatic or germ cells is sufficient to label the compound "mutagenic". As shown in Table 1, a total of 86 compounds were found to have both teratology data and results of in vivo cytogenetic assays. A summary of this information is presented in Table 2. The combined positive and negative correlation (62%) is only slightly greater than by chance alone. From this, it is clear that the general predictive value of in vivo cytogenetic tests for teratogenic activity is not very high. However, the data in Table 2 suggest that compounds which have cytogenetic activity are highly likely to be teratogenic also. From Table 2, 34 of 40 compounds (85%) with positive cytogenetic activity also possessed teratogenic activity. The conclusion reached is that positive activity in in vivo cytogenetics is highly predictive of teratogenicity.

## C. In Vitro Cytogenetics Versus Teratology

The sensitivity of in vivo cytogenetic models for monitoring induced gross chromosomal damage may be diminished by such physiologic factors as absorption, distribution, and excretion of the test substance. Cytogenetically active substances negative in in vivo assessment because they never reach the cytogenetic target cell may nonetheless have access to the fetus where chromosome damage and terata may result. This probable insensitivity of in vivo cytogenetic models has been partially overcome with the development of in vitro procedures where mammalian cells are exposed directly to the test substances without complicating physiologic or pharmacologic factors. Although the extrapolation of data from these tests to issues of human genetic health is not clear-cut, these tests do provide the opportunity to test, under the most rigorous possible conditions, the intrinsic ability of the substance to induce chromosome damage. Additional sensitivity can be achieved by the incorporation of metabolic capabilities in the form of microsomal enzymes (NATARAJAN et al. 1976) or cocultivated metabolically competent cells (HOLDEN et al. 1980a). These modifications permit detection of agents which require activation.

For this survey, the literature was examined for substances which have been tested for both teratogenic activity and cytogenetic activity, as defined by in vitro models. Table 3 is the listing of compounds which have been evaluated for both end points. The in vitro cytogenetic data is limited to studies on the effect of the compound on chromosome structure in cultured mammalian cells. Established cell

**Table 3.** Literature survey of compounds studied for both teratology and in vitro cytogenetic effects

| Compound | Teratology | | | | | | In vivo cytogenetics | |
|---|---|---|---|---|---|---|---|---|
| | Mouse | Rat | Hamster | Rabbit | Primate | Human | Teratogenic? | Mutagenic? |
| Actinomycin D | | +[1] | | +[2] | | | Yes | Yes[3] |
| Adriamycin | –[4] | +[5] | | –[5] | | | Yes | Yes[6] |
| Aflatoxin | | | +[7] | | | | Yes | Yes[8] |
| Aldrin | +[9] | | +[9] | | | | Yes | Yes[10] |
| Aminopyrene | +[11] | –[12] | | | | | Yes | No[13] |
| 1-β-D-Arabinofuranosylcytosine | | +[14] | | +[15] | | | Yes | Yes[16] |
| Arsenic | +[17] | +[18] | +[19] | | | | Yes | Yes[20] |
| Asbestos | –[21] | | | | | | No | Yes[22] |
| Azathioprine | –[23] | –[23] | | +[23] | | | Yes | Yes[24] |
| Barbitol | +[25] | +[26] | | +[27] | | –[28] | Yes | Yes[13] |
| Benzene | +[29] | –[30] | | | | | Yes | Yes[31] |
| Benzo[a]pyrene | –[32] | –[33] | | | | | No | No[34] |
| 5-Bromo-2′-deoxyuridine (BRdU) | +[35] | +[36] | +[37] | –[38] | | | Yes | Yes[39] |
| Butylhydroxyanisole | –[40] | –[40] | | | | | No | No[13] |
| Cadmium | | +[41] | +[42] | | | | Yes | Yes[43] |
| Caffeine | +/–[44] | +/–[44] | | +/–[44] | | +/–[44] | Inc. | Yes[45] |
| Captan | | –[46] | –[46] | –[47] | –[48] | | No | No[49] |
| Carbaryl | | –[50] | –[51] | –[51] | | | No | Yes[13] |
| Chlorambucil | | +[14] | | | | | Yes | Yes[52] |
| Chloramphenicol | –[53] | –[53] | | –[53] | –[54] | | No | No[55] |
| Chlordiazepoxide | | | | | | –[56] | No | No[57] |
| Chlorpromazine | | –[58] | | | | –[58] | No | No[59] |
| Cyclohexylamine | –[60] | | | | | | No | No[61] |
| Cyclophosphamide | +[62] | +[63] | | +[64] | +[65] | | Yes | Yes[66] |
| Danomycin | | +[5] | | | | | Yes | Yes[67] |
| DDT | –[72] | –[73] | | –[74] | | | No | Yes[75] |
| Diazepam | +[68] | –[69] | | | | +[70] | Yes | No[71] |
| Diethylnitrosamine | | –[76] | | | | | No | Yes[77] |
| Diethylstibesterol | | | | | | +[78] | Yes | Yes[13] |
| Dimethylbenzanthracene | +[79] | +[80] | | | | | Yes | Yes[81] |

| | | | | | | | | |
|---|---|---|---|---|---|---|---|---|
| Diphenylhydantoin | +[82] | | | | | +[83] | Yes | No[84] |
| Ergotamine | –[85] | –[85] | | –[85] | | | No | Yes[86] |
| Ethanol | +[87] | –[88] | | | | Inc.[44] | Inc. | No[34] |
| *N*,*N*-Ethylenethiourea | | +[89] | | +[89] | | | Yes | Yes[90] |
| *N*-Ethyl-*N*-nitrosourea | | +[91] | | | | | Yes | Yes[13] |
| 5-Fluorouracil | +[92] | +[14] | | | | | Yes | Yes[93] |
| Hycanthone | +[94] | | | | | | Yes | Yes[95] |
| Hydroxyurea | | +[96] | | | | | Yes | Yes[97] |
| Imipramine | –[98] | –[98] | | –[98] | –[99] | –[100] | No | No[101] |
| Lead | +[102] | +[102] | +[102] | | | | Yes | No[103] |
| Methotrexate | +[104] | | | –[105] | | | Yes | Yes[106] |
| *N*-Methyl-*N*-nitro-*N*-nitrosoguanidine | +[107] | | | | | | Yes | Yes[13] |
| *N*-Methyl-*N*-nitrosourea | | +[108] | | | | | Yes | Yes[13] |
| Methylurea | +[109] | +[110] | | | | | Yes | No[13] |
| Mitomycin C | +[111] | –[14] | | | | | Yes | Yes[112] |
| Naphthy-*N*-Methyl carbamate | | –[113] | –[113] | –[113] | | | No | Yes[13] |
| Nicotine | +[114] | –[115] | | | | | Yes | No[116] |
| Nitrogen mustard | +[14] | +[14] | | | | | Yes | Yes[117] |
| Patulin | –[118] | | | | | | No | Yes[119] |
| Phenylbutazone | | –[120] | | –[120] | | | No | No[121] |
| Procarbazine | | +[122] | | | | | Yes | Yes[123] |
| Progesterone | –[124] | –[125] | | | | | No | No[126] |
| Rifampicine | +[127] | +[127] | | –[127] | | | Yes | Yes[128] |
| Saccharin | –[129] | –[130] | | | | | No | Yes[131] |
| Sodium nitrate | –[132] | –[132] | –[132] | –[132] | | | No | Yes[13] |
| Tetracycline | | +/–[44] | | | | | Yes | Yes[133] |
| Thioguanine | | +[134] | | | | | Yes | Yes[135] |
| Thiotriethylenephosphoramide (thio-TEPA) | +[136] | +[137] | | | | | Yes | Yes[138] |
| Triethylene phosphoramide (TEPA) | | +[139] | | | | | Yes | Yes[140] |
| Urethane | +[141] | +[142] | | | | | Yes | Yes[13] |

Inc. = inconclusive

[1] Wilson 1966; [2] Tuchmann-Duplessis and Mercier-Parot 1960; [3] Ostertag and Kersten 1965; [4] Ohgurs et al. 1973; [5] Thompson et al. 1978; [6] Vig 1971; [7] Elias and DiPaolo 1967; [8] Dolimpo et al. 1968; [9] Ottolenghi et al. 1974; [10] Georgian 1975; [11] Nomura et al. 1977; [12] Loosli et al. 1964; [13] Ishidate and Odashima 1977; [14] Chaube and Murphy 1968; [15] Ohkuma et al. 1973; [16] Wobus 1976; [17] Hood and Bishop 1972; [18] Beaudoin 1974; [19] Ferm et al. 1971; [20] Patton and Allison 1972; [21] Schneider and Maurer 1977; [22] Huang et al. 1978;

**Table 3** (continued)

[23] TUCHMANN-DUPLESSIS and MERCIER-PAROT 1968; [24] HAMPEL et al. 1971; [25] SETALA and NYYSSONEN 1964; [26] PERSAUD 1965; [27] MCCOLL et al. 1967; [28] SHAPIRO et al. 1976; [29] WATANABE and YOSHIDA 1970; [30] GREEN et al. 1978; [31] KOIZUMA et al. 1974; [32] MACKENZIE et al. 1979; [33] RIGDON and RENNELS 1964; [34] ABE and SASAKI 1977; [35] DIPAOLO 1964; [36] CHAUBE and MURPHY 1968; [37] RUFFOLO and FERM 1965; [38] ADAMS et al. 1961; [39] LAMBERT et al. 1976; [40] CLEGG 1965; [41] BARR 1973; [42] FERM and CARPENTER 1967a; [43] ROHR and BAUCHINGER 1976; [44] SHEPARD 1980; [45] WEINSTEIN et al. 1973; [46] KENNEDY et al. 1968; [47] FABRO et al. 1966; [48] VONDRUSKA et al. 1971; [49] RAPOSA 1978; [50] WEIL et al. 1973; [51] ROBENS 1969; [52] LAWLER and LELE 1972; [53] FRITZ and HESS 1971a; [54] COURTNEY and VALERIO 1968; [55] JENSEN 1972; [56] HARTZ et al. 1975; [57] STAIGER 1969; [58] KALTER 1968; [59] KAMADA et al. 1971; [60] BECKER and GIBSON 1970; [61] GREEN et al. 1970; [62] GIBSON and BECKER 1968; [63] CHAUBE et al. 1967; [64] FRITZ and HESS 1971b; [65] WILK et al. 1978; [66] BISHUN 1971; [67] VIG et al. 1969; [68] Miller and BECKER 1975; [69] BEALL 1972; [70] SAXEN 1975; [71] STAIGER 1970; [72] WARE and GOOD 1967; [73] OTTOBONI 1969; [74] HART et al. 1971; [75] MAHR and MUTENBERGER 1976; [76] DRUCKREY 1973a; [77] NATARAJAN et al. 1976; [78] MCLACHLAN and DIXON 1977; [79] LAMBERT and NEBERT 1977; [80] CURRIE et al. 1970; [81] O'BRIEN et al. 1971; [82] HARBINSON and BECKER 1969; [83] MONSON et al. 1973; [84] ALVING et al. 1976; [85] GRAUWILER and SCHON 1973; [86] ROBERTS and RAND 1977; [87] CHERNOFF 1977; [88] SANDOR and AMELS 1971; [89] RUDDICK and KHERA 1975; [90] SEILER 1977; [91] DRUCKREY et al. 1966; [92] DAGG 1960; [93] HAMPEL and GEBHARTZ 1965; [94] MOORE 1972; [95] RAY et al. 1975; [96] CHAUBE and MURPHY 1966; [97] OPPENHEIM and FISHBEIN 1965; [98] HARPER et al. 1965; [99] HENDRICKX 1975; [100] BANISTER et al. 1972; [101] FU and JARVIK 1977; [102] FERM and CARPENTER 1967b; [103] SCHMID 1973; [104] SKALKO and GOLD 1974; [105] ADAMS et al. 1961; [106] MURCIA and NOMBELA 1972; [107] INOUYE and MURAKAMI 1978; [108] NAPALKOV and ALEXANDER 1968; [109] CROS et al. 1972; [110] VON KREYBIG et al. 1969; [111] TANIMURA 1968a; [112] NOWELL 1964; [113] ROBENS 1969; [114] NISHIMURA and NAKAI 1958; [115] ESSENBERG et al. 1940; [116] BISHUN et al. 1972; [117] NASJLETI and SPENCER 1966; [118] REDDY et al. 1978; [119] UMEDA et al. 1977; [120] SCHARDEIN et al. 1969; [121] GEBHART and WISSMUELLER 1973; [122] TUCHMANN-DUPLESSIS and MERCIER-PAROT 1967; [123] RUTISHAUSER and BOLLAG 1963; [124] JOHNSTONE and FRANKLIN 1964; [125] REVERZ et al. 1960; [126] NAKANISHI and MAKINO 1964; [127] TUCHMANN-DUPLESSIS and MERCIER-PAROT 1969; [128] ROMAN and GEORGIAN 1977; [129] LORKE 1969; [130] FRITZ and HESS 1968; [131] KRISTOFFERSSON 1972; [132] FOOD and Drug Research Laboratories 1972; [133] TSUTSUI et al. 1976; [134] THIERSCH 1957a; [135] ENGEL et al. 1967; [136] TANIMURA 1968b; [137] MURPHY et al. 1958; [138] BENEDICT et al. 1977; [139] THIERSCH 1957b; [140] STURELID 1971; [141] SINCLAIR 1950; [142] TAKAORI et al. 1966

**Table 4.** Teratology versus in vitro cytogenetics

| | |
|---|---|
| A. Positive teratology, positive cytogenetics | 33 |
| B. Negative teratology, negative cytogenetics | 10 |
| C. Positive teratology, negative cytogenetics | 6 |
| D. Negative teratology, positive cytogenetics | 9 |
| E. Inconclusive teratology or cytogenetics | 2 |
| F. Total compounds surveyed | 60 |
| Total correlation [(A+B)/F × 100)] | 72% |

lines such as the CHO or DON-C lines derived from Chinese hamsters have been most frequently used for this purpose. These lines have a high mitotic index and a low number of large chromosomes. However, significant work has also been done on other established lines, e.g., human fibroblasts or lymphoblasts, and on primary cultures of human lymphocytes. The latter provide a convenient means to examine a relatively synchronous population of genetically normal cells of human origin. A total of 60 compounds has been examined in both teratology and in vitro cytogenetics. A summary profile of these data is presented in Table 4. The general correlation derived from this survey is 72%; a slight increase over the in vivo cytogenetics general correlation. However, as with the in vivo data, there is a higher correlation of positive cytogenetic activity with teratogenicity. In this case, 33 of 42 compounds (80%) with positive activity in in vitro cytogenetics were also positive in teratology.

## D. Teratogenicity and Microtubule Disruption

Chromosomal mutations may be classified as either structural or numerical. Whereas the previous sections have dealt primarily with gross changes in chromosome structure, the importance of numerical aberrations as they relate to teratology should be recognized. The impact of such changes on the human genetic disease burden in general and on reproductive problems in particular has been well documented (JACOBS 1972). The etiology of numerical changes has, however, not been well defined. Most are believed to arise by disturbance of the normal disjunctive process which occurs at anaphase of mitosis or meiosis. Because of the mechanistic role of spindle fibers in the disjunction of chromosomes, it is reasonable to assume that agents which induce changes in microtubules may have severe genetic consequences by inhibiting the equal distribution of chromosomes to the daughter cells. If such numerical aberrations occur in the germ cells prior to fertilization, or in the early stages of embryonic cell proliferation, malformations may result.

Models for the detection of spindle disruptive properties of chemicals have, for various reasons, not been widely used, especially in the area of safety assessment. Nonetheless, a considerable data base is available concerning the discovery, serendipitous in many cases, of spindle disruptive properties of many compounds. This data base originates from three lines of research. First, cytologic observations of metaphase arrest in dividing mammalian cells. This phenomenon, called "C-metaphase" because of its original association with colchicine, is characterized by

**Table 5.** Teratogenicity of compounds with microtubule disruptive properties

| Compound | Teratogenic? | Evidence for microtubule disruption |
|---|---|---|
| Arsenic | Yes [1,2,3] | 4 |
| Benzimidazoles | | |
| Isopropyl 2-(4-thiazalyl)-5-benzimidazole-carbamate (cambendazole) | Yes [5] | 5 |
| Methylbenzimidazole carbamate | Yes [6] | 7 |
| Methyl-5-benzoyl-2-benzimidazole carbamate (mebendazole) | Yes [5] | 8 |
| Methyl-1-(butylcarbomyl)-2-benzimidazole carbamate (benomyl) | No [6] | 9 |
| Methyl-5-butyl-2-benzimidazole carbamate (parbendazole) | Yes [5] | 8 |
| Methyl-5-(4-fluorobenzolyl)-2-benzimidazole carbamate (flubendazole) | No [10] | 11 |
| Methyl-5-(phenylthio)-2-benzimidazole carbamate (fenbendazole) | No [12] | 8 |
| Chloroform | Yes [13] | 14 |
| Chlorpromazine | No [15] | 16 |
| Colchicine | Yes [17] | 18 |
| Diethylstilbesterol | Yes [19] | 20 |
| Diphenylhydantoin | Yes [21] | 22 |
| Ether | Yes [23] | 24 |
| Griseofulvin | Yes [25] | 26 |
| Heparin | No [27] | 28 |
| 5-(4-hydroxyphenyl)-5-phenylhydantoin | No [29] | 30 |
| Podophyllin | No [31] | 32 |
| Procaine | No [33] | 34 |
| Sodium cacodylate | Yes [35] | 36 |
| Vinblastine | Yes [27] | 26 |
| Vincristine | Yes [27] | 37 |

[1] HOOD and BISHOP 1972; [2] BEAUDOIN 1974; [3] FERM et al. 1971; [4] LUDEFORD 1936; [5] DELATOUR et al. 1976; [6] DELATOUR and RICHARD 1976; [7] DAVIDSE 1975; [8] HOLDEN et al. 1980b; [9] KAPPAS et al. 1974; [10] THIENPONT et al. 1978; [11] BORGERS et al. 1975; [12] BAEDER et al. 1974; [13] MURRAY et al. 1979; [14] DEYSSON 1948; [15] KALTER 1968; [16] QUINN 1975; [17] MORRIS et al. 1967; [18] EIGSTI and DUSTIN 1955; [19] MCLACHLAN and DIXON 1977; [20] SAWADA and ISHIDATE 1978; [21] MONSON et al. 1973; [22] MACKINNEY et al. 1978a; [23] SCHWETZ and BECKER 1970; [24] GAVAUDAN 1945; [25] KLEIN and BEALL 1972; [26] MALAWISTA et al. 1968; [27] SHEPARD 1980; [28] DEYSSON 1965; [29] HARBINSON and BECKER 1969; [30] MACKINNEY et al. 1978b; [31] THIERSCH 1963; [32] MATUROVA et al. 1959; [33] BAKER 1960; [34] HASCHKE et al. 1974; [35] HARRISON et al. 1980; [36] DUSTIN 1939; [37] DEYSSON 1975

random dispersal of chromosomes throughout the mitotic cell rather than an equatorial orientation, and by excessive contraction of the chromosomes. In addition, cells are arrested and accumulate in this C-metaphase configuration, thus giving rise to a higher than normal mitotic index. Second, spindle disruption can be recognized by use of eukaryotic models specifically designed to detect nondisjunction. Models employed for this purpose include the D6 strain of *Saccharomyces cerevisiae* (PARRY 1978), *Neurospora crassa* (GRIFFITHS and DELANGE 1977), and *As-*

*pergillus niger* (KAFER et al. 1976). Finally, physicochemical techniques have been refined which measure the interaction of isolated microtubule proteins with a test chemical (DAVIDSE 1975). Because of the heterogeneous nature of this data base, much of the evidence for spindle disruptive properties is indirect. However, for the purpose of this survey, the ability of an agent to produce a response in any of these models will be assumed to indicate the ability to disrupt spindle formation in mitotic mammalian cells.

Table 5 is a compilation of chemicals which have been evaluated for teratogenic activity, and which are also known to possess the ability to interact with microtubules. All teratology data in this table comes from rodents. Of the 22 compounds with microtubule disruptive properties, 14 (64%) are positive teratogens. Although the data base for this correlation is too limited to permit widespread conclusions, it does suggest that agents which interact with microtubules have a greater than even chance of also being teratogenic. Another approach to this correlation would be to determine the extent of teratogenic activity of agents known to be *inactive* in microtubule models. Unfortunately, this data base is even more limited, since negative results of this nature would seldom appear in the literature. However, a study of several benzimidazole analogs in a mammalian cell culture model indicates that, even among closely related analogs, the ability to produce metaphase arrest is not necessarily predictive of teratogenicity (HOLDEN et al. 1980b).

# E. Carcinogens as Mutagens and Teratogens

The Ames *Salmonella*/S9 metabolic activation system is used extensively to screen compounds for mutagenic potential. The test monitors mutation at the histidine locus in genetically defined strains of *Salmonella typhimurium*. A rat liver homogenate mixture is employed to approximate in vivo mixed function oxidase metabolism. A compound active in this assay produces an increase in the number of histidine-independent colonies in a defined cell population. Since the correlation between mutagenesis in this assay and in vivo carcinogenesis has been high, and some carcinogens are teratogens, it is worthwhile to identify any useful relationship between the mutagenic and teratogenic activity of these compounds. The 60 carcinogens in Table 6 were selected on the basis of available mutagenic and mammalian teratogenic data, principally in RINKUS and LEGATOR (1979) and SHEPARD (1980) respectively.

Table 7 summarizes the correlation of response. Cadmium and vinyl chloride have been excluded from calculations, owing to contradictory teratology data from mammalian and human reports. Of the remaining 58 carcinogens, 46 (79%) are reported to be teratogenic in one or more species. Of these 46 carcinogens/teratogens, 35 gave a positive response in the *Salmonella* test. Conversely, 35 of the 38 known carcinogens (92%) with positive *Salmonella* results were also teratogens. Of the 12 carcinogens which were not teratogens, 9 were not active in the *Salmonella* test. The overall correlation of mutagenic and teratogenic activity was 76%. Cytogenetic data was available for 9 of the 11 compounds which were positive teratogens, but negative in the *Salmonella* test; 4 were clastogenic: actinomycin D, aldrin, procarbazine, and urethan, and 5 were negative.

**Table 6.** Literature survey of carcinogens studied for teratology and *Salmonella* point mutations

| Compound | Teratogenesis | | | | | | | Mutagenesis | | | |
|---|---|---|---|---|---|---|---|---|---|---|---|
| | Mouse | Rat | Hamster | Rabbit | Primate | Human | Other | Terato-genic?[1] | Salmo-nella | Point Mutagen?[2] | Cyto-genetics |
| Acetamide | | − | | | | | | No | − | No | |
| 2-Acetylaminofluorene | + | | | | | | | Yes | + | Yes | |
| Actinomycin D | | + | | + | | | | Yes | − | No | Yes |
| Adriamycin | − | + | | | | | | Yes | + | Yes | Yes |
| Aflatoxin | | + | + | | | | | Yes | + | Yes | |
| Aldrin | | + | + | | | | | Yes | − | No | Yes |
| 4-Aminofolic acid (aminopterin) | | + | | | | + | | Yes | − | No | No |
| Azaserine | | + | | | | | | Yes | + | Yes | |
| Azathioprine | − | − | | + | | | | Yes | + | Yes | Yes |
| Benzo[a]pyrene | | − | | | | | | No | + | Yes | Yes |
| Biphenyl | | − | | | | | | No | − | No | |
| Busulfan | | + | | | | | | Yes | + | Yes | Yes |
| Cadmium | | + | + | | | − | | Yes | +/− | Inc. | Yes |
| Captan | | − | − | | − | | −(Dog) | No | + | Yes | No |
| Carbon tetrachloride | | − | | + | | | | Yes | − | No | |
| Chlorambucil | | + | | | | + | | Yes | + | Yes | Yes |
| *p*-Chlorodimethyl aminoazobenzene | + | | | | | | | Yes | + | Yes | |
| Chromium | | | + | | | | | Yes | + | Yes | |
| Cyclophosphamide | + | + | | + | + | + | | Yes | + | Yes | Yes |
| Daunomycin | | + | | | | | | Yes | + | Yes | Yes |
| 2.4-Diaminotoluene | + | − | | | | | | Yes | + | Yes | |
| Dieldrin | − | + | + | | | | —(Pig) | Yes | − | No | No |
| 1,2-Diethylhydrazine | | +[3] | | | | | | Yes | + | Yes | |
| *trans*-α,α′-Diethyl-4,4′-stilbene-diol (DES) | | + | | | | + | Yes | Yes | − | No | No |
| *N*,*N*-Dimethyl-4-amino-azobenzene | + | + | | | | | | Yes | + | Yes | |
| 7,12-Dimethylbenz[a]anthracene (DMBA) | + | + | | | | | | Yes | + | Yes | Yes |
| 1,2-Dimethyl hydrazine | | − | | | | | | No | − | No | |
| Ethionine | | − | | | | | | No | − | No | |
| Ethylenethiourea (Imidazole) | | + | | + | | | | Yes | + | Yes | Inc. |
| Ethylnitrosourea (ENU) | | + | | | | | | Yes | + | Yes | Yes |

| | | | | | | | | | |
|---|---|---|---|---|---|---|---|---|---|
| *m*-Fluorodimethyl aminoazobenzene | + | | | | | | Yes | + | Yes | |
| Furylfuramide (AF-2) | +[4] | | | | | | Yes | + | Yes | |
| Griseofulvin | | + | | | | | Yes | – | No | No |
| Hycanthone methane sulfonate | + | | | | | | Yes | + | Yes | Yes |
| 7-Hydroxymethyl-12-methylbenz[a]-anthracene | | + | | | | | Yes | + | Yes | |
| *N*-Hydroxyurethan | | + | | | | | Yes | + | Yes | Yes |
| Kanechlor 500 (polychlorinated biphenyl compounds) | | – | | | | | No | – | No | |
| Lead | | + | + | | | | Yes | – | No | No |
| Lindane | | – | | – | | | No | – | No | |
| METEPA | | + | | | | | Yes | + | Yes | Yes |
| *N*-Methyl-4-aminoazobenzene | + | | | | | | Yes | + | Yes | |
| Methylazoxy-methanol | | | | | | + (Guinea pig) | Yes | + | Yes | |
| 3-Methylcholanthrene | Inc. | + | | | | | Yes | + | Yes | Yes |
| 4-Methylethylene thiourea | | + | | | | | Yes | + | Yes | |
| 2-Methyl-4-nitro-1-(4-nitrophenyl)imidazole | – | – | | | | – (Dog) | No | + | Yes | |
| *N*-Methyl-*N*′-nitro-*N*-nitrosoguanidine (MNNG) | + | | | | | | Yes | + | Yes | Yes |
| *N*-Methyl-*N*-nitrosourea | | + | | | | | Yes | + | Yes | Yes |
| Mirex | | + | | | | | Yes | – | No | |
| Mitomycin C | + | – | | | | | Yes | + | Yes | Yes |
| Nitrogen mustard HCl | | + | | | | | Yes | + | Yes | |
| 1-Phenyl-3,3-dimethyltriazene | | + | | | | | Yes | + | Yes | No |
| Piperonyl butoxide | | – | | | | | No | – | No | |
| Procarbazine | | + | | | | | Yes | – | No | Yes |
| Saccharin | – | – | | | | | No | – | No | |
| Thio-TEPA | + | + | | | | | Yes | + | Yes | Yes |
| 1,1,1-Trichloro-2,2-bis-(4-chlorophenyl)ethane (*p,p*′-DDT) | – | – | | – | | | No | – | No | No |
| Triethylenemelamine (TEM) | + | + | | | | | Yes | + | Yes | Yes |
| Uracil mustard | | + | | | | | Yes | + | Yes | No |
| Urethan (ethyl carbamate) | + | + | | | | | Yes | – | No | Yes |
| Vinyl chloride | | – | | | Inc. | | Inc. | + | Yes | |

Inc. = inconclusive
[1] SHEPARD 1980; [2] RINKUS and LEGATOR 1979; [3] DRUCKREY 1973a; [4] KONDO et al. 1975

**Table 7.** Teratology and *Salmonella* results for carcinogens

| | |
|---|---|
| A. Positive teratology, positive *Salmonella* | 35 |
| B. Negative teratology, negative *Salmonella* | 9 |
| C. Positive teratology, negative *Salmonella* | 11 |
| D. Negative teratology, positive *Salmonella* | 3 |
| E. Inconclusive teratology | 2 |
| F. Total compounds surveyed (conclusive results) | 58 |
| G. Total compounds surveyed | 60 |
| Total correlation [(A + B)/F × 100] | 76% |

False negatives in the *Salmonella* assay may be due to inadequate metabolic activation, as in the case of carbon tetrachloride, or failure of the system to detect chemicals which form short-lived active species, or for which activation requires several enzymatic steps in vivo, such as procarbazine (LEE and DIXON 1978) or urethan (RINKUS and LEGATOR 1979). As reported by AMES and MCCANN (1976) the *Salmonella* system is not sensitive with or without metabolic activation to steroids (diethylstilbestrol) or steroid antagonists, antimetabolites (aminopterin), polychlorinated hydrocarbons (Mirex, dieldrin), or inorganics (arsenic, lead). Antimitotic agents which inhibit normal cell division by spindle disruption or other mechanisms are negative in assays to identify chromosome breakage and point mutation, but are likely to be active carcinogens. This class includes griseofulvin (STEELMAN and KOCSIS 1978; MALAWISTA et al. 1968), colchicine and derivatives (DIPAOLO and KOTIN 1966), chloridine (DYBAN et al. 1976), and podophyllotoxin (WIESNER et al. 1958).

Benzo[*a*]pyrene, captan, and 2-methyl-4-nitro-1-(4-nitrophenyl)imidazole were the three carcinogens found positive in the *Salmonella* test which did not induce fetal malformations. Benzo[*a*]pyrene does induce increased lethality in rat embryos and chromosome breakage in rat somatic cells. Captan causes dominant lethal mutations in rats and mice, demonstrated by increased fetal mortality, and transmissible second generation effects in mice, probably due to polygenic point mutations (BRIDGES 1975).

From Table 7, it is interesting that of the 58 carcinogens evaluated, 11 not active in the *Salmonella* test were teratogenic, while 3 were not teratogenic, despite mutagenic activity. In the more limited context of the 12 carcinogens that were *not* teratogens, 9 were *not* active in the *Salmonella* test and 3 were active, maintaining a 3:1 predictive ratio. Of the 3 active compounds, at least 2, benzo[*a*]pyrene, and captan, demonstrate fetotoxic activity. This suggests that positive results in the *Salmonella* test may indicate broader reproductive effects.

## F. Discussion

Traditionally, the human genetic disease burden has been defined by such diverse end points as specific metabolic disorders, congenital defects based on chromosome anomalies, fetal wastage, and carcinogenicity. The role of mutations in another end point. teratogenicity, has been the subject of considerable debate, ranging from claims of direct association of teratology and mutagenicity to the opposite view that any association is purely coincidental. It is most reasonable to assume that the true relationship lies somewhere between these extremes. Efforts to characterize this relationship more accurately have, for the most part, suffered from a limited data base and/or an overly restricted definition of mutation. This latter problem is particularly acute when only a relatively insensitive test model is selected as the basis for defining genetic activity. The relative sensitivities of genetic test models will be discussed in more detail in the rest of this section.

## I. Teratology Correlated with Chromosome Alteration

The present survey suggests that agents which produce chromosome damage in in vivo or in vitro models have a high predictive value of teratogenicity (85% and 80%, respectively). The correlation is even greater (90%) when mutagenically active carcinogens were examined for teratogenic activity. However, for compounds which are negative in these test systems, the likelihood of predicting teratogenic potential is no greater than chance. The incidence of discordance in the range of 25%–30% indicates that although the relationship of mutagenesis to teratogenesis is not fortuitous, the sensitivity of these assay systems is not sufficient to afford overall predictability.

The sensitivity of cytogenetic assays varies considerably from model to model. Even within the present grouping for in vivo assessments, it is generally agreed that the sensitivities can be ranked as follows: metaphase assay > micronucleus assay > germ cell cytogenetics > dominant lethal test > heritable translocation test.

In the latter three models, negative results must be regarded with caution, since many known mutagenic agents give "false negative" results in terms of intrinsic chromosomal activity in these assays. In the present survey, fully one-third of the compounds tested in both somatic and germ cell assays are negative in germ cell models, but positive in somatic cells. Attention is drawn to this point because the insensitivity of these assays in general and the germ cell assays in particular may be partly responsible for reducing the correlation with teratology. Another factor which undoubtedly diminishes the power to predict is the fact that many electrophilic species generated in the maternal liver, although possibly mutagenic and teratogenic per se, do not elicit an effect in the fetus, simply because the reactive species is retained in the maternal liver, is highly labile, or is unable to cross the placental barrier. A strong example of the latter is 3-methylcholanthrene which has been shown to be teratogenic only when injected directly into the amnion (ALEXANDROV 1973). On the other hand, some agents may have access to the fetus and thus be teratogenic, yet be restricted from bone marrow or germ cells by physical or chemical barriers. In terms of teratogenic activity, these compounds would give "false negatives" in the in vivo cytogenetic assays.

For the study of the direct effect of a substance on mammalian chromosome structure, in vitro cytogenetic assays offer a number of attractive features. In these models, precise control of the exposure of the target cell to the test substance is practical. Moreover, the suitability of the material for cytogenetic analysis can be optimized by such technical procedures as enrichment of the mitotic population by synchronization or harvesting techniques. The target cells themselves can be selected from a variety of cytogenetically attractive species (e.g., lines derived from the Chinese hamster which has a low number of large chromosomes). In practice, in vitro cytogenetic models have been shown to be a highly sensitive means for measuring chemically induced chromosome damage. However, this applies primarily to agents which are direct acting mutagens. A serious drawback in these models is the fact that metabolic capabilities of the target cells are generally minimal. In the absense of exogenous metabolic activation, many otherwise potent mutagens go undetected in these assays (AU et al. 1980). Addition of rodent liver microsomal enzymes has met with limited success, primarily because of the severe toxic effect on mammalian cells (BIMBOES and GREIM 1976). More recently, studies have suggested that cocultivation with intact metabolically competent cells may be a significant improvement in this procedure (HOLDEN et al. 1980a). Nonetheless, most of the literature base used in the present survey involves unactivated systems. This undoubtedly serves to decrease the correlation between in vitro cytogenetic results and teratology.

The relationship between microtubule disruption and teratology is somewhat more tenuous than chromosome damage. However, if one considers that many reproductive effects are due to chromosome alterations, whether numerical or structural, it is not surprising that the incidence of correlation is similar in relating teratogenic activity with microtubule disruption (numerical changes), and with clastogenic activity (structural changes). The present survey indicates that the overall correlation with both these genetic end points is approximately 65%. The data base for the microtubule disruption is too limited to permit further conclusions, especially in the absence of solid data on inactive compounds. Furthermore, since the existing literature includes little in vivo data, the survey on microtubule disruption suffers from essentially the same limitations as the in vitro data base already discussed.

## II. Teratology Correlated with Carcinogen-Induced Point Mutations

The Ames *Salmonella*/S9 metabolic activation system is purported to achieve an 85% or greater correlation between mutagenesis and carcinogenesis for all chemical classes evaluated (MCCANN et al. 1975). A more recent compilation by RINKUS and LEGATOR (1979) demonstrated that for 465 compounds assigned to 35 chemical classes, the overall correlation for the predictive value of the *Salmonella* assay was 77%. Poorly detected categories of carcinogens included polychlorinated aromatics, cyclics and aliphatics, steroids, antimetabolites, symmetrical hydrazines, and compounds which are bactericidal, volatile, that cross-link DNA or inhibit mitosis.

However, the correlation of *Salmonella* test results for classes of chemicals that are ultimate electrophiles or chemicals that can be activated by liver microsomes to electrophilic species is 94%. The ability of such compounds to alter DNA, RNA, or protein is due to the reaction of the electrophile with nucleophilic sites on the target molecule. CONNER (1975) and later HARBISON (1978), have suggested that the electrophilic action of cytotoxic agents provides a common mechanism for mutagenicity and teratogenicity. Mutagenically active carcinogens, such as nitroso compounds, polycyclic aromatic hydrocarbons, and aromatic amides are known to cross the placenta and induce both tumors and malformations in the fetus (ALEXANDROV 1973).

Teratogenic responses and transplacental tumor induction are mediated by the chemical reactivity of a compound, the ability of the compound to cross the placenta, and the time of exposure of the active moiety to the fetus. Methylnitrosourea (MNU) is a potent, direct acting teratogen in the rat fetus when administered intravenously to the dam on day 10 or day 14 of gestation. However, tumors are induced by MNU only when administered on the last day of gestation (ALEXANDROV 1969; DRUCKREY 1973a, b). For carcinogens which must be metabolically activated, it is uncertain whether the proximate carcinogen in transplacental events originates in the maternal organism or in the fetus. Maternally derived proximate carcinogens must be sufficiently stable to cross the placental barrier. DRUCKREY (1973) cites nitrosamines as potent carcinogens in adult rats although they do not induce tumors in the fetus when administered on day 15 of gestation. He concludes that although the highly reactive carbonium ion is formed in the adult rat liver it is too unstable to reach the fetus and that the fetus, although sensitive at this stage, cannot independently activate nitrosamines. A short-lived, highly reactive molecule such as 2-acetylaminofluorene may induce tumors in adult livers, but never realize teratogenic potential. Nitrosomethylurethane (NMUt) fails to induce malformations in the fetus when administered to pregnant rats, although it is metabolized in exactly the same way as the potent teratogen MNU, by undergoing hydrolysis with the formation of diazomethane. However, if NMUt is injected directly into the placenta of rat embryos on day 13 gestation, 91% of the embryos exhibit microcephaly, micrognathia, cleft palate, and anomalies of the extremities. NMUt is less stable than MNU and is likely to be inactivated before reaching the embryo (ALEXANDROV 1973).

The placenta, once considered a protective barrier for the developing embryo, demonstrates variable permeability and metabolic activity during embryonic development. Passage is mediated by lipid solubility, molecular weight of the compound, and the age of the placenta. Compounds with a molecular weight of less than 600 daltons cross the placenta with little difficulty (HARBISON 1978). High molecular weight polycyclic hydrocarbons such as 1,2,5,6-dibenzanthracene, 3,4-benzpyrene, or 3-methylcholanthrene are not teratogenic because they are unable to cross the placental barrier. However, when 3-methylcholanthrene is injected into the amnion of mouse embryos on day 10 of gestation, some malformations are produced (ALEXANDROV 1973).

Some transplacental carcinogens produce tumors in offspring of treated animals, but are not teratogenic. ALEXANDROV (1973) reported that treatment of pregnant rats with the symmetric dialkylnitrosamines, dimethyl-, diethyl-, or dibutylnitrosamine resulted in increased prenatal mortality, but did not induce malformations. The maternal toxicity induced by high doses of these compounds was considered responsible for increased embryolethality. He theorized that if these compounds act indirectly via an alkylating metabolite formed by enzymatic demethylation in certain organs, a lack of these enzymes in the embryo at the time of sensitivity to teratogens resulted in lack of malformations. This concurs with the statement by DRUCKREY (1973b) that the failure of diethylnitrosamine to induce tumors transplacentally, unless administered on the last day of gestation, is due to a lack of development of relevant metabolic processes in the fetus until just prior to birth. The role of the developing fetal metabolic system cannot be overlooked in evaluating teratogenicity. GILLETTE et al. (1973) reported that enzymes which catalyze the reduction of nitro compounds such as nitrofurozone exist in the fetal liver and may participate in drug-induced fetotoxicity.

The importance of appropriate metabolic activation for both in vitro and in vivo systems used to identify biologic activity is further illustrated by data from YAGI et al. (1976) for the phthalate ester, di-2-ethylhexyl phthalate (DEHP). DEHP induces fetal death and skeletal and soft tissue malformations when administered to mice on day 7 or 8 of gestation, respectively. DEHP induces dominant lethal mutations (DILLINGHAM and AUTIAN 1973), but it is not positive in bacterial screening tests. Although the in vitro metabolic activating system appears inadequate to transform DEHP to a mutagenically active species, a monoester metabolite tested separately demonstrated a positive mutagenic response in *Escherichia coli*. KONDO et al. (1975) reported that furylfuramide (AF-2) was mutagenic in *Salmonella* and *E. coli* and weakly teratogenic in mice. In 1976, NOMURA and KONDO reported enhancement of teratogenic properties of AF-2 in mouse embryos following pretreatment of the pregnant dam with phenobarbital to activate metabolic enzymes. In this instance, a compound found positive in microbial systems warranted reevaluation in a mammalian in vivo system, resulting in elucidation of metabolic activation of AF-2.

Although a variety of physical and biologic factors impede the utility of applying a point mutation assay to identify teratogenic as well as carcinogenic potential, a 76% correlation between teratogenesis and mutagenesis for a group of 60 carcinogens has been established. Alkylating agents such as cyclophosphamide, *N*-methyl-*N*-nitro-*N*-nitrosoguanidine, and nitrogen mustard make up the largest class of active teratogens. Various sites on the DNA molecule react with alkylating agents, the N-7 and O-6 sites on guanine being the most sensitive. Alkylation of guanine results either in its depurination and eventual removal from DNA, or the induction of transition mutations by incorrect pairing of guanine with thymine rather than cytosine. Mitomycin C is one of a number of polyfunctional alkylating agents which also cross-link DNA and inhibits replication. Arylating agents such as aflatoxin, 7,12-dimethylbenz[*a*]anthracene, or 3-methylcholanthrene, the second largest group of active compounds, bind covalently to DNA via existing reactive functional groups or by metabolically induced reactive groups. Polycyclic compounds in this category also intercalate with DNA, causing frameshift mutations and abnormal gene products. Three teratogenically active carcinogens, actinomycin D, daunomycin, and hycanthone are intercalating agents. They distort the normal DNA structure by wedging into the DNA helix, resulting in addition or deletion of bases during replication. Enzyme inhibitors (azaserine) and folic acid inhibitors (aminopterin) induce both mutation and malformations or cell death by disrupting formation of enzymes involved in the biosynthesis of normal nitrogenous bases, inhibiting function of repair enzymes, or altering normal protein synthesis.

## III. Mutation and Abnormal Development

In Vol. 1 of the Handbook of Teratology, WILSON (1977) proposes nine mechanisms by which teratogens induce abnormal development. Six of these events – gene mutation, chromosomal alteration, mitotic disruption, altered nuclei acid integrity or function, lack of normal precursors or substrates, and enzyme inhibition – can be initiated by compounds with measurable mutagenic activity. However, numerous maternal and fetal physiologic factors intervene between the occurrence of a genetic event in vivo in a mature animal and similar expression in a developing embryo. The basic process of mutagenesis and carcinogenesis involves the alteration of a single cell. If the event occurs in a germ cell, it is transmissible to subsequent generations sired by the affected parent, expressed in fetal wastage, familial malformations or diseases, sterility, or heritable neoplasms (e.g., bilateral retinoblastoma). If the event occurs in a somatic cell, the result may be cell death or the formation of daughter cells which produce altered gene products or tumors. Teratogenesis requires insult to a critical number of cells in a population designated to form specific tissues or organs (WILSON 1973) at a critical stage in development. Thus, a mutagenic event inducing proliferation of a significant population of altered daughter cells can result in malformations.

Environmental factors, such as dietary deficiencies, extremes of temperature, and a variety of chemicals may cause fetal death, increased incidence of spontaneously occurring malformations such as cleft palate, or unique malformations, without altering the genetic makeup of parental germ cells or subsequent unexposed offspring. However, as many as 50% of all human early spontaneous abortions possess chromosomal abnormalities (CARTER 1977), suggesting a potential etiologic relationship between chromosome damage and fetal wastage. Nonetheless, it is clear that individual mutagenic events may initiate or contribute to the developmental disruption which result in terata, without being the sole cause. In fact, it is probable that several organizational stages may intervene between a mu-

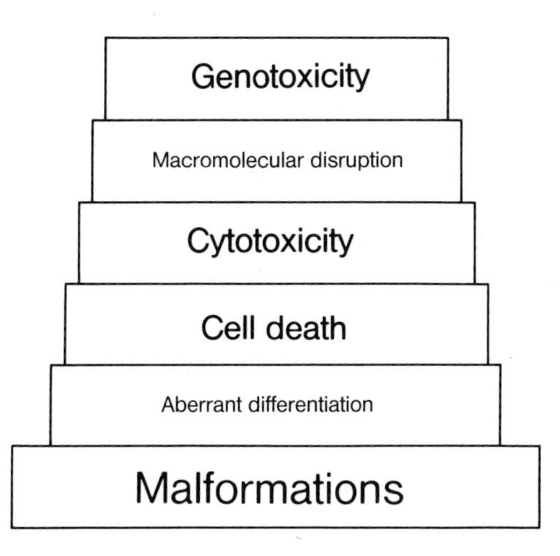


**Fig. 1.** Organizational stages leading from a genotoxic event to fetal malformation

tagenic event and its ultimate expression as a malformation. Each stage may itself be susceptible to nongenetic disruption which may later be expressed as malformation. This concept is presented diagrammatically in Fig. 1. Clearly, most but not all malformations are attributable to aberrant differentiation; the remainder to a poorly defined mixture of other factors. Likewise, a major but not exclusive cause of aberrant differentiation is cell death. However, some aberrant differentiation may be attributable to other causes. As this progression is followed to the top of the diagram in Fig. 1, two conclusions can be reached. First, genotoxicity has a significant but indirect impact on malformations and second, a variety of nongenetic factors also contribute to the induction of malformation.

A relationship has been demonstrated between the function of compounds as genotoxic agents or compounds capable of inhibiting normal cellular metabolism by blocking biosynthetic pathways and their teratogenic activity. The 76% correlation with Ames *Salmonella* assay for point mutation and the overall correlation of 65% for cytogenetic assays are not adequate criteria to recommend these mutagenicity tests as general screening tests for teratogenesis. However, it is clear that the relationship between mutagenesis, carcinogenesis, and teratogenesis is not coincidental. Active electrophiles can cause point mutations in bacteria and malformed offspring in laboratory animals. A large fraction of compounds which break chromosomes or alter chromosome number are also teratogenic. Any compound capable of damaging DNA could cause malformations under proper conditions of exposure and metabolism. Therefore, a compound positive in the basic screening tests for mutagenicity should be considered a potentially active teratogen, and be promptly evaluated for reproductive activity.

## References

Abe S, Sasaki M (1977) Chromosome aberrations and sister chromatid exchanges in Chinese hamster cells exposed to various chemicals. J Natl Cancer Inst 58:1635–1641
Adams CE, Hay MF, Lutwak-Mann C (1961) The action of various agents on the rabbit embryo. J Embryol Exp Morphol 9:468–491
Adler ID, Ramarao G, Epstein S (1971) *In vivo* cytogenetic effects of trimethylphosphate and of TEPA on bone marrow cells of male rats. Mutat Res 13:263–273
Aeschbacher HO, Milon H, Wurzner H (1978) Caffeine concentrations in mice plasma and testicular tissue and the effect of caffeine on the dominant lethal test. Mutat Res 57:193–200
Alexandrov VA (1969) Transplacental blastomogenic effect of N-nitrosomethylurea on rat offspring (in Russian). V OPr Onkol 15:55–61
Alexandrov VA (1973) Embryotoxic and teratogenic effects of chemical carcinogens. In: Tomatis L, Mohr U, Davis W (eds) Transplacental carcinogenesis. International Agency for Research on Cancer Scientific Publ 4 IARC, Lyon, pp 112–174
Alving J, Jensen M, Meyer H (1976) Diphenylhydantoin and chromosome morphology in man and rat. A negative report. Mutat Res 40:173–176
Anderson D, McGregor D, Purchase I (1976) Dominant lethal studies with paraouat and diguat in male CD-1 mice. Mutat Res 40:349–358
Arrighi FE, Hsu TC (1965) Experimental alteration of metaphase chromosome morphology. Effect of actinomycin D. Exp Cell Res 39:305
Au W, Johnston D, Collie-Bruyere C, Hsu T (1980) Short-term cytogenetic assays of nine cancer chemotherapeutic drugs with metabolic activation. Environ Mutagenesis 2:455–464

Baeder C, Bahr H, Christ O, Duv D, Kellner H, Kirsch R, Loewe H, Schultes E, Schutz E, Westen H (1974) Fenbendazole: A new highly effective anthelmintic. Experientia 30:753–754

Baker J (1960) The effects of drugs on the fetus. Pharmacol Rev 12:37–90

Banister P, DaFoe C, Smith E, Miller J (1972) Possible teratogenicity of tricyclic antidepressants. Lancet 1:838–839

Baranov VS (1966) The specificity of the teratogenic effects of aminopterin as compared to other teratogenic agents. Bull Exp Biol 1:77–82

Barr M (1973) The teratogenicity of cadmium chloride in two stocks of Wistar rats. Teratology 7:237–242

Basler A, Rohrborn G (1976) Chromosome aberrations in oocytes of NMRI mice and bone marrow cells of Chinese hamster induced with 3,4-benzpyrene. Mutat Res 38:327–332

Beall J (1972) Study of the teratogenic potential of diazepam and SCH 12041. Can Med Assoc J 106:1061

Beaudoin A (1974) Teratogenicity of sodium arsenate in rats. Teratology 10:153–158

Becker B, Gibson J (1970) Teratogenicity of cyclohexylamine in mammals. Toxicol Appl Pharmacol 17:551–552

Beliles R, Korn N, Benson B (1973) Comparison of the effects of methyl methanesulfonate in various reproductive toxicity screening tests. Res Commun Chem Pathol Pharmacol 5:713–724

Benedict W, Banerjee A, Gardner A, Jones P (1977) Induction of morphological transformation in mouse C3H/10T½ clone 8 cells and chromosomal damage in hamster A(Tl)Cl-3 cells by cancer chemotherapeutic agents. Cancer Res 37:2202–2208

Bimboes D, Greim H (1976) Human lymphocytes as target cells in a metabolizing test system *in vitro* for detecting potential mutagens. Mutat Res 35:155–160

Bishun N (1971) The cytogenetic effect of cyclophosphamide on a Burkett tumor cell line (EE4) *in vitro*. Mutat Res 11:258–268

Bishun NP, Lloyd N, Raven RW, Williams DC (1972) The *in vitro* and *in vivo* cytogenetic effects of nicotine. Acta Biol Acad Sci Hung 23/2:175–180

Bishun N, Smith N, Eddie H, Williams D (1974) Lack of *in vivo* cytogenetic effects of imipramine in rats. Teratology 10:191–192

Bishun N, Smith N, Eddie H, Williams D (1977) Cytogenetic studies and diethylstibesterol. Mutat Res 46:211–212

Borgers M, DeNollin S, Verheyen A, DeBrabander M, Thienport D (1975) Effects of new anthelmintics on the microtubular system of parasites. In: Borgers M, DeBrabander M (eds) Microtubules and microtubule inhibitors. North-Holland/Elsevier, New York, pp 497–508

Brar B (1969) The effect of meprobamate on fertility gestation and offspring viability and development of mice. Arch Int Pharmacodyn 117:416–422

Brewen JG, Nettesheim P, Jones K (1970) A host-mediated assay for cytogenetic mutagenesis. Preliminary data on the effect of methyl methanesulfonate. Mutat Res 10:645–649

Bridges BA (1975) The mutagenicity of captan and related fungicides. Mutat Res 32:3–34

Brusick D (1980) Principles of genetic toxicology. Plenum, New York, 279 pp

Budreau C, Singh R (1973) Effect of fenthion and dimethoate on reproduction in the mouse. Toxicol Appl Pharmacol 26:29–38

Bus JS, Gibson J (1973) Teratogenicity and neonatal toxicity of ifosfamide in mice. Proc Soc Exp Biol Med 143:965–970

Carter CD (1977) The relative contribution of mutant genes and chromosome abnormalities to genetic ill-health in man. In: Scott D, Bridges B, Sobels F (eds) Progress in genetic toxicology. Elsevier/North Holland, Amsterdam, pp 1–14

Caujolle F, Caujolle D, Cros S, Calvet M (1967) Limits of toxic and teratogenic tolerance of dimethyl sulfoxide. Ann NY Acad Sci 141:110–125

Chaube S, Murphy ML (1966) The effects of hydroxyurea and related compounds on the rat fetus. Cancer Res 26:1448–1457

Chaube S, Murphy ML (1968) The teratogenic effects of the recent drugs active in cancer chemotherapy. In: Woollam D (ed) Advances in teratology, vol 3. Academic Press, New York, pp 204–205

Chaube S, Krury G, Murphy M (1967) Teratogenic effects of cyclophosphamide (NCA-26271) in the rat. Cancer Chemother Rep 51:363–376
Chaubey R, Kavi B, Chauhan P, Sundaram K (1977) Evaluation of the effect of ethanol on the frequency of micronuclei in the bone marrow of Swiss mice. Mutat Res 43:441–444
Chernoff G (1977) The fetal alcohol syndrome in mice. An animal model. Teratology 15:223–230
Clegg DJ (1965) Absence of teratogenic effect of butylated hydroxyanisole (BHA) and butylated hydroxytoluene (BHT) in rats and mice. Food Cosmet Toxicol 3:387–403
Conner TA (1975) Cytotoxic agents in teratogenic research. In: Posivello DE, Berry CL (eds) Teratology trends and applications. Springer, Berlin, pp 49–88
Courtney K, Valerio D (1968) Teratology in the *Macaca mulatta*. Teratology 1:163–172
Cros SB, Moisand C, Tollon Y (1972) Influence de la tetramethylurie sur le developpement embryonaire de la souris. Ann Pharm Fr 9:585–593
Currie AR, Bird CC, Crawford A, Sims P (1970) Embryopathic effects of 7,12-dimethylbenz(a)anthracene and its hydroxymethyl derivatives in the Sprague-Dawley rat. Nature 226:911–914
Dagg C (1960) Sensitive stages for the production of developmental abnormalities in mice with 5-fluorouracil. Am J Anat 106:89–96
Davidse LC (1975) Antimitotic activity of methyl benzimidazol-2-ylcarbamate in fungi and its binding to cellular protein. In: Borgers M, DeBrabander M (eds) Microtubule and Microtubule inhibitors. North Holland, Amsterdam, pp 483–495
Dean B, Thorpe E (1972) Cytogenetic studies with dichlorvos in mice and Chinese hamsters. Arch Toxicol 30:39–49
Delatour P, Richard Y (1976) Proprietes embryotoxiques et antimitotiques en serie benzimidazole. Therapie 31:505–515
Delatour P, Lorgue G, Lappas M, Richard Y (1976) Proprietes embryotoxiques et antimitotiques du parbendazole et du cambendazole. C R Acad Sci [D] (Paris) 282:517–518
Deysson G (1948) Thesis, Universitie de Paris
Deysson G (1965) Sur l'activite antimitotique des heparinoide: etude d'un polyester sulfurique de D-xylane (8061CB) à l'aide du test allium. C R Soc Biol (Paris) 159:125–127
Deysson G (1975) Microtubules and antimitotic substances. In: Borgers M, DeBrabander M (eds) Microtubules and microtubule inhibitors. North Holland, Amsterdam, pp 427–451
Dillingham EO, Autian J (1973) Teratogenic, mutagenic and cellular toxicity of phthalate esters. Environ Health Perspect 3:81–89
DiPaolo JA (1964) Polydactylism in the offspring of mice injected with 5 bromodeoxyuridine. Science 145:501–503
DiPaolo JA, Kotin P (1966) Teratogenesis-Oncogenesis: A study of possible relationships. Arch Pathol 81:3–23
Dix K, Van der Pauw C, McCarthy W (1977) Toxicity studies with dieldrin. Teratological studies in mice dosed orally with HEOD. Teratology 16:57–62
Dolimpo DA, Jacobson C, Legator M (1968) Effects of aflatoxin on human leukocytes. Proc Soc Exp Biol Med 127:559
Druckrey H (1973a) Specific carcinogenic and teratogenic effects of indirect alkylating methyl and ethyl compounds and their dependency on stages of oncogenic developments. Xenobiotica 3:271–303
Druckrey H (1973b) Chemical structure and action in transplacental carcinogenesis and teratogenesis. In: Tomatis L, Mohr U, Davis W (eds) Transplacental carcinogenesis. International Agency for Research on Cancer Scientific Publ 4 IARC, Lyon, pp 45–57
Druckrey H, Ivankovic S, Preussmann R (1966) Teratogenic and carcinogenic effects in the offspring after single injection of ethylnitrosourea to pregnant rats. Nature 210:1378–1379
Dustin A (1939) Some recent applications of caryoclastic poisons. Acta Brevia Neerl Physiol Pharmacol Microbiol 9:227–230
Dyban AP, Barilyak IR, Tikhodeeva II, Chebotak NA (1976) Correlation of the teratogenic and antimitotic activity of a series of derivatives of 2,4-diaminopyrimidine (in Russian). Ontogenez 7:55–63

Eigsti O, Dustin P (1955) *Colchicine*. Iowa State College Press, Ames, Iowa
Elias J, DiPaolo J (1967) Aflatoxin B1 induction of malformations. Arch Pathol 83:53–57
Emmerson JL, Thompson D, Strebing R, Gerbig C, Robinson V (1971) Teratogenic studies on 2,4,5-trichlorophenoxyacetic acid in the rat and rabbit. Food Cosmet Toxicol 9:395–404
Engel W, Krone W, Wolf U (1967) Die Wirkung von Thioguanin, Hydroxylamin und 5-Bromo-Desoxyuridin auf menschliche Chromosomen *in vitro*. Mutat Res 4:353–368
Epstein S (1969) A practical test for chemical mutagens in mammals. Toxicol Appl Pharmacol 14:653
Epstein S, Bass U, Bass W, Arnold E, Bishop Y, Joshi S, Adler I (1971) Sterility and semisterility of male progeny of male mice treated with the chemical mutagen TEPA. Toxicol Appl Pharmacol 19:134–146
Epstein S, Arnold E, Andrea J, Bass W, Bishop Y (1972) Detection of chemical mutagens by the dominant lethal assay in the mouse. Toxicol Appl Pharmacol 23:288–325
Essenberg J, Schwind J, Patras A (1940) The effects of nicotine and cigarette smoke on pregnant female albino rats and their offspring. J Lab Clin Med 25:708–716
Fabro S, Smith R, Williams R (1966) Embryotoxic activity of some pesticides and drugs related to phthalimide. Food Cosmet Toxicol 3:587–590
Ferm V (1966) Congenital malformations induced by dimethyl sulfoxide in the golden hamster. J Embryol Exp Morphol 16:49–54
Ferm VH, Carpenter SJ (1967a) Teratogenic effects of cadmium and its inhibitions by zinc. Nature 216:123
Ferm V, Carpenter S (1967b) Developmental malformations resulting from administration of lead salts. Exp Mol Pathol 7:208–21 3
Ferm V, Saxon A, Smith B (1971) The teratogenic profile of sodium arsenate in the golden hamster. Arch Environ Health 22:557–560
Food and Drug Research Laboratories Inc (1972) Teratologic evaluation of FDA 71-7 (sodium nitrate). National Toxicology Information Service PB-221-775
Frank DW, Trzos RJ, Good PI (1978) A comparison of two methods for evaluating drug induced chromosome alterations. Mutat Res 56:311–317
Fritz H, Hess R (1968) Prenatal development in the rat following administration of cyclamate, saccharin and sucrose. Experientia 24:1140–1141
Fritz H, Hess R (1971a) The effect of chloramphenicol on the prenatal development of rats, mice and rabbits. Toxicol Appl Pharmacol 19:667–674
Fritz H, Hess R (1971b) Effects of cyclophosphamide on embryonic development in the rabbit. Agents Actions 2:83–86
Fu TK, Jarvik LF (1977) The *in vitro* effects of imipramine on human chromosomes. Mutat Res 48:89–94
Gaines T, Kimbrough R (1966) The sterilizing, carcinogenic and teratogenic effects of Metepa on rats. Bull WHO 34:317–320
Gavaudan P (1945) Thesis, Universitié de Paris
Gebhart E, Wissmueller HF (1973) Investigations on the effect of phenylbutazone on chromosomes and mitosis in the bone marrow of rats. Mutat Res 17:283–286
Generoso W, Preston R, Brewen J (1975) 6-Mercaptopurine, an inducer of cytogenetic and dominant lethal effects in premeiotic and early meiotic germ cells of male mice. Mutat Res 28:437–447
Georgian L (1975) The comparative cytogenetic effects of aldrin and phosphamidon. Mutat Res 31:103–108
Gibson JE (1973) Teratology studies in mice with 2-sec-butyl-4,6-dinitrophenol (dinoseb.) Food Cosmet Toxicol 11:31–43
Gibson JE, Becker B (1968) Teratogenicity of cyclophosphamide in mice. Cancer Res 28:475–480
Gillette JR, Menard RH, Stripp B (1973) Active products of fetal drug metabolism. Clin Pharmacol Ther 14:680–692
Goetz P, Sram R, Dohnalova J (1975) Relationship between experimental results in mammals and man. Cytogenetic analysis of bone marrow injury induced by a single dose of cyclophosphamide. Mutat Res 31:247–254

Goldman A, Yakovac W (1964) Salicylate intoxication and congenital anomalies. Arch Environ Health 8:648–656
Grauwiler J, Schon H (1973) Teratological experiments with ergotamine in mice, rats and rabbits. Teratology 7:227–236
Green JD, Leong B, Laskin S (1978) Inhaled benzene fetotoxicity in rats. Toxicol Appl Pharmacol 46:9–18
Green S, Palmer KA, Legator MS (1970) *In vitro* cytogenetic investigation of calcium cyclamate, cyclohexylamine and triflupromazine. Food Cosmet Toxicol 8:617–623
Green S, Carr J, Sauro F, Legator M (1973) Effects of hycanthone on spermatogonial cells, deoxyribonucleic acid synthesis in bone marrow and dominant lethality in rats. J Pharmacol Exp Ther 187:437–443
Griffiths A, Delange A (1977) p-Fluorophenylalanine increases meiotic non-disjunction in a Neurospora test system. Mutat Res 46:345–354
Hampel KE, Gebhartz H (1965) Action of 5-fluorodeoxyuridine on human chromosomes. Antimicrob Agents Chemother 5:306
Hampel KE, Lackner A, Schulz G, Busse V (1971) Chromosomenmutationen durch Azathioprin bei menschlichen Leukozyten *in vitro*. Z Gastroenterol 9:47–51
Harbison RD (1978) Chemical-biological reactions common to teratogenesis and mutagenesis. Environ Health Perspect 24:87–100
Harbison R, Becker B (1969) Relations of dosage and time of administration of diphenylhydantoin to its teratogenic effect on mice. Teratology 2:305–312
Harper K, Palmer A, Davies R (1965) Effect of imipramine upon the pregnancy of laboratory animals. Arzneim Forsch 15:1218–1221
Harrison W, Frazier J, Mazzanti E (1980) Teratogenicity of disodium methanearsonate and sodium dimethylarsinate (Sodium Cacodylate) in mice. Teratology 21:43A
Hart M, Adamson R, Fabro S (1971) Prematurity and intrauterine growth retardation induced by DDT in the rabbit. Arch Int Pharmacodyn Ther 192:286–290
Hartz S, Heinonen O, Shapiro S, Siskind V, Slone D (1975) Antenatal exposure to meprobamate and chlordiazepoxide in relation to malformations mental development and childhood mortality. N Engl J Med 292:726–728
Haschke R, Byers M, Fink B (1974) Effects of lidocaine on rabbit brain microtubular protein. J Neurochem 22:837–843
Hastings S, Huffman K, Gallo M (1976) The dominant lethal effect of dietary triethylenemelamine. Mutat Res 40:371–378
Heinonen O, Slone D, Shapiro S (1977) Birth defects and drugs in pregnancy. Publishing Sciences Group, Littleton, Mass
Hendrickx A (1975) Teratologic evaluation of imipramine hydrochloride in bonnet (*Macaca mulatta*). Teratology 11:219–222
Holden HE, Ray VA, Wahrenburg MG, Zelenski JD (1973) Mutagenicity studies with 6-mercaptopurine: I. Cytogenetic activity *in vivo*. Mutat Res 20:257–263
Holden H, Ray V, Wahrenburg M, Ellis J, Florio J (1975) A comparative study of schistosomicides in cytogenetic and point mutation assays. Mutat Res 31:309–310
Holden H, Crider P, O'Brien E (1980a) A primary hepatocyte activation system for *in vitro* cytogenetic studies. Environ Mutagenesis 2:277
Holden H, Crider P, Wahrenburg M (1980b) Mitotic arrest by benzimidazole analogs in human lymphocyte cultures. Environ Mutagenesis 2:67–73
Hood R, Bishop S (1972) Teratogenic effects of sodium arsenate in mice. Arch Environ Health 24:62–65
Huang Sl, Saggioro H, Michelmann H, Malling HV (1978) Genetic effects of crocidolite asbestos in chinese hamster lung cells. Mutat Res 57:225–232
Inouye M, Murakami Y (1978) Teratogenic effect of N-methyl-N-nitro-N-nitrosoguanidine in mice. Teratology 18:263–268
Ishidate M, Odashima S (1977) Chromosome tests with 134 compounds on Chinese hamster cells *in vitro*. A screening for chemical carcinogens. Mutat Res 48:337–354
Itoi M, Gaften J, Kaneko N, Ishii Y, Ramer R, Gasset A (1975) Teratogenicities of ophthalmic drugs 2. Antiviral ophthalmic drugs. Arch Ophthamol 93:46–49

Jacobs P (1972) Chromosome mutations frequency at birth in humans. Hum Genet 17:61–64
Jensen MK (1972) Phenylbutazone, chloramphenicol and mammalian chromosomes. Hum Genet 17:61–64
Jensen M, Philip P (1971) The cytogenetic effects of rubidomycin *in vivo* in rats. Mutat Res 12:91–96
Jenssen D, Ramel C, Goethe R (1974) The induction of micronuclei by frameshift mutagens at the time of nucleus expulsion in mouse erythroblasts. Mutat Res 26:553–555
Johnstone E, Franklin R (1964) Assay of progestins for fetal virilizing properties in the mouse. Obstet Gynecol 23:359–362
Kafer E, Marshall P, Cohen G (1976) Well-marked strains of Aspergillus for tests of environmental mutagens. Identification of induced mitotic recombination and mutation. Mutat Res 38:141–146
Kageyama M, Nishimura H (1961) Developmental anomalies in mouse embryos induced by triethylene melamine (T.E.M.). Acta Med Univ Kyoto 37:318–327
Kalter H (1968) Teratology of the central nervous system. University of Chicago Press, Chicago
Kalter H (1971) Correlation between teratogenic and mutagenic effects of chemicals in mammals. In: Hollaender A (ed) Chemical mutagens, vol 1. Plenum, New York, pp 57–82
Kamada N, Brecher G, Tjio JH (1971) *In vitro* effects of chlorpromazine and meprobamate on blast transformation and chromosomes. Proc Soc Exp Biol Med 136:210–214
Kappas A, Georgopoulos G, Hastie A (1974) On the genetic activity of benzimidazole and thiophanate fungicides on diploid *Aspergillus nidulans*. Mutat Res 26:17–27
Kavlock R, Daston G, Grabowski C (1979) Studies on the developmental toxicity of ozone. 1. Prenatal effects. Toxicol Appl Pharmacol 48:19–28
Kawachi T, Yahagi T, Kada T, Tazima Y, Ishidate M, Sasaki M, Sugiyama T (1980) Cooperative programme on short-term assays for carcinogenicity in Japan. International Agency for Research on Cancer Sci Pub 27 IARC Lyon, pp 323–330
Kennedy GL, Fancher DE, Calandra JC (1968) An investigation of the teratogenic potential of Captan, Folpet and Difolatan. Toxicol Appl Pharmacol 13:420–430
Kennedy G, Frawley J, Calandra J (1973) Multigeneration reproductive effects of three pesticides in rats. Toxicol Appl Pharmacol 25:589–596
Khera K, Whitta L, Clegg D (1970) Embryopathic effects of diquat and paraquat. In: Deichmann WB, Radomski J, Penalver R (eds) Pesticides symposia, Interamerican congress on toxicology and occupational medicine. Halos & Assoc, Miami, pp 257–261
Klein M, Beall J (1972) Griseofulvin a teratogenic study. Science 175:1483–1484
Koizuma A, Dobachi Y, Tachibana Y, Tsuda K, Katsunuma H (1974) Cytokinetic and cytogenetic changes in cultured human leucocytes and HELA cells induced by benzene. Ind Health (Japan) 12:23–29
Kondo S, Ichikawa-Ryo H, Nomura T (1975) Mutagenesis in bacteria and teratogenesis in mouse by furylfuramide. Mutat Res 31:263–264
Kristoffersson U (1972) The effect of cyclamate and saccharin on the chromosomes of a Chinese hamster cell line. Hereditas 70:271–282
Kroes R, Peter D, Berkvens J, Verschuuren T, Van Esch G (1977) Long term toxicity and reproduction study (including a teratogenicity study) with cyclamate, saccharin, and cyclohexylamine. Toxicology 8:285–300
Lambert B, Hanson K, Lindsten J, Sten M, Werelius B (1976) Bromodeoxyuridine-induced sister chromatid exchanges in human lymphocytes. Hereditas 83:163–174
Lambert G, Nebert D (1977) Genetically mediated induction of drug-metabolized enzymes associated with congenital defects in the mouse. Teratology 16:147–154
Larsson KS, Erikkson M (1966) Salicylate-induced fetal death and malformations in two mouse strains. Acta Paediatr Scand 55:569–576
Lawler SD, Lele KP (1972) Chromosomal damage induced by chlorambucil in chronic lymphocytic leukaemia. Scand J Haematol 9:603–612
Lazarus S, Volk B (1963) Absence of teratogenic effect of tolbutamide in rabbits. J Clin Endocrinol 23:597–599

Lee IP, Dixon RL (1978) Mutagenicity, carcinogenicity and teratogenicity of procarbazine. Mutat Res 55:1–14
Legator M, Palmer K, Green S, Petersen K (1969) Cytogenetic studies in rats of cyclohexylamine, a metabolite of cyclamate. Science 165:1139
Leonard A, Leonard E (1978) Cytogenetic effects of myleran *in vivo* on bone marrow cells from male mice. Mutat Res 56:329–333
Loosli R, Loustalot P, Schalch W, Sievers K, Stenger E (1964) Joint study in teratogenicity research in some factors affecting drug toxicity. Proceedings of the European Society for the Study of Drug Toxicity. Toxicity 4:214–216
Lorke D (1969) Untersuchungen von Cyclamat und Saccharin auf embryotoxische und teratogene Wirkung an der Maus. Arzneim Forsch 19:920–922
Ludford R (1936) The action of toxic substances upon the division of normal and malignant cells *in vitro* and *in vivo*. Arch Exp Zellforsch 18:411–441
Lyon JP (1976) Mutagenicity studies with benzene. Diss Abstr B 36:5537
Machemer L, Lorke D (1976) Evaluation of the mutagenic potential of cyclohexylamine on spermatogonia of the Chinese hamster. Mutat Res 40:243–250
MacKenzie KM, Lucier E, McLachlan J (1979) Infertility in mice exposed prenatally to benzo-α-pyrene. Teratology 19:37A
MacKinney AA, Vyas R, Powers K (1978a) Morphologic effects of hydantoin drugs on mitosis and microtubules of cultured human lymphocytes. J Pharmacol Exp Ther 204:195–202
MacKinney AA, Vyas R, Walker D (1978b) Hydantoin drugs inhibit polymerization of pure microtubular proteins. J Pharmacol Exp Ther 204:189–194
Mahr U, Miltenburger HG (1976) The effect of insectides on Chinese hamster cell cultures. Mutat Res 40:107–118
Maier P, Schmid W (1976) Ten model mutagens evaluated by the micronucleus test. Mutat Res 40:325–338
Majumdar S, Hall R (1973) Cytogenetic effects of 2,4,5-T on *in vivo* bone marrow cells of mongolian gerbil. J Hered 64:213–216
Malawista SE, Sato H, Bensch KG (1968) Vinblastine and griseofulvin reversibly disrupt the living mitotic spindle. Science 160:770–771
Matter B (1976) Failure to detect chromosome damage in bone-marrow cells of mice and Chinese-hamsters exposed *in vivo* to some ergot derivative. J Int Med Res 4:382
Matter B, Grauwiler J (1974) Micronuclei in mouse bone marrow cells. A simple *in vivo* model for the evaluation of drug-induced chromosomal aberration. Mutat Res 23:239–249
Maturova M, Malinsky J, Santavy F (1959) The biological effects of some podophyllin compounds and their dependence on chemical structure. J Natl Cancer Inst 22:297–301
McCann J, Ames BN (1976) Detection of carcinogens as mutagens in the *Salmonella*/microsome test: Assay of 300 chemical, Part II. Proc Natl Acad Sci USA 73:950–955
McCann J, Choi E, Yamasaki E, Ames BN (1975) Detection of carcinogens as mutagens in the *Salmonella*/microsome test: Assay of 300 chemicals, part I. Proc Natl Acad Sci USA 72:5135–5139
McCarthy JF, Fancher D, Kennedy G, Keplinger M, Calandra J (1971) Reproduction and teratology with the insecticide Carbofuran. Toxicol Appl Pharmacol 19:370
McColl J, Robinson S, Glolus M (1967) Effect of some therapeutic agents on the rat fetus. Toxicol Appl Pharmacol 10:244–256
McKenzie W, Knelson J, Rummo N, House D (1977) Cytogenetic effects of inhaled ozone in man. Mutat Res 48:95–102
McLachlan JA, Dixon RL (1977) Teratologic comparison of experimental and clinical exposures to diethylstilbesterol during gestation. In: Thomas J, Singh R (eds) Regulator mechanisms affecting research. University Park, Baltimore, pp 309–336
Melnyk J, Duffy D, Sparkes E (1971) Human mitotic and meiotic chromosome damage following *in vivo* exposure to methotrexate. Clin Genet 2:28–31
Meretoja T, Vainio H, Sorsa M, Harkonen H (1977) Occupational styrene exposure and chromosomal aberrations. Mutat Res 56:193–197

Michelmann H, Maier P, Ficsor G, Feldman D (1977) Bone marrow and lymphocyte cytogenetics of monkeys (*Macaca mulatta*) treated with the clastogen, mitomycin C. Mutat Res 45:193–197

Milkovich L, Van den Berg B (1974) Effects of prenatal meprobamate and chlordiazepoxide hydrochloride on human embryonic and fetal development. N Engl J Med 291:1268–1271

Miller R, Becker B (1975) Teratogenicity of oral diazepam and diphenylhydantoin in mice. Toxicol Appl Pharmacol 32:53–61

Mitra A, Manna G (1971) Effect of some phenolic compounds on chromosomes of bone marrow cells of mice. Indian J Med Res 59:9

Monson R, Rosenberg L, Hartz S, Shapiro S, Heinonen D, Slone D (1973) Diphenylhydantoin and selected malformations. N Engl J Med 289:1049–1052

Moore J (1972) Teratogenicity of hycanthone in mice. Nature 239:107–109

Morris J, Van Wagenen G, Hurteau G, Johnston D, Carlsen R (1967) Compounds interfering with ovum implantation and development: alkaloids and antimetabolites. Fertil Steril 18:7–17

Muller D, Arni P, Fritz H, Langauer M, Strasser F (1978) Comparative studies of 14 mutagenic or carcinogenic substances in 7 mutagenicity test system. (Point mutation tests, cytogenetic test and the dominant lethal test). Mutat Res 53:235

Murcia CR, Nombela JA (1972) Cytological aberrations produced by methotrexate in mouse ascites tumors. Mutat Res 14:405–412

Murphy ML, Delmoro A, Lacon CR (1958) The comparative effects of five polyfunctional alkylating agents on the rat fetus with additional notes on the chick embryo. Ann NY Acad Sci 68:762–782

Murray F, John J, Balmer M, Schwetz B (1978) Teratologic evaluation of styrene given to rats and rabbits by inhalation and by gavage. Toxicology 11:335–343

Murray F, Schwetz B, McBride J, Staples R (1979) Toxicity of inhaled chloroform in pregnant mice and their offspring. Toxicol Appl Pharmacol 50:515–522

Nakanishi Y, Makino S (1964) Phase cinimatography studies on the effects of radiation and some chemicals on cells and chromosomes. Symp Int Soc Cell Biol 3:47

Napalkov NP, Alexandrov V (1968) On the effects of blastomogenic substances on the organism during embryogensis. Z Krebsforsch 71:32–50

Nasjleti CE, Spencer HH (1966) Chromosome damage and polyploidization induced in human peripheral leukocytes *in vivo* and *in vitro* with nitrogen mustard, 6-mercaptopurine and A-649. Cancer Res 26:2437–2443

Natarajan AT, Tates AD, Van Buul PPW, Meijers M, De Vogel N (1976) Cytogenetic effects of mutagens/carcinogens after activation in a microsomal system *in vitro*. Induction of chromosome aberrations and sister chromatid exchange by diethylnitrosamine (DEN) and dimethylnitrosamine (DMN) in CHO cells in the presence of rat liver microsomes. Mutat Res 37:83–90

Nelson C, Holson J, Green H, Gaylor D (1979) Retrospective study of the relationship between agricultural use of 2,4,5-T and cleft palate occurrance in Arkansas. Teratology 19:377–384

Newton M, Bohner B, Lilly L (1977) Chromosomal aberrations in rat lymphocytes treated *in vivo* with 1-phenyl-3, 3-dimethyltriazene and N-nitrosomorpholene. A further report on a possible method for carcinogenicity screening. Mutat Res 56:39–46

Nishimura H, Nakai K (1958) Developmental anomalies in offspring of pregnant mice treated with nicotine. Science 127:877–878

Nolen G, Klusman L, Black D, Buehler E (1971) Reproduction and teratology of trisodium nitrilotriacetate in rats and rabbits. Food Cosmet Toxicol 99:509–518

Nomura T, Isa Y, Tanaka H, Kanzaki T, Kimura S, Sakamoto Y (1977) Teratogenicity of aminopyrine and its molecular compound with barbital. Teratology 16:118

Nomura T, Kondo S (1976) The enhancement effect of phenobarbital on toxicity of furylfuramide in mouse embryo. Mutat Res 35:167–172

Nowell PC (1964) Mitotic inhibition and chromosome damage by mitomycin in human leukocyte cultures. Exp Res 33:445–449

O'Brien RL, Poon P, Kline E, Parker JW (1971) Susceptibility of chromosomes from patients with Down's syndrome to 7,12-dimethylbenz(α) anthracene-induced aberrations *in vitro*. Int J Cancer 8:202–210
Ohguro T, Hatano M, Imamura T, Shimizu M (1973) Toxicological studies on adriamycin-HCl 4, Teratological study. Med Treat (Tokyo) 6:1152–1164
Ohkuma H, Tsuyama F, Hirayama H (1973) Teratogenicity of cyclocytidine on rabbit or rat fetus. Teratology 8:102
Oppenheim JJ, Fishbein WN (1965) Induction of chromosome breaks in cultured normal human leukocytes by potassium arsenate, hydroxyurea and related compounds. Cancer Res 25:980
Ostertag W, Kersten W (1965) The action of proflavin and actinomycin D in causing chromatid breakage in human cells. Exp Cell Res 39:296–301
Ottoboni A (1969) Effect of DDT on reproduction in the rat. Toxicol Appl Pharmacol 14:74–81
Ottolenghi AD, Haseman J, Suggs F (1974) Teratogenic effects of aldrin, dieldrin and endrin in hamsters and mice. Teratology 9:11–16
Parkin R, Wayforth H, Magee P (1973) The activity of some nitroso compounds in the mouse dominant lethal mutation assay. Mutat Res 21:155–161
Parry J (1978) The detection of chromosome non-disjunction in the yeast *Saccharomyces cerevisiae*. Mutat Res 53:248
Partington M, Bateman A (1964) Dominant lethal mutations induced in male mice by methyl methanesulfonate. Heredity 19:191–200
Patton GR, Allison AC (1972) Chromosome damage in human cell cultures induced by metal salts. Mutat Res 16:332–336
Percy DH (1975) Teratogenicity effects of pyrimidine analogues 5-iododeoxyuridine and cytosine arabinoside in late fetal mice and rats. Teratology 11:103–108
Persaud T (1965) Tierexperimentelle Untersuchungen zur Frage der teratogenen Wirkung von Barbituraten. Data Biol Med Ger 14:89–90
Philip P, Jensen M (1970) Benzene induced chromosome aberrations in rat bone marrow cells. Acta Pathol Microbiol Scand [A] 78:489–490
Pilinskaya M (1974) Cytogenetic effect of the herbicide 2,4-D on human and animal chromosomes. Cytol Genet 8/3:6–10
Pushkina N, Gofmekler V, Klertsova G (1968) Changes in content of ascorbic acid and nuclei acids produced by benzene and formaldehyde. Bull Exp Biol Med 66:868–869
Quinn PJ (1975) The effect of microtubular-active agents on phosphatidylinositol phosphodiesterase activity. In: Borges M, De Brabander M (eds) Microtubules and microtubule inhibitors. North Holland, Amsterdam, pp 79–90
Raposa T (1978) Sister chromatid exchange studies for monitoring DNA damage and repair capacity after cytostatics *in vitro* and in lymphocytes of leukaemic patients under cytostatic therapy. Mutat Res 57:241–251
Ray VA, Holden HE, Ellis JH, Hyneck ML (1975) A comparative study on the genetic effects of hycanthone and oxamniquine. Toxicol Environ Health 1:211–227
Reddy C, Chan P, Hayes A (1978) Teratogenicity and dominant lethal studies of patulin in mice. Toxicology 11:219–223
Rees ED, Majumdar S, Shuck A (1970) Changes in chromosomes of bone marrow after intravenous injections of 7,12-dimethylbenz(a)anthracene and related compounds. Proc Natl Acad Sci 66:1228–1235
Revesy C, Chappel C, Gaudry R (1960) Masculinization of female fetuses in the rat by progestational compounds. Endocrinology 66:140–144
Richardson J (1974) A preliminary assessment of the cytogenetic effects of Metepa on mouse bone marrow using the micronucleus test. Mutat Res 26:391–394
Rigdon R, Rennels E (1964) Effect of feeding benz(a)pyrene on reproduction in the rat. Experientia 20:224–226
Rinkus SJ, Legator MS (1979) Chemical characterization of 465 known or suspected carcinogens and their correlation with mutagenic activity in the *Salmonella typhimurium* system. Cancer Res 39:3289–3318

Robens JF (1969) Teratologic studies of carbaryl, diazinon, norea, disulfiram and thiram in small laboratory animals. Toxicol Appl Pharmacol 15:152–163
Roberts G, Rand MJ (1977) Chromosomal damage induced by some ergot derivatives *in vitro*. Mutat Res 48:205–214
Rohr G, Bauchinger M (1976) Chromosome analyses in cell cultures of the Chinese hamster after application of cadmium sulphate. Mutat Res 40:125–130
Roll R (1971) Untersuchungen über die teratogene Wirkung von 2,4,5-T bei Mäusen. Food Cosmet Toxicol 9:671–676
Roman IC, Georgian L (1977) Cytogenetic effects of some anti-tuberculosis drugs *in vitro*. Mutat Res 48:215–224
Rothschild B, Levy G (1950) Action de la quinacrine sur la gestation chez la rat. C R Soc Biol (Paris) 144:1350–1352
Ruddick J, Khera K (1975) Pattern of anomalis following single oral doses of ethylenethiourea in pregnant rats. Teratology 12:277–282
Ruffolo PR, Ferm VH (1965) The embryocidal and teratogenic effects of 5-bromodeoxyuridine in the pregnant hamster. Lab Invest 14:1547–1553
Rutishauser A, Bollag W (1963) Cytological investigations with a new class of cytotoxic agents: Methylhydrazine derivatives. Experientia 19:131
Sandor S, Amels D (1971) The action of ethanol on the prenatal development of albino rats. Rev Roum Embryol Cytol Ser Embryol 8:105–118
Sawada M, Ishidate M (1978) Colchicine-like effect of diethylstilbesterol (DES) on mammalian cell *in vitro*. Mutat Res 57:175–182
Saxen I (1975) Associations between oral clefts and drugs taken during pregnancy. Int J Epidemiol 4:37–44
Schardien J, Blatz A, Woosley E, Kaup D (1969) Reproductive studies on sodium meclofenamate in comparison to aspirin and phenylbutazone. Toxicol Appl Pharmacol 15:46–55
Schmahl W (1978) Different teratogenic efficacy to mouse fetal CNS of 5-azacytidine in combination with x-irradiation depends on the sequence of successive application. Teratology 18:143
Schmid E, Bauchinger M (1973) Chromosomal analysis in mammalian cells after exposure to lead *in vitro* and *in vivo*. Mutat Res 21:48
Schmid W (1973) Chemical mutagen testing on *in vivo* somatic mammalian cells. Agents Actions 3:79–85
Schmid W, Arakari D, Breslau N, Culbertson JC (1971) Chemical mutagenesis. The Chinese hamster bone marrow as an *in vivo* test system. Cytogenetic results on basic aspects of the methodology obtained with alkylating agents. Hum Genet 11:103–118
Schneider U, Maurer R (1972) Asbestos and embryonic development. Teratology 15:273–280
Schupback M, Hummler H (1977) A comparative study on the mutagenicity of ethylenethiourea in bacterial and mammalian test systems. Mutat Res 56:111–120
Schwetz B, Becker B (1970) Embryotoxicity and fetal malformations of rats and mice due to maternally administered ether. Toxicol Appl Pharmacol 17:275
Schwetz B, Sparschu G, Gehring P (1971) The effect of 2,4-dichlorophenoxyacetic acid (2,4-d) and esters of 2,4-d on rat embryonal, foetal and neonatal growth and development. Food Cosmet Toxicol 9:801–817
Seiler JP (1976) The mutagenicity of benzimidazole and benzimidazole derivatives. Cytogenetic effects of benzimidazole derivatives in the bone marrow of the mouse and the Chinese hamster. Mutat Res 40:339–348
Seiler JP (1977) Nitrosation in vitro and in vivo by sodium nitrate, and mutagenicity of nitrogenous pesticides. Mutat Res 48:225–236
Setala K, Nyyssonen O (1964) Hypnotic sodium pentobarbital as a teratogen in mice. Naturwissenschaften 51:412
Shapiro S, Hartz S, Siskind V, Mitchell A, Slone D, Rosenberg L, Monson R, Heinonen O, Idanpaan J, Haro S, Saxen L (1976) Anticonvulsants and prenatal epilepsy in the development of birth defects. Lancet 1:272–275

Shepard T (1980) Catalog of teratogenic agents, 3rd edn. John Hopkins Press, Baltimore
Sherman H, Culik R, Jackson RA (1975) Reproduction, teratogenic and mutagenic studies with benomyl. Toxicol Appl Pharmacol 32:305–315
Shimada T, Watanabe T, Endo A (1976) Potential mutagenicity of cadmium in mammalian oocytes. Mutat Res 40:389–396
Sinclair JG (1950) A specific transplacental effect of urethane in mice. Tex Rep Biol Med 8:623–632
Skalko RG, Gold MP (1974) Teratogenicity of methotrexate in mice. Teratology 9:159–164
Smithberg M, Runner MN (1963) Teratogenic effects of hypoglycemic treatments in inbred strains of mice. Am J Anat 113:479–489
Soukup S, Au W (1975) Effect of ethylnitrosourea on chromosome aberrations in vitro and in vivo. Hum Genet 29:319–328
Staiger GR (1969) Chlordiazepoxide and diazepam: Absence of effects on the chromosomes of diploid human fibroblast cells. Mutat Res 7:109–115
Staiger GR (1970) Studies on the chromosomes of human lymphocytes treated with diazepam in vitro. Mutat Res 10:635–644
Steelman RL, Kocsis JJ (1978) Determination of the teratogenic and mutagenic potential of griseofulvin. Toxicol Appl Pharmacol 45:343–344
Sturelid S (1971) Chromosome breaking capacity of TEPA and analogs in *Vicia faba* and Chinese hamster cells. Hereditas 68:255–276
Sugiyama T (1973) Chromosomal aberrations and carcinogenesis by various benz(a)anthracene derivatives. Gan 64:637–639
Takaori S, Tanabe K, Shimamoto K (1966) Developmental abnormalities of skeletal system induced by ethylurethan in the rat. Jpn J Pharmacol 16:63–73
Takeuchi I, Murakami U (1978) Influence of cysteamine on the teratogenic action of 5-azacytidine. Teratology 18:143
Tanimura T (1968a) Effects of mitomycin C administered at various stages of pregnancy upon mouse fetuses. Okajimas Folia Anat Jpn 44:337–355
Tanimura T (1968b) Relationship of dosage and time of administration to teratogenic effects of thioTEPA in mice. Okajimas Folia Anat Jpn 44:203–253
Tezuka H, Teramoto S, Kaneda M, Henmi R, Murakami N, Shirasu Y (1978) Cytogenetic and dominant lethal studies on captan. Mutat Res 57:201–207
Thienpont D, Vanparijs O, Niemegeers C, Marsboon R (1978) Biological and pharmacological properties of Flubendazole. Arzneim Forsch 28:605–606
Thiersch JB (1952) Therapeutic abortion with folic acid antagonist 4-aminopteroylglutamic acid (4-amino P.G.A.) administered by oral route. Am J Obstet Gynecol 63:1298–1304
Thiersch JB (1957a) Effect of 2-6-diaminopurine (2-6-DP): 6-chloropurine (CLP) and thioguanine (THG) on rat litter in utero. Proc Soc Exp Biol Med 94:40–43
Thiersch JB (1957b) Effect of 2,4,6-triamin-S-triazine (TR), 2,4,6-tria (ethyleneimino)-S-triazine (TEM) and N,N,N-triethylenephosphoramide (TEPA) on rat litter in utero. Proc Soc Exp Biol Med 94:36–43
Thiersch J (1963) Effect of podophyllin (P) and podophyllotoxin (PT) on the rat litter in utero. Proc Soc Exp Biol Med 113:124–127
Thiersch JB (1971) Investigations into the differential effect of compounds on rat litter and mother. In: Tuchmann-Duplessis H (ed) Malformations Congenitales des Mammiferes. Masson et Cie, Paris, pp 95–113
Thompson DJ, Molello HA, Strebing RJ, Dyke IL (1978) Teratogenicity of adriamycin and daunomycin in the rat and rabbit. Teratology 17:151–158
Thorpe E, Wilson A, Dix K, Blair D (1972) Teratologic studies with dichlorvos vapour in rabbits and rats. Arch Toxicol 30:29–38
Thueraut J, Schaller K, Engelhardt E, Gossler K (1975) The cadmium content of the human placenta. Int Arch Occup Environ Health 36:19–27
Tjalve H (1972) A study of the distribution and teratogenicity of nitrilotriacetic acid (NTA) in mice. Toxicol Appl Pharmacol 23:216–221
Tsuchimoto T, Malter B (1977) Comparison of micronucleus test and chromosome examination in detecting potential chromosome mutagens. Mutat Res 46:240

Tsutsui T, Umeda M, Sou M, Maizume H (1976) Effect of tetracycline on cultured mouse cells. Mutat Res 40:261–268
Tuchmann-Duplessis H, Mercier-Parot L (1959) Influence de divers sulfamides hypoglycemiants sur le developpement de l'embryon. Etude experimentale chez le rat. Acad Natl Med (Paris) 143:238–241
Tuchmann-Duplessis H, Mercier-Parot L (1960) Influence de l'actinomycine D sur la gestation et le developpement foetal du lapin. C R Soc Biol (Paris) 154:914–916
Tuchmann-Duplessis H, Mercier-Parot L (1967) Production chez le rat de malformations oculaires et squelettiques par administration d'une methyl-hydrazine. C R Soc Biol (Paris) 161:2127–2131
Tuchmann-Duplessis H, Mercier-Parot L (1968) Foetopathes therapeutiques: production experimentale de malformations des membres. Union Med Can 97:283–288
Tuchmann-Duplessis H, Mercier-Parot L (1969) Influence d'un antibiotic, la rifampicine, sur le developpement prenatal des ronguers. C R Acad Sci [D] (Paris) 269:2147–2149
Turner G, Collins E (1975) Fetal effects of regular salicylate ingestion during pregnancy. Lancet 2:338–339
Umeda M, Tsutsui T, Saito M (1977) Mutagenicity and inducibility of DNA single strand breaks and chromosome aberrations by various mycotoxins. Gan 68:619–625
Van Wagenen G, Deconti R, Handschumacker R, Wade M (1970) Abortifacient and teratogenic effects of triacetyl-6-azauridine in the monkey. Am J Obstet Gynecol 108:272–281
Veninga T (1967) Toxicity of ozone in comparison with ionizing radiation. Strahlentherapie 134:469–477
Vig BK (1971) Chromosome aberrations induced in human leukocytes by the antileukemic antibiotic adriamycin. Cancer Res 31:32–38
Vig BK, Kontras SB, Aubele AM (1969) Sensitivity of G1 phase of the mitotic cycle to chromosome aberrations induced by daunomycin. Mutat Res 7:91–97
Vogin E, Oser B (1969) Effects of cyclamate: saccharin mixture on reproduction and organogenesis in rats and rabbits. Fed Proc 28:2709
Vondruska JF, Fancher DE, Calandra JC (1971) An investigation into the teratogenic potential of captan, folpet and difolatan in non-human primates. Toxicol Appl Pharmacol 18:619–624
Von Kreybig T, Preusmann R, Von Kreybig I (1969) Chemische Konstitution und teratogene Wirkung bei der Ratte. II. N-alkylharnstoffe, N-alkylsulfonamide, N,N-dialkylacetamide, N-methylthioacetamid, Chloracetamide. Arzneim Forsch 19:1073–1076
Ware G, Good E (1967) Effects of insecticides on reproduction in the laboratory mouse. II. Mirex, tetodrin and DDT. Toxicol Appl Pharmacol 10:54–64
Warkany J, Takacs E (1959) Experimental production of congenital malformations in rats by salicylate poisoning. Am J Pathol 35:315–331
Watanabe G, Yoshida S (1970) The teratogenic effect of benzene in pregnant mice. Acta Med Biol 17:285–291
Weil C, Woodside M, Bernard J, Condra N, King J, Carpenter C (1973) Comparative effect of carbaryl on rat reproduction and guinea pig teratology when fed either in the diet or by stomach intubation. Toxicol Appl Pharmacol 26:621–638
Weinstein D, Mauer I, Katz ML, Kazmer S (1973) The effect of caffeine on chromosomes of human lymphocytes. A search for the mechanism of action. Mutat Res 20:115–125
Weinstein L (ed) (1976) Teratology and congenital malformations: A comprehensive guide to the literature. Plenum, New York
Wiesner BP, Wolfe M, Yudkin J (1958) The effects of some antimitotic compounds on pregnancy in the mouse. Proc Soc Study Fertil 9:129–136
Wild D (1978) Cytogenetic effects in the mouse of 17 chemical mutagens and carcinogens evaluated by the micronucleus test. Mutat Res 56:319–327
Wilk A, McClure H, Horigan E (1978) Induction of craniofacial malformations in the rhesus monkey with cyclophosphamide. Teratology 17:24A
Wilson JG (1966) Effects of acute and chronic treatment with actinomycin D on pregnancy and the fetus in the rat. Harper Hosp Bull 24:109–118
Wilson JG (1973) Environment and birth defects. Academic Press, New York

Wilson JG (1977) Current status of teratology. In: Wilson JG, Fraser FC (eds) Handbook of teratology: Plenum, New York, pp 47–74

Wobus AM (1976) Clastogenic activity of cytosine arabinoside and 3-deoxy-3-fluorothymidine in Ehrlich ascites tumor cells in vitro. Mutat Res 40:101–106

Yagi Y, Tutikawa K, Shimoi N (1976) Teratogenicity and mutagenicity of a phthalate ester. Teratology 14:259–260

Yashuda M (1972) Teratologic evaluation of Tsumacide/n-tolymethylcarbamate in rats. Bochu-Kagaku 37:161–165

# Adverse Effects on Function

CHAPTER 10

# Behavioral Testing Procedures: A Review

R. P. JENSH

## A. Introduction

Behavioral teratology, a multidisciplinary science which is less than two decades old, is concerned with the identification of agents which cause abnormal behavior in offspring, and the assessment of functional consequences of an insult during prenatal development. This area of investigation also includes subtle biochemical and anatomic disturbances which produce functional abnormalities. One of the basic premises of behavioral teratology is that functional alterations, usually deficits, may be present even when no morphological abnormalities are observed (BARLOW and SULLIVAN 1975; RODIER 1978). Behavioral teratology has been defined by WERBOFF and GOTTLIEF (1963) as the study of "deleterious changes in the behavior of animals, attributed to teratogenic agents administered during prenatal development." This definition is too limited, however, since an agent must be predetermined to be a teratogen according to classical morphological standards (JENSH 1980; WERBOFF and GOTTLIEB 1963).

Behavioral teratology has often been considered a subdividion of behavioral toxicology, which is a subclass of functional toxicology. Behavioral toxicology, however, is concerned with the study of agents which cause deleterious toxic behavioral effects in exposed organisms, but have no therapeutic effect. Functional toxicology is concerned with functional changes induced by toxic agents which are not readily related to biochemical or morphological defects. Functional effects are often reversible and may be indicators which precede irreversible structural damage. Although behavioral teratology may, in some instances, be considered part of functional toxicology, it has matured into a separate specialty, concerned with the postnatal behavioral effects of any suspect agent to which an organism is prenataly exposed.

The term "behavior" has been defined in many ways. SKINNER (1938) defined behavior as "what an organism is doing – or more accurately, what it is observed by another organism to be doing. By behavior, then, I mean the movement of an organism or its parts in a frame of reference provided by the organism itself or by various external objects." KANDEL (1976) defined behavior simply as "all observable processes by which an animal responds to perceived changes in the internal state of its body, or in the external world." P. SILVERMAN (1978), however, considers behavior to be the constantly fluctuating relationship of an organism to its environment, and the adjustments made to maintain that relationship, LIVINGSTON (1978) has attempted to define behavior differently, by relating behavior to evolution. He states that evolution is "a progressive and creative selection procedure acting on the basis of behavior that..." shapes successful genetic lines, and that behavior, successful adaption to the environment, is selected, while perception and sensory processes are only secondarily selected. He further points out that the latter are often in error, but that the organism is not compromised as long as the behavior (adaptive response) is successful (LIVINGSTON 1978). For the purposes of this chapter, it is most productive to define behavior in the broadest terms. Therefore, behavior will be considered to be an integrated action or reaction (response) within an organism's environment.

Behavioral alterations may be some of the earliest and most subtle abnormalities that can be observed. SPYKER (1975) has stated that "behavioral measurements may serve as the earliest indicators that some, as yet covert, toxic action has occurred" since "toxic effects may manifest as subtle disturbances of behavior long before any classical symptoms of poisoning become apparent." BUTCHER et al. (1975) and RODIER (1978) agree, stating that in a number of instances function has been shown to be a more sensitive indicator of teratogenic effects than physical malformation. VERNADAKIS and WEINER (1974) pointed out that, although testing for subtle behavioral effects of an agent is much more difficult than evaluating gross malformations, many recent studies have indicated that behavioral deviations in early childhood and adolescence may be due to subtle biochemical alterations which occurred during critical periods of brain tissue development and/or differentiations. COYLE et al. (1976) have stated that behavioral changes can be the most sensitive indicators of teratogenic action and that behavioral testing is now a necessary adjunct to morphological analysis as well as biochemicl assays. Some teratologists feel that subtle functional alterations in the offspring of exposed mothers may be the most sensitive indicators of toxicity. Such alterations include not only deviations in behavior, but also delays in the attainment of certain kinds of behavior in early life. COYLE et al. (1976) have stated that in some instances such delays could be more sensitive indicators of toxicity than evaluation of adult behavior.

The "no effect level" (NEL) of an agent was defined by the FAO/WHO Joint Committee on Food Additives as "the level of a substance that can be included in the diet of animals without toxic effects". An in-depth discussion of implications and ramifications related to this concept are beyond the purpose of this chapter. From this concept, however, came the term "acceptable daily intake" (ADI), which was calculated from the NEL as "that amount of a chemical which can be taken without harm for the whole life." The NEL and ADI are based on the tenets that all chemicals affect biologic systems in a dose–response relationship, ant that there is a threshold below which there are no effects (ZBINDEN 1979). Determination of the NEL is greatly dependent upon the skill and sophistication of the investigator. Behavioral teratologists have become increasingly aware that the traditional tests utilized to determine NELs may no longer be valid.

Although individual investigators were conducting behavioral teratology studies as early as the 1930s and 1940s (BIEL 1939; HARNED et al. 1940), it was not until the 1960s that behavioral teratologic investigations were begun in depth. In 1962, WERBOFF and his associates published the results of studies of behavioral alterations produced by both tranquilizers and X-rays (WERBOFF 1962; WERBOFF and HAVLENA 1962; WERBOFF et al. 1962). In less than two decades, the number nd variety of test procedures used and the level of sophistication of workers in the field have increased greatly. With the growing awareness of problems, limitations, and realistic expectations to be attained by behavioral testing, has come the knowledge that no single test can fully evaluate a suspect agent. As VORHEES et al. (1979a) have pointed out, "No single positive treatment could be expected to affect all types of behavior"; so, too, no single test should be expected to reveal all treatments which cause any behavioral alterations. In addition, negative results in a single behavioral test yield no conclusive information, while positive results may be difficult to interpret. Therefore, a multiple test series must be utilized to test for a wide range of functions following an insult (FURCHTGOTT 1973; WERBOFF 1970). Thus the concept of a "battery" was developed.

Behavioral testing may be considered as a rapid technique for determining the existence of subtle abnormalities. Although no single test gives a comprehensive behavioral assessment, the pattern of results in a multitest procedure permits a degree of localization of the lesion within the organism. Several single function tests are generally preferable to one complex multifunction test which requires considerable time and expertise. For a multitest procedure to be effective, there are a number of criteria which must be achieved. The following have been suggested (BUELKE-SAM and KIMMEL 1979; KIMMEL 1977; LASAGNA 1979; RODIER 1978; P. SILVERMAN 1978; SPYKER and AVERY 1976; VORHEES et al. 1979b):

1. The tests should be simple
2. The tests should be comprehensive, examining a variety of behavioral functions (global)
3. The tests should be sensitive to slight alterations in the organism's functions, as well as to alterations produced by a number of different agents
4. The behavioral schedule should be simple, to minimize the training time of personnel
5. The tests should take a minimum amount of time
6. The tests should be reliable, reproducible, and valid in the same laboratory as well as in the laboratories of other investigators
7. The tests should have a proven past history of positive results
8. The tests should be economical in terms of financial expense and utilization of animals
9. The tests should be within the framework of existing guidelines
10. The protocol should move in graded steps from elementary to more sophisticated tests
11. Data should be quantifiable
12. The tests should be predictive of effects in humans.

SPYKER (1975) adds another criterion: longitudinality. Since the organism changes during its life, a type of personal evolution, testing must be possible at various stages of the life cycle of the organism. She also maintains that since it is generally impossible to predict, a priori, behavioral changes due to exposure to a suspect agent, the battery must include a variety of maturational and behavioral tests applicable throughout life. COYLE et al. (1976) addressed this problem when they stated that "the major difficulty in administering a battery of tests is the differential sensitivity of the subjects at different ages to the various tests," but they still strongly advocate testing over a period of time.

The objective of using a battery of tests as a screening system differs from the goals of the traditional behavioralist. BUELKE-SAM and KIMMEL (1979) described the procedure as "apical testing." They stated that the use of behavioral evaluations which test integrated behavior rather than discrete function might be most valuable since apical testing is concerned with gross evaluations rather than the mechanisms causing the alterations. RODIER (1978) agrees, stating that the tests need not be easily interpreted in terms of anatomic origin or adaptive functions, unless the investigator whishes to persue the mechanism behind the behavior. The apical testing procedure is used to determine "Is there an abnormality, yes or no". RODIER (1978) has stated that some tests may be inappropriately subtle for use in a screening procedure. Furthermore, teratologists should not feel compelled to interpret observed behavioral alterations or to rank one type of behavior as being more or less meaningful than another.

There is a great deal of controversy concerning behavioral testing in general and specifically which tests should be included in a battery. RODIER et al. (1979) have stated that the results of their investigations indicated that a slightly different test battery could have yielded a different pattern of results, which would have led to entirely different conclusions. In addition, balance must be maintained between thoroughness and utility; time and money. Perhaps the most important consideration should be *standardization* of the test procedures, as stated by KIMMEL (1977).

Another area of concern is that of intertest interaction: the effects of one or more previous test experiences on the behavior of an animal in a new test situation. Although investigators disagree on this point, it appears that the influence of one test experience upon another depends at least on the tests involved and the time period between them (BARLOW and SULLIVAN 1975; JENSH et al. 1978b; JENSH et al. 1980b; LEVINE and BOADHURST 1963). Although many investigators believe there is a positive interaction, few of those using a multitest battery randomize the order of tests to correct for this situation.

Behavioral testing procedures are not meant to be used instead of morphological studies or other classical methodologies. Behavioral assessment is an adjunct to the more static methods, and may reveal deficits that other methods do not. The results of behavioral tests can be more valuable and meaningful when analyzed in conjunction with biochemical, anatomic, or physiologic data. Behavioral analysis offers a sensitive but indirect way to determine damage, since function, not damage, is monitored by behavioral testing (ALTMAN and SUDARSHAN 1975; JENSH 1980; NORTON 1978; RODIER 1978).

There are a number of texts which describe a variety of behavioral measures altered by specific changes in the central nervous system. There is also a vast amount of literature concerning the interrelations of other systems with the central nervous system, resulting in behavioral alterations. Investigators have stressed caution when attempting to interpret behavioral data, although correlative studies have been completed in many areas (RODIER 1978; THOMPSON et al. 1972). There are several reviews which may be of interest to the reader (BARLOW and SULLIVAN 1975; BLISS et al. 1972; BUELKE-SAM and KIMMEL 1979; JOFFE 1969; MOGENSON 1977; RODIER 1978; P. SILVERMAN 1978; SPROTT and STAATS 1979).

Many tests are currently used by investigators, ranging from the very simple to the highly complex. This chapter describes in detail those most commonly used.

References are included for some procedures not fully described. The rat has been extensively studied as a model of mammalian behavior. Therefore, unless otherwise stated, the present review is limited primarily to studies concerning the rat. Various testing situations and desired responses may require the use of different species (ALTMAN and KATZ 1979; BARNETT 1975).

## B. Morphological Development of the Central Nervous System

The central nervous system is a highly diversified system undergoing multitudinous development and maturation, the sequencing and developmental continuum being highly unique to each subsystem. Although there are regional differences, the cells of the central nervous system are formed over an extensive period of time. They are vulnerable to interference at many stages, such as the proliferative, migrational, and differentiative stages. There are excellent reviews (ALTMAN 1975; GOLDMAN 1976) as well as numerous texts concerning neural development. One basic premise is that among all mammalian species there occurs the same basic progression of brain development, with the major variations in maturation being primarily those of brain size and cell number (GOLDMAN 1976; LANGMAN et al. 1975).

DAVISON and DOBBING (1968) have presented a general sequence of neurologic development which is supportive of the rationale for longitudinal studies, a concept that has been advocated by RODIER (1978) and others. They list four primary stages. Stage I is primarily in utero and is defined as the time of organogenesis and neuronal proliferation. Stage II is referred to as the "growth spurt" and is divided into axonal and dendritic growth, and glial proliferation and myelinization. This stage is primarily postnatal. Stage III refers to the mature brain, while stage IV is the period of senile regression. The rat's central nervous system approximates that of a mature adult at about 4 weeks of age, having attained a rich behavioral repertoire by this age (RUDY and CHEATLE 1977). These investigators maintain that, although the timing may vary among species, the sequence is the same. They summarize a comparative chronology of brain growth. They conclude that parturition is irrelevant when considering exposure times; neuronal growth and development timing should be the basis for treatment times (DAVISON and DOBBING 1968; WEISS 1976).

SHERWOOD and TIMIRAS (1970) indicated that the rat brain is relatively undifferentiated at birth. They maintained that the critical period in brain maturation is during the first 21 postnatal days as opposed to other mammals, where the analogous critical period occurs in utero. They asserted that the early period of brain development occurs from postnatal days 1 to 10, and that day 21 marks a transition period to slower functional maturation, with adult levels being attained by 39 days of age. They observed shifts in nuclei and in fiber tracts during this period. They showed that myelinization was almost nonexistent at 10 days of age, although the first signs of myelinization occurred at 2 days of age in the spinal cord (WATSON 1903). Myelinization was largely present by 3 weeks of age, although adult levels were not attained until after 39 days of age (JACOBSON 1963; SHERWOOD and TIMIRAS 1970; WAGNER and GAVOUTTE 1963). These studies were completed from a neuroanatomist's point of view and may be disputed by embryologists. BIRCH

(1974) has cautioned against too specific an interpretation of the structure–function relationship. Of importance is the subtle interplay of the environment with nervous tissue, and the constantly altering relationship among the sense systems which in turn involve the development of the entire sensory organizational interrelationship.

The sequence of the mouse brain stem development has been reviewed by FRIEDE (1975). The time of origin of nuclei is from fetal days 10 to 13, with completion by day 14; cranial motor nuclei originate somewhat earlier, while cochlear nuclei appear later. The nuclei of the mouse cerebral cortex appear about day 13, with deeper nuclei appearing earlier and more superficial ones later (ANGEVINE and SIDMAN 1962). Autoradiographic studies indicate cellular activity on day 15 (LANGMAN et al. 1975). In general, corticogenesis occurs within 1 week, and is essentially completed by parturition (ANGEVINE and SIDMAN 1961; GOLDMAN 1976; HICKS and D'AMATO 1968). Thalamic nuclei "arrive" from days 10 to 15 (mean = 13) in the mouse (ANGEVINE 1970). Nuclei of the hypothalamus have a high level of proliferative activity on day 15 (LANGMAN et al. 1975). The hippocampal nuclei are present by day 12.5 (ANGEVINE 1965), although some nuclei are not present until later. Nuclei in other areas of the central nervous system "arrive" as late as postnatal day 20 (HINDS 1966). Autoradiographic analyses indicate that prenatal day 15 is a peak period for cellular activity in a number of other areas, including the corpus striatum, olfactory areas, amygdala, and other areas of the midbrain. Peak periods of activity for the dentate gyrus and olfactory bulbs occur on fetal day 19 and postnatal day 3 respectively (LANGMAN et al. 1975). BAYER and ALTMAN (1974) have shown that 85% of the granule cells in the dentate gyrus are of postnatal origin; 45% of which are present within the first week, with other small granule cells appearing during the second week.

Cerebellum nuclear origin in rodents occurs between prenatal days 10 and 15, with some granule cells and small cells appearing as late as the second week of postnatal life (ALTMAN 1967; FRIEDE 1975). LANGMAN et al. (1975) have observed positive labeling in mice on prenatal day 19 and postnatal day 3. ALTMAN et al. (1971) stated that, in the rat, most of the cerebellar cortex, including primary basket, stellate, and granule cells, is formed after birth, with neurogenesis ending by postnatal day 21. Purkinje cells are formed prenatally (CLARK et al. 1970). The development and structure of the cerebellum have been described extensively. Its cytoarchitecture and circuit patterns have been described more precisely than any other subsystem. Two important reviews are those of ALTMAN (1975) and GOLDMAN (1976). The former describes in detail the development of the rat cerebellum. The latter emphasizes the interrelationship of structure and function, the neuronal basis of behavioral development, and the biologic constraints among species cencerning when and what features of the environment will be effective stimuli.

A number of studies have been completed, comparing humans and rats, concerning areas of the brain most responsible for specific functions (MAES 1979). Although there are many differences between the two, there are also many interspecies similarities, some of which are: visual discrimination, associated with the occipital region (GLONING et al. 1968); maze learning with the hippocampus and subthalamus (MEIER and STORY 1967; MILNER et al. 1968); aggressiveness with the septal area (ZEMAN and KING 1958; ZBINDEN 1979); locomotor alterations with the cerebellum (SYPERT and ALVORD 1975); and somnolence with the lateral hypothalamus (SANO et al. 1970).

A number of agents have been shown to cause alterations in central nervous system cytoarchitecture. Agents which interfere with central nervous system cellular proliferation include vitamin A (excess), 5-fluorodeoxyuridine, methylazoxymethanol, hydroxyurea, colcemid, viruses, and zinc (deficiency) (LANGMAN et al. 1975). Prenatal and postnatal nutritional deficiencies, such as protein malnutrition, affect anatomic, physiologic, biochemical, and behavioral growth and development (RESNICK et al. 1979). X-irradiation can cause a reduction in cerebellar cell number during infancy and adulthood (ALTMAN and ANDERSON 1971 a). Alterations in exercise in mice during the late postnatal period can also alter cerebellar morphology (PYSH and WEISS 1979). Changes in the environment can cause morphological alterations. Enriched environments have caused behavioral changes which have been correlated with a heavier cerebral cortex, increased cholinesterase activity, and altered brain amines (ROSENZWEIG 1971). Environmental experience during early life in monkeys also has been correlated with altered cerebellar Purkinje cell structure (FLOETTER and GREENOUGH 1979).

THOMPSON (1978) has completed an extensive study of the relationship of behavioral alterations to anatomic changes in the central nervous system. His results indicate that no single structure is solely and individually responsible for the expression of a given behavior or response. Instead, a specific group of nuclei are involved in each response. It is a combined activity, and this multiple involvement partially explains the phenomenon of extensive recovery following brain damage. He observed that some types of behavior were more susceptible to interference by brain damage than others, that no deficits are unique to the neocortex, and that cortical processes do not necessarily take precedence over subcortical processes in the performance of any learned activity (OAKLEY 1971; BJURSTEN et al. 1976; NORTON 1978). He rejected the "center" concept as misleading, and preferred the theory of the combined activity of a number of areas (THOMPSON 1978). MYERS (1974) has agreed, stating that a particular area of the brain is not necessarily the center for a specific function, although it may be important as a link in the system. He replaced the work "center" with "primary monitoring zone."

LYNCH (1976) has discussed the "distance effect." Alterations may occur in brain areas far removed from the lesion site, contributing more significantly to behavioral alterations than the loss of neural tissue would indicate. It therefore becomes increasingly difficult to interpret behavioral changes simply from local brain damage (ISSACSON 1976). However, it has been established that some areas of the brain are more directly involved than others in the expression of certain behaviors, although the localization–nonlocalization controvery continues (THOMPSON 1978). Unique syndromes associated with specific brain areas suggest that no two brain areas are identical in their functional roles. There is no consensus concerning the relationship of specific behavioral syndromes to damage to a specific area o f the brain, since a great deal of contradictory evidence exists. Many variables influence the behavioral outcome of local brain damage. There is currently general agreement that discrete behavioral functions depend upon nuclear groups which may be dispersed throughout the nervous system (LURIA 1966; THOMPSON 1978). Multiple species must be used to elucidate areas of disagreement. MYERS (1974) has pointed out that "to accept or reject a hypothesis about an integrated function on the basis of one species alone is anatomically foolhardy."

Specific areas of the central nervous system control specific functions, within the context of the interaction of multiple centers: the limbic system mediates emotional experience and behavior; vision is the province of the retinogeniculo striate system (THOMPSON 1978); thermoregulation occurs in the rostral portion of the hypothalamus; the ascending brain stem reticular system regulates attention and arousal; and the medial forbrain bundle system controls reward and pleasure (MYERS 1974; THOMPSON 1978). The lateral hypothalamus seems to be related secondarily to a number of functions, from influencing heart rate and blood pressure, respiration, temperature control, and feeding behavior, to motor response, learning, motivational levels, and many other activities. The amygdala also appears to subserve other primary centers by contributing to the control and/or alteration of emotionality, aggression, drinking and feeding, autonomic activity, sexual behavior, etc. (MYERS 1974; THOMPSON 1978).

The brain has considerable structural redundancy, which further complicates the interpretation of the structure–function interrelationship. The redundancy may explain why normal function can occur during structural damage, how compensatory "learning" occurs following brain damage, and why behavioral deficits change with age (NORTON 1978; RODIER 1978).

With all these variables, the functional, i.e., behavioral, tests are extremely important as they allow observation of the intact organism, where invasive techniques may be impractical or impossible. The basic concept is that physical, chemical, and biologic alterations underlie functional changes. Behavioral testing may prove to be more sensitive in detecting anomalous development, owing to central nervous system redundancy, duplication, and compensatory mechanisms. Behavioral testing adds dimension for obtaining the most precise information concerning the action of a toxic substance on the exposed organism (NORTON 1978).

## C. Variables in Behavioral Teratologic Testing

### I. Examples of Behavioral Teratogens

Many environmental variables can affect an organism's response to a situation. Clinical studies have related cerebral palsy, mental retardation, and various vision and motor problems to maternal complications during pregnancy (JOFFE 1969). Behavioral problems in offspring have also been related to maternal stress (ARCHER and BLACKMAN 1971), smoking (BUTLER and GOLDSTEIN 1973), nutrition (HARREL et al. 1955), and socioeconomic status (STOTT 1957).

There are many agents which can be classified as behavioral teratogens, based on experimental studies. Such agents include intrauterine infections (DUDGEN 1973), pesticides and pollutants (MILLER 1974; SHARDEIN 1976; SPYKER and SMITHBERG 1971; SPYKER and SMITHBERG 1972; SPYKER et al. 1972; WOGAN 1976a, b), psychotropic drugs (DESMOND et al. 1969), tranquilizers (CLARK et al. 1970; HOFFIELD et al. 1968; WERBOFF 1970; WERBOFF and HAVLENA 1962), salicylates (BUTCHER et al. 1972; SHARDEIN 1976), barbiturates (ARMITAGE 1952), methazoxymethanol (Ciofalo et al. 1971; Langman et al. 1975; Rabe and Haddad 1972), hormones (Joffe 1969; Sara and Lazarus 1974; Schapiro 1971), and radiation (Furchgott and Echols 1958; Langman et al. 1975; Wallace and Altman 1970). Myers (1974) has presented a table of 42 chemicals which have caused behavioral alterations among five species when given at specific sites in the brain. Dietary deficiencies (Dobbing and Smart 1973; Patel et al. 1973; Simonson et al. 1971; Smart and Dobbing 1971 a, b; Tachibana 1979; Wehmer and Hafez 1975; Young 1964; Zemanof et al. 1968; Zeman 1970; Zimmerman and Zimmerman 1972), as well as vitamin excesses (Butcher et al. 1970) are also behavioral teratogens.

## II. Premating and Prenatal Variables

There are a number of prenatal variables which must be considered in the design of a behavioral teratologic study. The species to be used in the study is one variable (Barlow and Sullivan 1975; Coyle et al. 1976). Stanton (1978) has suggested that there are several factors to be considered when selecting a species as a model: (a) the rate of intrauterine development and maturation, as there is great variation among species, both functionally and morphologically; (b) the degree of neonatal adaptation; and (c) maternal characteristics. The choice of a species is also dependent upon the tests to be used and the sophistication of the results desired, as well as the timing of the treatment. Growth spurts and resultant "vulnerable periods" of systems such as the central nervous system vary among species (Altman 1970). Mice and rats have similar developmental chronologies, but may react differently when given identical treatment (Thompson and Olian 1961), as may rabbits and rats (Velayuhan 1974).

Once a species is chosen, the strain of the animal must be considered. Animals can be selected on the basis of specific morphological, functional, and behavioral characteristics (Broadhurst 1960; Ward 1980; Yanai 1979). There are also individual differences which may be based in part on the experience of previous generations (Coyle et al. 1976). Postnatal behavioral and morphological development and maturation are determined not only by the interaction of the individual's genetic constitution with its immediate environment, but also by the experience of previous generations; a phenomenon referred to as "the nongenetic transmission of information" (Denenberg and Rosenberg 1967). This influencing factor has been documented in studies of the effects of psychotropic drugs through three generations (Gauron and Rowley 1971, 1973), as well as in handling and stress studies (Becker and Kowell 1977; Denenberg and Whimbey 1963; Wehmer and Hafez 1975; Wehmer et al. 1970). Rearing conditions, a possible cause of prenatal stress, and maternal health are also variables which must be controlled (Broadhurst 1960; Meisel et al. 1979; Politch and Herrenkohl 1979; Thompson 1957; Ward and Weisz 1980; Young 1964).

The type of agent used is a variable owing to the nature and mechanism of its action. An agent may alter behavior in one or a combination of actions, such as mutation, chromosomal aberration, interference or alteration of nucleic acid synthesis, alterations in production and/or availabilities of enzymes, substrates or precursors, and changes in cellular metabolism or membrane permeability (Coyle et al. 1976). Other drug-related variables include drug dosage, method of administration, and time of treatment; i.e., the developmental stage of the organism at the time of exposure (BARLOW and SULLIVAN 1975; COYLE et al. 1976; SPYKER and AVERY 1976). Restriction of exposure to the period of embryogenesis is inadequate for behavioral teratologic studies. Agents may affect different aspects of brain development at various stages. Rats, mice, and rabbits can be affected from day 6 through weaning (BARLOW and SULLIVAN 1975). Other varibles include the duration of exposure and individual sensitivity (COYLE et al. 1976).

## III. Postnatal Variables

Many postnatal variables, mostly environmental, must be considered in behavioral studies. The organism's behavior is affected by the size of the litter. AKUTA (1979) has shown that preweaning litter size and postweaning group size differentially affect various aspects of open-field behavior, while ROBINSON (1976) reported similar findings using the T-maze (ROBINSON 1976). Growth rates and maturation vary with litter size. Although there is still disagreement as to what extent behavior is altered, several investigators have reported altered emotionality related to litter size in mice and rats (CARLSON 1961; DENENBERG 1961; LORE and AVIS 1970; MILKOVIC et al. 1976; PRIESTNALL 1973; SEITZ 1954).

Rearing conditions, including lactation, nesting behavior, or general maternal care, such as recognition of pups and their normality (MEIER and SCHULTZMAN 1968; READING 1966), as well as nutritional status exert a behavioral influence on the offspring (MISANIN et al. 1979). Other rearing conditions include temperature, humidity, noise level, lighting, cage size and design, diet, handling procedures, cage cleaning procedures, and animal husbandry techniques, as well as other laboratory routines (BARLOW and SULLIVAN 1975; BRAIN and BENTON 1979; COYLE et al. 1976; DENENBERG 1961; EINON and MORGAN 1978; JENSH et al. 1976; RESNICK et al. 1979; SHERROD et al. 1977; WILL et al. 1979).

Several investigators have shown that the mother's behavior is interrelated with offspring behavior (BELL 1979; GRAHAM and LETZ 1929; SALES 1979). As a result the concept of fostering has developed. SPYKER and AVERY (1976) have stated that fostering procedures may not be required for an initial screening procedure, depending upon the study objectives. SPYKER (1975) does state, however, that it may be desirable to eliminate the maternal variable through such a procedure. Therefore, groups must include fostered (within experimental and control groups), cross-fostered (across groups), and nonfostered offspring, as the results must account for possible effects of the fostering procedure itself. RODIER (1978) has pointed out that this is often impractical. She stated that there are alternatives, such as fostering only to control mothers, depending on the information the investigator needs to derive from the experiment. Fostering is not necessary if the sole conclusion required is the risk of hazard of a given treatment. She further stated that the fostering procedure is not necessary until there is some evidence that an offspring is affected by a suspect agent. BARLOW and SULLIVAN (1975) offered another alternative, mixed fostering. In this instance, all offspring of various groups are fostered in a mix within litters to mothers of a single type, with appropriate identification procedures. Although initially complicated, this procedure does offer a cost-effective balance.

The experience of grandmothers appears to be a variable (CLARK et al. 1970; COYLE et al. 1976; SHARDEIN 1976). There are also well-documented paternal effects on perinatal and postnatal alterations in offspring (FRIEDLER 1974; FRIEDLER and WHEELING 1979; JOFFE 1979). The experience of the offspring itself during infancy can affect its development and maturation. Frequent handling has been shown to alter reactivity to stress (LEVINE et al. 1967) as well as emitionality and learning (LEVINE and BOADHURST 1963). Enriched environments also affect behavior (ROSENZWEIG 1971). The sex of the offspring is a behavioral variable. Females and males have been shown to be differentially reactive as a function of the agent (HUGHES and SPARBER 1978; HUTCHINGS et al. 1979; MEIER and SCHULTZMAN 1968; WERBOFF et al. 1962), as well as age (SCHULTZE 1976; VALLE and BOLS 1976). Some sex differences are apparently due to cyclic rhythms (BIRKE et al. 1979), although YANAI (1979) has also shown sex differences in the morphology of the rat brain.

There are variables which relate to the testing procedure itself; test conditions, criteria, and the time of day during which the animals are tested (MAYERSBACH 1979; WOOD and ROSE 1979). The time span between exposure and testing may affect test results. As RODIER (1978) has stated, as the time between exposure and evaluation increases, so does the impingement of a progressively greater number of variables (RODIER 1978). Another variable which has been shown to affect test results is the organism's age at the time of testing (MARSHALL and BERVIOS 1979; NIEMI and THORPSON 1980; SCHULTZE 1976). Finally, one of the most subtle variables is the "experimenter effect"; i.e., the unconscious bias that an investigator may bring to the test environment by previous knowledge of the animal's individual history (JOHNSON 1976). The effects must be accounted for in the design, procedures, and protocol, and in the analysis of the results of the experiment.

## D. Postnatal Assessment

Evaluation of an organism during postnatal life can be classified into three areas. The first area is anatomic and includes weights and weight gain, and morphological measures, including gross and microscopic analysis. The second area is biochemical assessment. Changes in body chemistry is a result of exposure to an agent are measured, e.g., permanent alterations in 5-hydroxytryptamine (5-HT), noradrenaline, and dopamine due to prenatal exposure to methylamphetamine and chlorpromazine (TONGE 1973a, b), or the effects of stress on 5-HT levels (BLISS et al. 1972).

The third area of analysis is behavioral evaluation, which is essentially a functional profile of the organism. BARLOW and SULLIVAN (1975) have emphasized that this area must include physical and functional development to avoid misinterpretation of complex behaviors. SIMONSON et al. (1969) have divided the testing procedures into four areas; anatomic development, reflex appearance, neuromotor function, and social interaction. BARLOW and SULLIVAN (1975) maintained that data acquisition must include weights, anatomic development, reflex development, sensory maturation, strength and motor coordination, endocrine status, sexual maturation, and physiologic parameters such as blood pressure, heart rate, and respiratory rate, as well as behavioral evaluations. They realize that such a complete analysis is often impractical and unrealistic, especially with a large population. However, the very nature of a behavioral screening procedure requires a large sample size.

IRWIN (1968), in an attempt to attain maximal information in minimal time, devised a comprehensive systematic assessment procedure. According to IRWIN, the advantages to the methodology are that it can be learned quickly, has good interobserver and intraobserver consistency, and produces 52 separate items of information on each animal (mouse) within 3 min. One of the limitations to the procedure, however, is that much of the information, gathered at one time point, is of a similar nature, providing a narrow base.

STEHOUWER and CAMPBELL (1978) stated that habituation and sensitization are among the most primitive forms of learning, and may be the substructure for many other evolutionarily more complex learning processes. Therefore, they contend that these parameters should be a major consideration in the behavioral test procedure. The investigators stated that mammalian tests should meet three requirements: (1) the response should be easily and readily elicitable; (2) the responses and stimuli should be well defined; (3) the underlying neuronal circuitry should be known. They have used forelimb flexor withdrawal in their studies as it fulfills these criteria, and its developmental sequence correlates with the development of the spinal cord regarding increase in size and number of synaptic contacts (STEHOUWER and CAMPBELL 1978; STELZNER 1971).

Behavioral studies are further complicated by age dependency. Not only is there great variation with respect to rates of attainment and levels of competence at a given age among organisms, but these indices also fluctuate within the individual according to the age at which testing is initiated (BIRCH 1974). Currently, a wide variety of tests are being used. Most of these are being administered to offspring within the first 30–40 days of postnatal life, the majority involving reflex development, motor coordination, and locomotor activity (Buelke-Sam and KIMMEL 1979). BARLOW and SULLIVAN (1975) indicated that, in general, the most useful type of test for a screening procedure is one that will measure several types of behavior in a short period of time, e.g., open-field, rather than one behavioral characteristic over a long period of time, e.g., conditioned avoidance response.

Since no single test provides a comprehensive behavioral assessment of an organism, difficulties arise in selecting from the wide variety of tests available. BUELKE-SAM and KIMMEL (1979) suggested that, when designing a multitest screen, the protocol should include tests which can indicate toxicity at an early age through such parameters as reflex development, physiologic landmarks, growth patterns, etc. The tests should be easily correlated with physical or functional deficits later in life. The combined analysis of behavioral, morphological, and functional data will lead to more complete interpretation. SPYKER (1975) suggested that test series should include: (a) morphology and physical characteristics; (b) growth and growth rates; (c) specific responses such as reflexes and sensory–motor capacities; (d) activity levels; (e) neuromotor ability; (f) learning measures; (g) measures of emotionality; (h) motivational factors; (i) Sexual development; (j) psychopathologic behavior related to the central nervous system; and (k) physiologic rhythms.

A number of investigators have developed and refined batteries of tests, attempting to create a screening procedure which maximizes information retrieval and minimizes cost and time-and-effort input (ALTMAN et al. 1971; ALTMAN and SUDARSHAN 1975; BRUNNER et al. 1978; DEMERS and KIROUDC 1978; FOX 1965; JENSH 1980; VORHEES et al. 1978; ZAGON and MCLAUGHLIN 1978). Each of these batteries has limitations and omissions. There is no agreement concerning a standardized battery. The Committe on Postnatal Evaluation of Animals Subjected to Insult during Development, funded by the U.S. National Institutes of Health, was set up with the specific goals of determining whether there was a battery of behavioral tests which could be universally agreed upon and, if so, to determine what would be the consequences of the use of such a battery. The Committee developed an approach to such a screening procedure, but it was careful to state that this was only one recommended approach (KIMMEL 1977).

This chapter describes the more commonly used tests which have been utilized, either singly or as part of a behavioral test battery. The tests most often employed will be described in greater detail. The tests have been divided into two catagories: physical development, and behavioral analyses. The behavioral analyses section has been further divided into four catagories: (1) reflex development tests; (2) motor and coordination tests; (3) spontaneous or nonforced behavioral tests; and (4) forced behavioral tests. These catagories have been designed as an aid to the reader only, and do not represent an inviolable classification.

## I. Physical Development

The time of initiation of observation and the time at which the physical parameter is achieved varies with the investigator. Differences are related to the techniques employed to make the assessments. Times presented here serve only as guides. Primary sources should be consulted for the technique utilized and the criteria that were established by the investigator.

### 1. Pinna Detachment

Observations may be initiated on postnatal day 1 or 2; detachment usually occurs between days 3 and 4 (JENSH 1980; KIMMEL 1977; VORHEES et al. 1979b).

### 2. Incisor Eruption

Observations may start as early as day 1 or as late as day 6 or 7. Criterion is usually considered to be achieved with the eruption of both upper and lower incisiors. Superior maxillaries erupt by day 11, while inferior maxillary tooth eruption is completed by day 13. Tooth eruption should be completed during the second week (KIMMEL 1977; LAPOINTE and NOSAL 1979; VORHEES et al. 1979b).

### 3. Eye Opening

This test may commence from days 10 to 14. Criterion is generally considered to be achieved when both eyes of all littermates are open. Criterion is usually achieved by day 16 (JENSH 1980; KIMMEL 1977; LAPOINTE and NOSAL 1979; VORHEES et al. 1979b).

### 4. Ear Unfolding and Opening

Occurs on day 19, which coincides with achievement of sensory reaction (LAPOINTE and NOSAL 1979).

### 5. Testes Descent

May be observed on day 25 (KANDEL 1976).

### 6. Vaginal Opening

May be observed on day 30 (KANDEL 1976).

### 7. Development of Fur

Occurs approximately on day 17 (LAPOINTE and NOSAL 1979).

## II. Behavioral Analyses

### 1. Reflex Development Tests

Some of these reflexes include complex motor activity.

a) Crossed Extensor

The crossed extensor is a reflex that occurs during the first week. This reflex should disappear by day 6 (LAPOINTE and NOSAL 1979). The test consists of pinching the dorsal surface of the hindpaw and noting flexion of the stimulated limb and extension of the contralateral hindlimb (ZAGON and MCLAUGHLIN 1978).

b) Flexor Dominance

This primitive reflex also should disappear during the first 10 days, usually on day 10 (KANDEL 1976).

c) Rooting Reflex

This is also a primitive reflex which should cease about day 10 (KANDEL 1976).

d) Limb Withdrawal

In this test, the animal is suspended in a harness and the withdrawal response of the forelimb to a shock is amplified and recorded. Response intensity and rate are evaluated at different ages and as a function of treatment (STEHOUWER and CAMPBELL 1978; STELZNER 1971).

e) Forelimb Placing

The dorsal aspect of the forelimb is lightly brushed against an object. A positive response is a flexion of the limb and a placing of the paw (RODIER 1978). Achievement varies from day 4 (FOX 1965) to 5 (LAPOINTE and NOSAL 1979). SIKOV et al. (1960) have scaled this response in their studies of the effects of X-irradiation on neural development (SHIMADA and LANGMAN 1970).

f) Hindlimb Placing

The same procedure is used as in forelimb placing (RODIER 1978). FOX (1965) observed a positive reflex as early as day 6, but LAPOINTE and NOSAL (1979) did not record a positive response until day 11.

g) Forelimb and Hindlimb Grasp

LAPOINTE and NOSAL (1979) have separated the grasp reflex from the placing reflex. The forelimb grasp reflex occurs about day 11. The hindlimb grasp reflex occurs at a variable time, but at greater than 21 days of age in the rat.

h) Suckling Ability

This reflex becomes evident on day 2 (LAPOINTE and NOSAL 1979).

i) Tail Hang

ZAGON and MCLAUGHLIN (1978) described this reflexive behavior as a twisting flexion of the torso in an attempt to elevate the head when the animal is held by the tail during the 15-s trial period.

j) Vibrissae Stroking

Vibrissae are stroked alternately on each side for 10 s with a cotton swab. A turn toward the swab in an attempt to grasp it is considered a positive response (ZAGON and MCLAUGHLIN 1978).

k) Ear Twitch

This reflex response occurs about 18 days of age (LAPOINTE and NOSAL 1979).

l) Tail Pinch

The tail of the animal is pinched, inducing a consummatory reaction. ANTELMAN and SZECHTMAN (1975) states that this is a highly reliable test in which a positive response is eating, gnawing, or licking in 98% of trials following a 20-s pinch on the tail with a foam-rubber-tipped hemostat. The intensity is minimal, does not cause vocalization, and does not appear causally related to pain mechanisms. It is dependent upon brain dopamine levels. Other investigators have used different procedures with similar results (ANTELMAN and SZECHTMAN 1975; KOOB et al. 1976).

m) Tremors

A reflexive motor spasm normally not present, tremors have been observed from prenatal treatment on day 15 with 5-azacytidine as well as with X-irradiation (BRUNNER and ALTMAN 1973; LANGMAN et al. 1975).

n) Surface Righting

This test consists of placing the offspring in a supine position and determining its ability to turn over and place all four feet on the surface. A time limit of about 2 s for each trial is usually imposed. This test is generally initiated on postnatal days 1 or 2. Criterion varies, but often is considered to be achieved on the day when all members of the entire litter achieve positive responses in three of three trials, generally about days 9 to 11. There is great variation among investigators concerning criterion levels (ALTMAN and SUDARSHAN 1975; BRUNNER et al. 1978; DEMERS and KIROUDC 1978; KIMMEL 1977; LANGMAN et al. 1975; LAPOINTE and NOSAL 1979; RODIER 1978; RODIER et al. 1979; VORHEES et al. 1979a, b; YAMAZAKI et al. 1960; ZAGON and MCLAUGHLIN 1978).

o) Air Righting

During this test, the animal is held by its limbs or body in a supine position a variable distance (20–60 cm) above a flat surface and then released. A positive response is indicated when the animal lands on all four feet. Testing is usually initiated between days 12 and 14. Criterion is the attainment of a positive response in three of three daily trials for all members of the litter (day 16–19), although there is much variation in criterion levels among investigators (ALTMAN and SUDARSHAN 1975; BRUNNER et al. 1978; DEMERS and KIROUDC 1978; KIMMEL 1977; LAPOINTE and NOSAL 1979; RODIER 1978; RODIER et al. 1979; SMART and DOBBING 1971b; WERBOFF et al. 1961; ZAGON and MCLAUGHLIN 1978).

p) Auditory Startle

There is great variability in the design of the auditory startle test. In some instances a stabilimeter, located in a sound-attenuated room, has been used to measure the reflex jerk reaction to the sound of an automobile horn, while other designs are more simplistic, using a variety of sound devices. Trials are initiated about day 7, with positive criterion being attainment of a positive response by the entire litter (about day 14–18) (BRUNNER et al. 1978; KIMMEL 1977; LAPOINTE and NOSAL 1979; VORHEES et al. 1979b; ZAGON and MCLAUGHLIN 1978).

q) Negative Geotaxis

This procedure tests the reflex ability of the animal to turn away from gravity when placed on an inclined plane. The incline angle varies from 25° to 45°, as does the time allowed for the animal to make the 180° turn (generally 15–30 s). The number of daily trials ranges from one to five, but criteria are usually considered to be attained at the entire litter level. Positive response is generally achieved from day 9–11 (ALTMAN and SUDARSHAN 1975; DEMERS and KIROUDC 1978; LAPOINTE and NOSAL 1979; RODIER 1978; VORHEES et al. 1979a).

r) Visual Placing

Usually initiated about day 16; the rat is held by the tail and lowered toward a horizontal bar or taut rope, care being taken to avoid vibrissae touching. A positive response is recorded when the animal reaches toward the bar or rope. Generally at least two trials a day are given. Criterion is achievement of positive responses by the entire litter (about 16–24 days, as there is great variability) (KIMMEL 1977; LAPOINTE and NOSAL 1979; VORHEES et al. 1979b).

s) Vibrissae Placing

This procedure is similar to the previous one, except that the vibrissae touch the object. There is a great deal of variation in procedural design among investigators. Achievement of a positive response occurs at about 12 days of age (LAPOINTE and NOSAL 1979).

t) Cliff Avoidance

During this test, the animal is placed at the edge of a table or other surface, and its reaction within a specified time limit is observed. Turning or backing away from the edge is a positive response. The test is started on day 1–4; criterion is a positive response by all littermates, about day 8 (ALTMAN and SUDARSHAN 1975; BRUNNER et al. 1978; DEMERS and KIROUDC 1978; LAPOINTE and NOSAL 1979; RODIER 1978; VORHEES et al. 1979b; ZAGON and MCLAUGHLIN 1978).

u) Pain Reflex Reaction

The hindpaws are grasped with forceps and reaction is observed for 10 s. Alternate paws are stimulated each day. A rotation or withdrawal of the paw constitutes a positive response (ZAGON and MCLAUGHLIN 1978).

v) Olfactory Reflex

Cedar oil and warm chocolate have been used to test the offspring's reaction to olfactory stimulation. A positive response is the turning of the head toward the stimulus (ZAGON and MCLAUGHLIN 1978).

## 2. Motor and Coordination Tests

These tests primarily include forced, complex activities.

a) Bar Holding

The ability of a rat to hold onto a bar first occurs about day 16, depending on the test conditions (LAPOINTE and NOSAL 1979).

b) Forelimb Hanging

This test may be considered an extension of the previous test. The animal's ability to hang, the length of time it does hang, and its activity while hanging are observed (RODIER 1978; WERBOFF et al. 1962).

c) Visual Orientation

This test consists of passing a white cardbord square (1.0 × 1.0 cm) with black vertical bands, through the visual fields at a 10-cm distance, five times in either direction. Tracking of the head in the direction of the stimulus constitutes a positive response (ZAGON and MCLAUGHLIN 1978).

d) Inclined Plane

The ability of an animal to remain on an inclined plane is tested by placing the animal on an incline of about 25° for 30 s, and increasing the angle of incline at discrete time intervals until the animal cannot maintain its position. The angle of the inclined plane at this point is a measure of motor skill (ABEL and DINTCHEFF 1978; RODIER 1977; SPYKER 1975; SPYKER and AVERY 1976; WECHKIN et al. 1961).

e) Rotarods

This test can be initiated as early as 20 days of age in the rat, although it is commonly administered during adult life. A drum of variable diameter (10–20 cm) is rotated at about 4 rpm. The rotation speed is increased until the rat falls off the drum. When the increase in velocity is controlled, the time interval from start until the animal falls becomes a measure of motor ability. Usually the animals are previously exposed to the drum during a nontest trial. This basic test has many variations. Generally, rats do not achieve minimal levels until at least 21 days of age, but comparisons among investigators are difficult, owing to the variety of experimental conditions (ABEL and DINTCHEFF 1978; KIMMEL 1977; RODIER 1978; SPYKER and AVERY 1976; VORHEES et al. 1979b).

f) Parallel Bars

This test is one of many variations requiring the animal to walk a narrow ledge or ledges. Alterations can be made in the thickness of the parallel rods, texture, and distance between them (RODIER 1978).

g) Ascending Wire Mesh

A 13-mm wire mesh 31 cm long is placed in a container of water at a 75° angle. The rat is placed with its hind quarters and tail in the water. The rat must climb to the top of the mesh within 30 s. LAPOINTE and NOSAL (1979) listed achievement age as day 13 for a similar screen climb test, however the variety of test methodologies compromise comparisons. A variation of this test is the "vertical grid" test; 6.5-mm wire mesh may be used. The rat is given ten trials; five trials when it is placed on the grid head down and five trials with its head up. The grid may also be rotated to add a further variant (ALTMAN and SUDARSHAN 1975; DEMERS and KIROUDC 1978; LAPOINTE and NOSAL 1979; SPYKER 1975).

h) Ascending a Vertical Rod

A 17-mm diameter wooden rod is placed in the center of a container filled with 15 °C water. A platform is placed at the top, 22.5 cm above the surface of the water. The rat is placed at the base of the rod and must climb to the platform within 180 s. A variant of this procedure is the use of a rope in place of a rod, as well as varying the time criterion (ALTMAN et al. 1971; BRUNNER and ALTMAN 1973; RODIER 1978).

i) Clinging to and Descending a Vertical Rope

A 15-mm diameter rope is held taut in a vertical position. The rat is placed at the top of the rope and must descend the rope to a sawdust-filled box at the bottom.

Distance traveled, time limitation, cling time, and frequency of falling can be monitored (ALTMAN et al. 1971).

j) Swimming

A tank of variable size, filled with water at about 27 °C, is used. A platform is placed at one end of the tank. The animal is placed at the opposite end of the tank and must swim to the platform. Swimming behavior and swimming time are observed and recorded. A series of 10–20 trials with no intertrial interval (ITI) constitutes one test session. There are several variations to this procedure, and the age at which the test is given may vary from as early as postnatal day 6 to well into adulthood (BRUNNER et al. 1978; Jensh 1980; Rodier 1978; Schapiro et al. 1970; SPYKER 1972; VORHEES et al. 1979b).

## 3. Spontaneous or Nonforced Behavior Tests

These tests may include some motor evaluations.

a) Spontaneous Motor Behavior

In this type of test, the animal is generally placed in an open area and observed for a number of motor characteristics. In one test, the animal was placed on a cloth-covered table top and observed for 2 min/day for the following 11 parameters; (1) unilateral head turning with no return; (2) head turn right and return; (3) head turn left and return; (4) raising of the head; (5) pivoting less than 360°; (6) pivoting more than 360°; (7) simultaneous movement of the head and forelimbs; (8) simultaneous movement of the forelimbs and hindlimbs; (9) simultaneous movement of the head, forelimbs and hindlimbs; (10) crawl with forward movement; (11) walking–forward, with abdomen raised above the surface (ZAGON and MCLAUGHLIN 1978).

b) Head Elevation

This motor skill is generally first observed on the second postnatal day, and consists of keeping the head raised above the surface. The activity decreases, and then increases at about day 10. The first day of increase of this behavior during half of the 1-min observation time is generally recorded (ALTMAN and SUDARSHAN 1975; DEMERS and KIROUDC 1978; RODIER and REYNOLDS 1977).

c) Head Pointing

This action consists of raising the head more than 45°, and is recorded on the first day the activity is observed at least once (ALTMAN and SUDARSHAN 1975; DEMERS and KIROUDC 1978).

d) Hindlimb Elevation

Occurring during the second half of the second week, this action involves lifting of the hindlimbs and pelvis during at least half of the 1-min trial time (ALTMAN and SUDARSHAN 1975; DEMERS and KIROUDC 1978).

e) Rearing

This action occurs during the second and third weeks. Related to this observational test are tests which include: (a) elevation of the head, which first appears on the second day of postnatal life, decreases, then peaks at about day 10; (b) elevation of the forelimbs and shoulders during the first week; and (c) elevation of the hindlimbs and pelvis during the second half of the second week (ALTMAN and SUDARSHAN 1975; DEMERS and KIROUDC 1978; RODIER and REYNOLDS 1977).

f) Pivoting

This activity involves circular movements with no forward or backward propulsion. Observations are generally made once daily from days 2 to 12, and for a discrete length of time. The number of 90° turns, as well as the relative time spent turning, can be recorded. This activity normally disappears early in the second week (ALTMAN et al. 1971; ALTMAN and SUDARSHAN 1975; BRUNNER et al. 1978; DEMERS and KIROUDC 1978; KIMMEL 1977; LANGMAN et al. 1975; RODIER 1978; SHIMADA and LANGMAN 1970; VORHEES et al. 1979 b).

g) Gait

Walking patterns can be easily observed. Analysis can be judgmental or can involve inking of the footpads with different colors and measuring the angles and changes in stride (LANGMAN et al. 1975; MULLENIX et al. 1975; SPYKER and AVERY 1976).

h) Crawl

This activity begins during the second week and consists of forward motion with no elevation of the trunk (ALTMAN et al. 1971; ALTMAN and SUDARSHAN 1975; DEMERS and KIROUDC 1978; VORHEES et al. 1979 b).

i) Walk

Walking action commences about day 12 and consists of forward motion with forelimbs and hindlimbs fully supporting a raised trunk (ALTMAN et al. 1971; ALTMAN and SUDARSHAN 1975; DEMERS and KIROUDC 1978; VORHEES et al. 1979 b).

j) Backward Walking

This type of motor activity is rarely seen in adults, and may be considered aberrant behavior. It has been observed in animals treated with methylmercury (RODIER 1978; SPYKER 1972).

k) Grooming

This multiple activity includes the use of the head, tongue, and forelimbs by the animal in the process of cleaning various parts of the body (RODIER 1977).

l) Circling Behavior

This is an aberrant form of behavior which occurs owing to an imbalance of the nigrostriatal pathways on each side. The animal rotates toward the less-stimulated side. This test can be automated using a rotometer which records full left and right turns separately as a function of time (THIEBOT and SOUBRIE 1979).

m) Sleeping and Somnolence

The time spent sleeping or showing the inclination to sleep, i.e., drowsiness, an activity associated with the lateral hypothalamus, can be observed (SANO et al. 1970; THOMPSON 1978).

n) Hopping

This activity involves the animal's ability to raise its entire body off the surface, with a slight forward movement (RODIER 1978).

o) Home Cage Emergence

This test consists of observing the time required for the animal to emerge from or leave its home cage (RODIER 1978).

p) Resistance to Handling

The animal's negative reaction to being handled, including vocalization, is observed in this more subjective test. A scoring system can be adopted. Results may be interpreted as a function of the emotional state of the animal, although such interpretations should be made cautiously. As with many subjective tests, there is a high degree of variability associated with this test (RODIER 1978).

q) Feeding

Feeding behavior can be monitored during a given trial period. In one study, rats were placed in a dimly lit isolation area, exposed to white noise, and were observed from behind a window. Food pellets (300 g) were scattered over a dense layer of wood shavings or placed in a 15-cm diameter cup. The animal was deprived of food before testing. Generally, one 15-min test a day was given. The test was repeated several times. The animal was scored for feeding latency (time to start feeding) and total eating time. Other feeding behaviors observed included digging, scanning (rearing but not sniffing), sniffing walls, sniffing litter, sniffing food, sniffing while walking, walking or running to food, walking or running away from food, dropping food, transporting food, and other general activities, grooming, sitting, etc. (MAES 1979).

r) Undisturbed Behavior

This test is completed without disturbing the animals (home cage) and consists of observing general types of activity. The test, generally 1–4 min, may be repeated as many as nine times a day at 1-h intervals during the preweaning period, and can consist of recording the number of pups nursing, the number of pups with the mother, the number of pups not nursing, pups with other pups, and pups alone. Such home cage studies may also include observations of fedding behavior, grooming, investigative bahavior of familar surroundings (ecotaxis), and social interaction (CAUL et al. 1979; NORTON 1976).

s) Spontaneous and General Activity

Spontaneous activity may be monitored during the preweaning period. Generally, specific ages are chosen, such as at 5 and 10 days of postnatal life, and activities such as pivoting, crawling, walking, rearing, etc., are monitored during a 5-min test period. Spontaneous activity also may be monitored automatically using an activity meter. One such meter is a rocker platform to which microswitches are attached. The home cage can be put on the platform and the general activity of the animal can be recorded as a function of the number of times the microswitches are activated. Animals may be monitored throughout the day or for a predetermined time span. This type of test has usually been used when the animal is several months old. Another type of activity meter makes use of infrared beams. The monitoring principles are the same for both types of meters. Other general activity (see individual behaviors previously discussed) can be monitored at various ages and for specific lengths of time (ALTMAN and SUDARSHAN 1975; BARLOW and SULLIVAN 1975; BORNSCHEIN et al. 1980; DEMERS and KIROUDC 1978; LASKY et al. 1977; MAES 1979; RODIER et al. 1979; VELAYUHAN 1974; VORHEES et al. 1978).

t) Nose Poke

This novel test has been developed more recently. At 29 days of age, the rat was placed in a lightproof, sound-attenuated chamber. On one wall was a small hole to which a cylinder was attached on the outside. If the head poked into the hole, an infrared beam was broken, activating a counter and timer. Frequencies and duration of pokes during each 60-s trial could be measured (RILEY et al. 1979).

u) Head Dip

This test consists of placing the rat in an isolation chamber in which there are four holes in the floor. Cylinders extend outside the chamber from each hole. Light, food, or other objects may be introduced in some of the cylinders. If the head dips 1.5 cm into the hole, an infrared beam is broken, and frequencies and duration may be recorded for each hole entered during the trial period (RILEY et al. 1979).

v) Step-Down Test

In this test, the animal is placed on a small platform which is elevated above a grid floor. Five trials are given, during which the time taken for the rat to step down onto the floor is recorded. The last three trials are averaged as a score for this test (LASKY et al. 1977).

w) Thirst Test

This exploratory test has been proposed as a screening test. The rat is deprived of water overnight and then placed in an unfamiliar cage for one 5-min trial on two successive days. During the trial period, motor activity is recorded as the number of pauses in 1 min, including rearing and sniffing, and the time taken to find water. The first drink of greater than 10 s, or time to take the first ten licks may also be recorded (A. P. SILVERMAN 1978).

### x) Maternal Behavior

Maternal behavior in the preweaning cage has been used as a nonforced test. Behaviors recorded include pup retrievals, grooming, nursing, and pup contacts. This observational test generally is of 5 min duration and may be repeated ad libitum (CAUL et al. 1979). A variation of this test records the development of maternal behavior. In this test, a young adult female is placed in a cage and four 3–5-day-old pups are presented in front of the cage for 15 min, then left with her for 1 h. Observations are made on the basis of pup-oriented versus nonoriented behavior. The former include pup sniffing, any contact behavior, nest building, pup carrying, and crawling over the pups, while the latter include several activities such as grooming, rearing, sitting, eating, and drinking (MAYER et al. 1979; MAYER and ROSENBLATT 1979).

### y) Open-Field

This test is one of the most widely used behavioral tests. There are more technical variations to this norforced behavioral test than any other test. The basic structure is an enclosed area divided into a grid pattern of equal subunits into which the animal is placed. The animal is observed for a specified period of time and scored for a number of variables such as the number and distribution of squares (or subunits) entered, number of rearings, number of sniffings, number of urinations, and number of fecal boli. The field has varied in size and shape from square to circular and been subdivided into squares or concentric rings of equal size. It consists of wood, plexiglass, wallboard, etc., illuminated with various light sources and commonly painted black or gray. Trials may be conducted for various time periods from 2 min on one day only to several trials of 15 min or more over many days. This test is generally given to adult animals, although some investigators have tested rodents shortly after weaning. The test results indicate the degree of activity in a novel environment and emotionality. This test has some inherent difficulties. The area must be clean, as there is a definite "predecessor effect". Extraneous influences yield high levels of variability. Some activities are age dependent, i.e., defecation, and sex dependent, i.e., general activity. Finally, the general conditions of the test are important since the behavior observed is the result of a combination of curiosity, i.e., active behavior, and fearfulness, i.e., inhibitory behavior (ALTMAN et al. 1971; AULICH and VOSSEN 1978; BARLOW and SULLIVAN 1975; BOND and DIGIUSTO 1977; CANDLAND and CAMPBELL 1962; CAUL et al. 1979; CHAPMAN and STERN 1979; CLARK et al. 1970; COYLE et al. 1976; DENENBERG 1969; FURCHTGOTT et al. 1968; JENSH et al. 1978a, 1979, 1980a, c; LASKY et al. 1977; LEYLAND et al. 1979; NORTON 1978; ORDY et al. 1966; RABE and HADDAD 1972; RODIER 1978; RUSSELL and CHALKLY-MABER 1979; SPYKER 1975; SPYKER and AVERY 1976; VORHEES et al. 1979a, b).

### z) Activity Wheel

This is one of the oldest and most commonly used quantitative tests of nonforced activity. The unit generally consists of a vertical activity wheel, to which a counter is attached, and from which a door leads to a small cage. Test conditions vary greatly among investigators, from single 10-min trials to trials which may last from

1 day to several weeks with variable access to the cage. Access to food and water are also manipulated. This test is generally conducted on adult animals, but most investigators avoid using females, since their activity is correlated with their estrous cycle. Data are generally analyzed on the basis of the number of revolutions in each unit of time (BORNSCHEIN et al. 1980; HOFFIELD et al. 1968; JENSH et al. 1978a, 1979, 1980a, c; NORTON 1976; RODIER 1978; VORHEES et al. 1979b).

## 4. Forced Behavioral Tests

These tests primarily include learning skills. The term "learning" can be defined as a relatively permanent change in behavior which occurs because of previous experience (BARLOW and SULLIVAN 1975). It is a rather vague concept, therefore many investigators prefer to speak in terms of performance. Learning, or performance, is influenced by many factors, one of which is motivation. The motivational state is often erroneously referred to as emotionality. Motivational state is dependent upon the interaction of the individual's experiential history, genetic makeup, and immediate environment, including the minute-by-minute reactivity and responsiveness of that individual (RODIER 1978). MOGENSON (1977) has defined motivation as an unsatisfactory word which "refers to a heightened level of consciousness or arousal resulting from alterations in central nervous system activity and usually accompanied by responses of the whole animal in its external environment (behavioral changes)." He further characterized motivated behavior according to five criteria; purposive (goal-oriented), adaptive, self-regulatory, persistent, and periodic. It can be influenced by such factors as thermoregulation, hunger, thirst, emotion, sleep–wake rhythms, hormones, etc. Many reviews are available, including discussions concerning the place of operant learning techniques in teratology (MOGENSON 1977; WEISS 1976).

### a) Mazes

A wide variety of mazes exists, each of which demands a specific set of tasks (e.g. BOLLIES and WOODS 1964; BARLOW and SULLIVAN 1975; CLARK et al. 1970; HADDAD et al. 1969; LANGMAN et al. 1975; NORTON 1976; RODIER 1978). Following are some of the more commonly used mazes. The conditions of the reinforcement, as well as light, texture of the reinforcer, and other discriminative stimuli vary considerably among investigators:

*α) T-Maze.* Of variable size, the T-maze is generally constructed of wood, plexiglass, metal, or other suitable material, painted a neutral color such as gray or black. The maze has one long stem with a right and left arm. The rat is usually deprived of food for 24 h preceding the text period and then trained in the T-maze to choose the correct side (food pellets are present) to a specific criterion level, e.g., 85% correct choices during several testing days. Rats may be trained as early as 24 days of age. Retesting for retention varies greatly. In addition, the number of errors, latency time, and retracing errors can be recorded. Generally 1–3 tests/day are given, each test comprising 1–20 or more trials. Maze learning is related to hippocampal activity (BUTCHER et al. 1973; CLARK et al. 1970; JENSH et al. 1978a, 1979, 1980a; MILNER et al. 1968; PETERS 1979; RODIER 1978; THOMPSON 1978; VOR-

HEES et al. 1979a). VORHEES et al. (1978b) have designed a modified T-maze, which incorporates the home cage environment, as well as a double-ended T-maze for appetitive position discrimination. One variant of this maze is the water T-maze, in which the animal swims to escape from the water. An advantage of this maze is that no preconditions, such as food deprivation, are necessary. It has also been used for shape and brightness discrimination tests using circles versus triangles and white versus black (THOMPSON et al. 1979; ZENICK et al. 1978). In 1939, BIEL designed a multiple water T-maze which had six choice points. Animals were pretrained in a simple T-maze and then given two daily sessions of four trials each. Animals can be given this test as soon as the eyes of each member of the entire litter are open (ABEL 1979; BIEL 1939).

*β) Y-Maze.* This maze is generally composed of three symmetrical equidistant arms. It can be completely automated and can be used in a variety of avoidance and reward tests (CAUL et al. 1979; FOX et al. 1977; KIMMEL 1977).

*γ) Hebb–Williams Maze.* This maze requires the use of somatokinesthetic and visual cues for the animal to maneuver around barriers to locate a reward. It is valuable, in that scoring can be of a graded variety by adjusted the difficulty of the problems presented. It is insensitive to subjective differences in food motivation and emotionality, and requires extensive pretraining (CELEBON and COLOMBO 1979; HEBB and WILLIAMS 1946; RODIER 1978; WEHNER and HAFEZ 1975).

*δ) Lashley III Maze.* This is a spatial learning test in which running time and error counts are used to judge learning capacity (RODIER 1978; SPYKER 1975).

*ε) Olton Maze.* This eight-arm radial maze is used to observe and score the strategy the animal uses in investigating each arm. The animal is usually given one or more pretrials, followed by a test trial in which the number of reward as well as nonreward arms entered, is recorded. A variety of situations and criteria can be devised (RODIER et al. 1979).

### b) Operant Conditioning Tests

The major types of tests used, several brief comments about them, and references which may be reviewed by the reader for more detailed description are listed. The majority of tests have been conducted on young adults. These tests are generally not used by behavioral teratologists as they are complex, the equipment is expensive, and the protocols require extensive pretraining (autoshaping) (HUGHES and SPARBER 1978; HUTCHINGS et al. 1973; RODIER 1978; WALKER and FURCHTGOTT 1970; WOGAN 1976a, b).

*α) Bar-(Lever-)Press.* In this test, the animal is trained to press a bar for which it will receive a reward, usually food or water. Many variations can be incorporated, involving test intervals, bar-press pressure, sound, and light (CLARK et al. 1970; FALK 1969; FOWLER et al. 1962; HUGHES and SPARBER 1978; HUTCHINGS et al. 1979).

*β) Avoidance Testing.* Avoidance tests can incorporate a number of shock schedules. The strength and quality (a.c. or d.c.) of the shock are variables which must be taken into account when designing the test (DIETER 1976; LAWRY et al. 1978). It is important to describe the type of current, a.c. or d.c., the amperage, and the voltage, to describe fully the nature of the shock being administered. One of the most commonly used tests is the active avoidance or conditioned avoidance response (C.A.R.) test. An automated shuttle box is used, in which the animal is generally presented with a sound and/or a light stimulus for a given period of time. The animal must move to the opposite side of the shuttle box in order to avoid being shocked. One crossover, either avoidance or escape (after being shocked) constitutes one trial. Generally, a series of trials are given daily for several consecutive days. A variety of schedules or environmental conditions may be used to test short-term or long-term memory. Several variations to the design of the shuttle box are also available (ABEL 1979; HARRIS and CASE 1979; JENSH 1980a; JENSH et al. 1978a, 1979, 1980a; NIEMI and THORPSON 1980; RODIER 1977a; RODIER et al. 1979; TAMAKI and IHOUYE 1976; TAMAKI et al. 1976; VORHEES et al. 1979a, b; YEN-KOO et al. 1978).

The passive avoidance response test is the opposite of the previous test. In this instance, the animal is punished (shocked) for showing a particular bevavior. The animal shows a behavior spontaneously or is taught to elicit a behavior. It is then punished for that response and is scored on the basis of decreasing responsiveness (extinction). Pretraining may take as little as 1 day, depending on the schedule and variables being used (RODIER 1977; RODIER et al. 1979; VORHEES et al. 1979a, b). A modified passive avoidance test, which requires no previous training sessions, has been developed for use with the mouse by GLICK (1976). This test takes advantage of spontaneous locomotor activity. An open-field area is divided into four quadrants. Each quadrant is separately wired. Initial locomotor activity can be measured by the number of quadrants entered. Passive avoidance can be evaluated by giving a shock to the animal each time it attempts to move to another quadrant during a second trial (GLICK 1976). KIMMEL (1977) has also developed an open-field modified passive avoidance test (KIMMEL 1977). Alterations in active and passive avoidance performance have been reported to be associated with hippocampal lesions (RODIER, 1977, 1978).

*γ) Discrimination Reversal Learning*. This test is of limited value within the context of this chapter, since it requires extensive acquisition of learning to control for fear responses to novelty, and for emotionality (WEHMER and HAFEZ 1975; ZIMMERMAN and ZIMMERMAN 1972). Several other tests have been used, including the latch box test (THOMPSON et al. 1979), the brightness discrimination test (CARLSON 1961), and the jump-up escape/avoidance test (BORNSCHEIN et al. 1980). Tests also have been devised for sleep alteration (SHARDEIN 1976; KIYONO et al. 1973), as well as mating behavior (KIYONO et al. 1973; SHARDEIN 1976), and aversion (RUDY and CHEATLE 1977).

## E. Conclusions

This chapter is concerned with the multidisciplinary science of behavioral teratology. The relationship between function and morphology, testing procedures, and variables which must be considered when designing protocols have been presented.

It is unrealistic to expect that a single test or a few tests can evaluate central nervous system function in a comprehensive manner. The central nervous system is unlike any other organ system in its multiplicity of functions and complexity of organization. Such a system requires multiple analyses, since the pattern of results of a comprehensive behavioral assessment procedure permits a degree of localization of damage within the organism.

A battery of tests provides a comprehensive study of maturational and behavioral assessments. The results of such testing procedures will alter many present concepts of tetratogenic activity, and will necessitate the reevaluation of concepts applied to the human condition (SHARDEIN 1976). The use of a battery of tests also aids in the correlation between structure and function. It has been difficult to make such correlations, as RODIER (1978) pointed out, since: (a) lesions are seldom restricted to one specific area; (b) cellular development and migration in various areas occur at differing and overlapping times; (c) fetal and neonatal response to a lesion may differ from the adult; (d) the extent of structural damage may not directly relate to the severity of functional damage; and (e) some areas of the central nervous system have greater reparative powers than others (RODIER and REYNOLDS 1977b; RODIER 1978).

Behavioral testing is not meant to be totally sufficient, either as an apical testing technique, such as in screening procedures, or as the sole method for understanding the mechanisms of behavior modification. The full tetratogenic profile of a suspect agent inculdes prenatal, perinatal, and postnatal analyses of morphological, physiologic, biochemical, and behavioral parameters.

Specific tests to be adopted for use with any suspect agent must be carefully chosen. At the present time, standardization of test procedures is of paramount importance. It has been shown that testing techniques may vary so greatly as to obviate the comparison of results from different investigators. The individual researcher must presently choose the behavioral tests most suited to the experimental design. The investigator needs to have access to a standardized procedure for each of the chosen tests, including experimental protocols, construction designs, techniques, past results, and interpretative implications and limitations.

Behavior has been broadly defined as the action or reaction of an organism within its environment. Behavioral testing is a method of observing and quantitating the responses of an organism. Interpretation of those responses and the significance of the behavioral activity rely on the testing system. The validity of each test depends upon its reproducibility, and therefore standardization. The acquisition of behavioral data, coupled with other approaches, histologic, biochemical, etc., can provide a more complete profile of the tetratogenic activity of a suspect agent.

## References

Abel EL (1979) Prenatal effects of alcohol on adult learning in rats. Pharmacol Biochem Behav 10:239–243

Abel EL, Dintcheff BA (1978) Effects of prenatal alcohol exposure on growth and development in rats. J Pharmacol Exp Ther 207:916–921

Akuta T (1979) Effects of rearing conditions on the behavior of mothers and on the offspring in the mouse. Jpn J Psychol 50:73–81

Altman J (1967) Postnatal growth and differentiation of the mammlian brain, with implications for a morphological theory of memory. In: Quarton GC (ed) The Neurosciences. Rockefeller Press, NY, pp 723–743
Altman J (1970) Postnatal neurogenesis and the problem of neural plasticity. In: Himwich WA (ed) Developmental Neurobiology. CC Thomas, Chicago, p 197
Altman J (1975) Effects of interference with cerebellar maturation on the development of locomotion. In: Buchwald ND, Brazier MA (eds) Brain mechanisms in mental retardation. Academic Press, New York, p 41–91
Altman J, Anderson WJ (1971) Irradiation of the cerebellum in infants rats with low-level x-ray: Histological and cytological effects during infancy and adulthood. Exp Neurol 30:492–509
Altman J, Sudarshan K (1975) Postnatal development of locomotion in the laboratory rat. Anim Behav 23:896–920
Altman J, Anderson WJ, Strop M (1971) Retardation of cerebellar and motor development by focal x-irradiation during infancy. Physiol Behav 7:143–150
Altman PL, Katz DD (eds) (1979) Inbred and genetically defined strains of laboratory animals. I. Mouse and rat. Federation of American Society of Experimental Biology, Bethesda, Md
Angevine JB Jr (1965) Time of origin in the hippocampal region. Exp Neurol [Suppl] 2:1–70
Angevine JB Jra (1970) Time of origin in the diencephalon of the mouse. An autoradiographic study. J Comp Neurol 139:129–188
Angevine JB, Sideman RL (1961) Autoradiographic study of cell migration during histogenesis of cerebral cortex in the mouse. Nature 192:766–768
Angevine JB Jr, Sideman RL (1962) Autoradiographic study of histogenesis in the cerebral cortex of the mouse. Anat Rec 142:210 A
Antelman SM, Szechtman H (1975) Tail pinch induces eating in sated rats which appears to depend on nigrostriatal dopamine. Science 189:731–733
Archer JE, Blackman DE (1971) Prenatal psychological stress and offspring behavior in rats and mice. Dev Psychobiol 4:193
Armitage SG (1952) The effects of barbiturates on the behavior of rat offspring as measured on leaning and reasoning situations. J Comp Physiol Psychol 45:146
Aulich D, Vossen JMH (1978) Behavioral conflict in two strains of rat: home cage preference versus dark preference. Behav Proc 3:325–334
Barlow SM, Sullivan FM (1975) Behavioral teratology. In Berry CL, Poswillo DE (eds) Teratology: trends and applications. Springer, Berlin Heidelberg New York, pp 103–120
Barnett SA (1975) The rat: A study in behavior. Chicago Press, Chicago
Bayer SA, Altman J (1974) Hippocampal development in the rat: cytogenesis and morphogenesis examined with autoradiography and low-level x-irradiation. J Comp Neurol 157:55–80
Becker A, Kowell M (1977) Crucial role of the postnatal maternal environment in the expression of prenatal stress effects in the male rat. J Comp Physiol Psychol 91:1432–1446
Bell RW (1979) Ultrasonic control of materal behavior: developmental implications. Am Zool 19:413–418
Biel WC (1939) The effects of early inanition on a developmental schedule in the albino rat. J Comp Phychol 28:1–15
Birch HG (1974) Some ways of viewing studies in behavioral development. Pre- and postnatal development of the human brain. Mod Probl Paediatr 13:320–329
Birke LIA, Andrew RJ, Best SA (1979) Distractibility change during the oestrous cycle of the rat. Anim Behav 27:597–601
Bjursten LM, Horrsell K, Norrsell U (1976) Behavioral repertory of cats without cerebral cortex from infancy. Exp Brain Res 25:115–130
Bliss EL, Thather W, Ailion J (1972) Relationship of stress to brain serotomin and 5-hydroxyindoleacetic acid. J Psychiatr Res 9:71
Bolles RC, Woods PJ (1964) The ontogeny be behavior in the albino rat. Anim Behav 12:427–441
Bond N, DiGiusto E (1977) Open-field behavior a function of age, sex, and repeated trials. Psychol Rep 41:571–574

Bornschein RL, Hastings L, Manson JM (1980) Behavioral toxicity in the offspring of rats following maternal exposure to dichloromethane. Toxicol Appl Pharmacol 52:29–37
Brain P, Benton D (1979) The interpretation of physiological correlates of differential housing in laboratory rats. Life Sci 24:99–116
Broadhurst PL (1960) Experiments in psychogenetics: applications of biometrical genetics to the inheritance of behavior. In: Eysenk HJ (ed) Experiments in personality, vol 1. Routledge & Kegan Paul, London, p 1
Brunner RL, Altman J (1973) Locomotor deficits in adult rats with moderate to massive retardation of cerebellar development during infancy. Behav Biol 59:169–188
Brunner RL, McLean M, Vorhees CV, Butcher RE (1978) A comparison of behavioral and anatomical measures of hydroxyurea induced abnormalities. Teratology 18:379–384
Buelke-Sam J, Kimmel CA (1979) Development and standardization of screening methods for behavioral teratology. Treatology 20:17–30
Butcher RE, Brunner RL, Roth T, Kimmel CA (1970) A learning impairment associated with maternal hypervitaminosis-A in rats. Life Sci 2:141–145
Butcher RE, Vorhees CV, Kimmel CA (1972) Learning impairment from maternal salicylate treatment in rats. Nature 237:211–212
Butcher RE, Scott WJ, Kazmaier K, Ritter EJ (1973) Postnatal effects in rats of pretreatment with hydroxyurea. Teratology 1:161–165
Butcher RE, Hawver K, Burbacher J, Scot W (1975) Behavioral effects antenatal exposure to teratogens. In: Ellis NR (ed) Aberrant development in infancy; human and animal studies. Erlbaum, Hillsdale, NJ, pp 161–167
Butler HR, Goldstein H (1973) Smoking in pregnancy and subsequent child development. Br Med J 4:573
Candland DK, Campbell BA (1962) Development of fear in the rat as measured by behavior in the open-field. J Comp Physiol Psychol 55:593–596
Carlson PV (1961) The development of emotional behavior as a function of didactic mother-young relationships. Ph.D. thesis, Purdue University
Caul WF, Osborne GL, Fernandez K, Henderson GI (1979) Open-field and avoidance performance of rats as a function of prenatal ethanol treatment. Addict Behav 4:311–322
Celebon JM, Colombo M (1979) Effects of chlordiazepoxide on maze performance of rats subjected to undernitrition in early life. Psychopharmacologie 63:29–32
Chapman RH, Stern JM (1979) Failure of severe material stress on ACTH during pregnancy to effect emotionality of male rat offspring; implications of litter effects for prenatal studies. Dev Psychobiol 12:255–267
Ciofalo VB, Latranyi M, Taber RI (1971) Effect of prenatal treatment of methylazoxymethanol acetate on motor performance, exploratory activity, and maze learning in rats. Commun Behav Biol 6:223–226
Clark CVH, Gorman D, Vernakakis A (1970) Effects of prenatal administration of psychotropic drugs on behavior of developing rats. Dev Psychobiol 3:225–235
Coyle I, Wayner MJ, Singer A (1976) Behavioral teratogenesis: a critical evaluation. Pharmacol Biochem Behav 4:191–200
Davison AN, Dobbing J (eds) (1968) Applical neurochemistry. FA Davis, Philadelphia
Demers M, Kiroudc A (1978) Prenatal effects of ethanol on the behavioral development of the rat. Physiol Psychol 6:517–520
Denenberg VH (1961) Effects of early social experience on emotionalmotivational organization. Am Psychol 16:403
Denenberg VH (1969) Open-field behavior in the rat: What does it mean? Ann NY Acad Sci 159:852–859
Denenberg VH, Rosenberg KM (1967) Nongenetic transmission of information. Nature 216:549
Denenberg VH, Whimbey AE (1963) Behavior of adult rats is modified by the experiences their mothers had as infants. Science 142:1192
Desmond MM, Rudolph AJ, Hull RM, Clagtion JL, Dresser PR, Burghoff I (1969) Behavioral alterations in infants born to mothers on psychoactive medication during pregnancy. Farrell A (ed) Congenital mental retardation. University of Texas Press, Austin, P 235

Dieter S (1976) Continuity and intensity of shock in one-ray avoidance learing in the rat. Anim Learn Behav 4:303–307
Dobbing J, Smart JL (1973) Early undernutrition, brain development and behavior. In: Barnett SA (ed) Ethology and development. W Heinemann, London, p 16
Dudgen JA (1973) Chairman's summary. Intrauterine infections. Ciba Found Symp 10:200
Einon DF, Morgan MJ (1978) Early isolation produces enduring hyperactivity in the rat, but no effect upon spontaneous alteration. Q J Exp Psychol 30:131–156
Falk JL (1969) Drug effects on discriminative motor control. Physiol Behav 4:421–427
Floetter MK, Greenough WT (1979) Cerebellar plasticity: modification of purkinje cell structure by differential rearing in monkeys. Science 206:227–229
Fowler H, Hicks SP, D'Amato CJ, Beach FA (1962) Effects of fetal irradiation on behavior in the albino rat. J Comp Physiol Psychol 55:309–314
Fox KA, Abendschein DR, Lahcen RB (1977) Effects of benzodiazepines during gestation and infancy on Y-maze performance of mice. Pharmacol Res Commun 9:325–338
Fox WM (1965) Reflex-ontogeny and behavioral development of the mouse. Anim Behav 13:234–241
Friede RL (1975) Developmental neuropathology. Springer, Berlin Heidelberg New York, 1–524
Friedler G (1974) Morphine administration to male mice: effects on subsequent progency. Fed Proc 33:515
Friedler G, Wheeling HS (1979) Behavior effects in offspring of male mice injected with opioids prior to mating. Pharmacol Biochem Behav 11:23–28
Furchtgott E (1973) Behavioral effects of ionizing radiation: 1955–1961. Psychol Bull 60:167–199
Furchtgott E, Echols M (1958) Activity and emotionality in pre- and neonatally x-irradiated rats. J Comp Physiol Psychol 51:541–545
Furchtgott E, Taiken RS, Draper DO (1968) Open-field behavior and heart rate in prenatally x-irradiated rats. Teratology 1:201–206
Gauron EF, Rowley VN (1971) Cross-generational effects resulting from an early maternal chronic drug experience. Eur J Pharmacol 15:171
Gauron EF, Rowley VH (1973) Effects on offspring behavior of parental early drug experience and cross-fostering. Psychopharmacology (Berlin) 30:269
Glick SD (1976) Screening and therapeutics. In: Glick SD, Goldfarb J Behavioral pharmacology. CV Mosby, St Louis, pp 339–361
Gloning IK, Gloning K, Hoff H (1968) Neuropsychological symptoms and syndromes in lesions of the occipital lobe. Gauthier-Vallays, Paris
Goldman PS (1976) Maturation of the mammalian nervous system and the ontogeny of behavior. In: Rosenblatt JS, Hind RA, Shaw E, Beer C (eds) Advances in the study of behavior, vol 7. Academic Press, New York, pp 2–91
Graham M, Letz R (1929) Within-species variation in the development of ultrasonic signaling of preweanling rats. Dev Psychobiol 12:129–136
Haddad RK, Rube A, Laqeur GL, Spitz M, Valsamis P (1969) Intellectual deficit associated with transplacentally induced microcephaly in the rat. Science 163:88–90
Harned BK, Hamilton HC, Borrus JC (1940) The effect of bromide administration to pregnant rats on the learning ability of offspring. Am J Med Sci 200:846
Harrel RF, Woodyard LS, Gates RL (1955) The effects of mothers diets on the intelligence of offspring: A study of the influence of vitamin supplimentation of the diets of pregnant and lactating women on the intelligence of their children. Teachers College, Columbia University, New York
Harris RA, Case J (1979) Effects of maternal consumption of ethanol, barbital, or chlordiazepoxide on behavior of the offspring. Behav Neural Biol 26:234–247
Hebb DO, Williams KA (1946) A method of rating animal intelligence. J Genet Psychol 34:59
Hicks SP, D'Amato CJ (1968) Cell migration to the isocortex in the rat. Anat Rec 160:619–634
Hinds JW (1966) Autoradiographic study of histogenesis in the olfactory bulb and accessory olfactory bulb in the mouse. Anat Res 154:358–359

Hoffield DR, McNew, Webster RL (1968) Effect of tranquillising drugs during pregnancy on activity of offspring. Nature 218:357–358

Hughes JA, Sparber SB (1978) d-amphetamine unmasks postnatal consequences of exposure to methylmercury in utero: Methods for studying behavioral teratogenesis. Pharmacol Biochem Behav 8:365–375

Hutchings DE, Gibbon J, Kaufman MA (1973) Maternal vitamin A excess during the early fetal period: effects on learning and development in the offspring. Dev Psychobiol 6:445–457

Hutchings DE, Towey JP, Gorinson HS, Hunt HF (1979) Methadone during pregnancy: assessment of behavioral effects in the rat offspring. J Pharmacol Exp Ther 208:105–112

Irwin S (1968) Comprehensive observation assessment: 1a. systematic quantitative procedure for assessing the behavioral and physiologic state of the mouse. Psychopharmacology (Berlin) 13:222

Isaacson RL (1976) Experimental brain lesions and memory. In: Rosenzweig MR, Bennett EL (eds) Neural mechanisms of learning and memory. MIT Press, Cambridge MA, pp 521–543

Jacobson S (1963) Sequences of myelinization in the brain of the albino rat. A cerebral cortex, thalamus, and related structures. J Comp Neurol 121:5–29

Jensh RP (1980) Behavioral tetatology: application to low dose chronic microwave irradiation studies. In: Persaud TUN (ed) Advances in the study of burth defects, vol 4. Neural and behavioralteratology. International Medical, London, pp 135–162

Jensh RP, Vogel WH, Brent RL (1976) The teratologic and postnatal behavioral effects on rat offspring of maternally restricted food and water and isolution. Teratology 13:26 A

Jensh RP, Ludlow J, Weinberg I, Vogel WH, Rudder T, Brent RL (1978 a) Studies concerning the postnatal effects of protracted low doese prenatal 915 MHz microwave irradiation. Teratology 17:21 A

Jensh RP, Magaziner A, Sattel AB, Vogel WH (1978 b) Interactions among postnatal behavioral test results in rats exposed to multiple testing procedures. Teratology 17:21 A

Jensh RP, Ludlow J, Vogel WH, McHugh T, Weinberg I, Brent RL (1979) Studies concerning the effects of non-thermol protracted prenatal 915 MHz microwave radiation on prenatal and postnatal development in the rat. Digest of the XIV International Microwave Symposium, Monaco, p 99–101

Jensh RP, Ludlow J, McHugh T (1980 a) Studies concerning the effects of protracted prenatal 6 GHz microwave irradiation on pre- and postnatal development in the rat. Teratol 21(2):46 A

Jensh RP, Magaziner A, Vogel WH (1980 b) Effects of material environment and postnatal multiple testing on weanling and adult response in rat. Submitted for publication

Jensh RP, Vogel WH, Ludlow J, McHugh T, Brent RL (1980 c) Studies concerning the effects of non-thermal protracted prenatal 2450 MHz microwave irradiation on postnatal development in the rat. Teratol 21(2):46 A

Joffe JM (1969) Prenatal determinants of behavior. Int Ser Monogr Exp Psychol 7:vii–366

Joffe JM (1979) Influence of drug exposure of the father on perinatal outcome. Clin Perinatol 6:21–35

Johnson RFQ (1976) The experimenter attributes effect. A methodological analysis. Psychol Rec 26:67–78

Kandel ER (1976) Cellular basis of behavior. WH Freeman, San Francisco, p viii-727

Kimmel CA (ed) (1977) Final report of the committee on postnatal evaluation of animals subjected to insult during development. National Institute of Health, Research Triangle Park, North Caroline

Kiyono S, Tamaki Y, Ito M, Yamamura H (1973) Behavioral study on the rats from the dam treated with phenylhydrazine during pregnancy. Teratology 8:970

Koob GF, Fray PJ, Iversen SD (1976) Tail-pinch stimulation: sufficient motivation for learning. Science 194:637–639

Langman J, Webster W, Rodier P (1975) Morphological and behavioral abnormalities caused by insults to the CNS in the perinatal period. In: Berry CL, Poswillo DE (eds), Teratology: trends and applications. Springer, Berlin Heildelberg New York, pp 182–200

Lapointe G, Nosal G (1979) A rat model of neurobehavioral development. Experientia 35:205–207
Lasagna L (1979) Toxicological barriers to providing better drugs. Arch Toxicol 43:27–33
Lasky DI, Zagon IS, McLaughlin PJ (1977) Effect of maternally administered heroin on the motor activity of rat offspring. Pharmacol Biochem Behav 7:281–284
Lawry JA, Lupo V, Overmier JJ, Kochevar J, Hollis KL, Anderson DC (1978) Interference with avoidance behavior as a function qualitative properties of inescapable shocks. Anim Learn Behav 6(2):147–154
Levine S, Boadhurst PL (1963) Genetic and otogenetic determinants of behavior, II. Effects of infantile stimulation on adult emotionality and learning in selected strains of rats. J Comp Physiol Psychol 56:423
Levine S, Haltmeyer AC, Karas GG, Denenberg VH (1967) Physiological and behavioral effects of infantile stimulation. Physiol Behav 2:55
Leyland CM, Guyther RJ, Rylands JM (1979) An improved method for detecting drug effects in the open field. Psychopharmacology 63:33–37
Livingston PB (1978) Sensory, processing, perception and behavior. Raven, New York, pp vii-106
Lore R, Avis H (1970) Effects of auditory stimulation and litter size upon subsequent emotional behaviour in the rat. Dev Psychobiol 2:212
Luria AR (1966) Higher cortical functions in man. Basic Books, New York
Lynch G (1976) Some difficulties associated with the use of lesion techniques in the study of memory. In: Rosenzweig MR, Bennet EL (eds) Neural mechanisms of learning and memory. MIT Press, Cambridge, MA London, pp 544–546
Maes H (1979) Time course transition analysis of the behavioral effects of microinjection of pentobarbital and noradrenaline into the ventromedial hypothalamus of the rat. Behav Processes 4:341–358
Marshall JF, Bervios H (1979) Movement disorders of aged rats: reversal by dopamine receptor stimulation. Science 206:477–479
Mayer AD, Rosenblatt JS (1979) Ontogeny of material behavior in the laboratory rat: Early origins in 18-to-27-day-old young. Dev Psychobiol 125:407–424
Mayer AD, Freeman NCG, Rosenblatt JS (1979) Ontogeny of maternal behavior in the laboratory rat: Factors underlying changes in responsiveness from 30 to 90 days. Dev Psychobiol 125:425–439
Mayersbach HV (1979) Circadian differences in swimming performance of rats. Chronobiologia 6:130
Meier GW, Schultzman LH (1968) Mother-infant interactions and experimental manipulations; confounding or misidentification. Dev Psychobiol 1:141
Meier MJ, Story JL (1967) Selective impairment of porteus maze test performance after right subthalamotomy. Neuropsychologia 5:181–189
Meisel RL, Dohanich GP, Ward IL (1979) Effects of prenatal stress on avoidance acquisition, open-field performance, and lordotic behavior in male rats. Physiol Behav 223:527–530
Milkovic K, Paunovic J, Joffe JM (1976) Effects of pre- and postnatal littersize reduction on development and behavior of rat offspring. Dev Psychobiol 94:365–375
Miller RW (1974) How environmental effects in child health are recognized. Pediatrics 5:792
Milner B, Corkins S, Teuber H-L (1968) Further analysis of the hippocampal amnestic syndrome: 14 year follow-up study of H M. Neuropsychologia 6:215–234
Misanin JR, Hommel MJ, Krieger WG (1979) Effect of pup under-nutrition on the retrieval behavior of the rat dam. Behav Neurol Biol 2:115–119
Mogenson CJ (1977) The neurobiology of behavior: an introduction. Lawrence Erlbaum, Hillsdale, NJ, pp v-334
Mullenix BP, Norton S, Culver B (1975) Locomotor damage in rats after x-irradiation in utero. Exp Neurol 48:310–324
Myers RD (1974) Handbook of drug and chemical stimulation of the brain: Behavioral, pharmacological, and physiological aspects. Van Nostrand Reinhold Co, New York, pp vii-759

Niemi RR, Thorpson WR (1980) Pavlovian excitation, internal inhibition, and their interaction with free operant avoidance as a function of age in rats. Dev Psychobiol 131:61–76
Norton S (1976) Social behavior and activity. In: Proceedings, Workshop on behavioral toxicology. DHEW Publication No (NIH) 76-1189, U.S. Dept. Health Education and Welfare, Washington DC, pp 1–10
Norton S (1978) Is behavior or morphology a more sensitive indicator of central nervous system toxicity? Environ Health Persect 26:21–27
Oakley DA (1971) Instrumental learning in neodecorticate rabbits. Nature (New Biol) 233:185–187
Ordy JM, Samorajski J, Collins RL, Rolsten C (1966) Prenatal chlorpromazine effects of liver, survival, and behavior of mice offspring. J Pharmacol 151:110–125
Patel AJ, Balazs R, Johnson AL (1973) Effect of undernutrition on cell formation in the rat brain. J Neurochem 20:1151
Peters DP (1979) Effects of prenatal nutritional deficiency on discrimination learing in rats: acquisition and retention. Psychol Rec 44:451–456
Politch JA, Herrenkohl LR (1979) Prenatal stress reduces maternal aggression by mice offspring. Physiol Behav 23:415–418
Priestnall R (1973) The effects of littersize and post-weaning isolation or grouping on adult emotionality in C 3H mice. Dev Psychobiol 6:217
Pysh JJ, Weiss GM (1979) Exercise during development induces an increase on perkinje cells dendritic tree size. Science 206:230–231
Rabe A, Haddad RK (1972) Methyloxymethanol-induced microencephaly in rats: behavioral studies. Fed Proc 31:1536–1539
Reading AJ (1966) Effect of material environment on the behavior of inbred mice. J Comp Physiol Psychol 62:437–440
Resnick O, Miller M, Forbes W, Hall R, Kempa T, Bronzino J, Morgane J (1979) Developmental protein malnutrition: Influences on the central nervous system of the rat. Neurosci Biochem Rev 3:233–246
Riley EP, Shapiro HR, Lochry EA (1979) Nose-poking and head-dipping behaviors in rats prenatally exposed to alcohol. Pharmacol Biochem Behav 11:513–519
Robinson E (1976) The effects of littersize and crowding on position learning by male and female albino rats. Psychol Rec 26:61–66
Rodier PM (1977a) Correlations between prenatally-induced alterations in CNS cell populations and postnatal function. Teratology 162:235–246
Rodier PM (1978) Behavioral teratology. In: Wilson JG, Fraser FC (eds) Handbook of teratology, vol 4. Research procedures and data analysis. Plenum, New York, pp 397–428
Rodier PM, Reynolds SS (1977) Morphological correlates of behavioral abnormalities in experimental congenital brain damage. Exp Neurol 57:81–93
Rodier PM, Reynolds SS, Roberts WH (1979) Behavioral consequences of interferance with CNS development in the early fetal period. Teratology 193:327–336
Rosenzweig MR (1971) Effects of environment on development of brain and behavior. In: Tobach E, Aronso L, Shaw E (eds) The biopsychology of development. Academic Press, New York, p 303
Rudy JW, Cheatle MD (1977) Odor-aversion learning in neonatal rats. Science 198:845–846
Russell PA, Chalkly-Maber CJW (1979) Effects of conspecific odor on rats position and behavior in an open field. Anim Learn Behav 73:387–391
Sales GD (1979) Strain differences in the ultrasonic behavior of rats (Rattus norvegicus). Am Zool 19:513–527
Sano K, Mayanagi Y, Sekino H, Ogashiwa M, Ishejima B (1970) Results of stimulation and destruction of the posterior hypothalamus in man. J Neurosurg 33:689–707
Sarą VR, Lazarus L (1974) Prenatal action of growth hormone on brain and behavior. Nature 250:257–258
Schapiro S (1971) Hormonal and environmental influences on rat brain development and behavior. In: Sterman MB, McGinty DJ, Adinolfi AM (eds) Development and behavior, Academic Press, New York, p 307

Schapiro S, Salas M, Vukovich K (1970) Hormonal effects on progeny of swimming ability in the rat: assessment of central nervous system development. Science 168:147–150
Schultze I (1976) Sex differences in the acquisition of appetitively motivated learning in rats. Physiol Behav 17:19–22
Seitz PFD (1954) The effects of infantile experiences upon adult behavior in animals subjects: I. Effects of littersize during infancy upon adult behavior in the rat. Am J Psychiatry 110:916–927
Shardein JL (1976) Drugs as teratogens. CRC Press, Cleveland, Ohio, pp 1–291
Sherrod KB, Meier GW, Connor WH (1977) Open-field behavior of prenatally irradiated and/or postnatally handled C57BL/6 mice. Dev Psychobiol 103:195–202
Sherwood HM, Timiras PS (1970) A stereotaxis atlas of the developing rat brain. University of California Press, Berkeley London, pp 3–209
Shimada M, Langman J (1970) Repair of the external granular layer of the hamster cerebellum after prenatal and postnatal administration of methyloxy-methanol. Teratology 3:119–134
Sikov MR, Meyer JS, Resta CF, Lofstrom JE (1960) Neurological disorders produced by prenatal x-irradiation of the rat. Radiat Res 12:472
Silverman AP (1978) A behavioral test applied in an acute toxicity screen. Br J Pharmacol 63:349–350
Silverman P (1978) Animal behavior in the laboratory. Pica, New York, pp xi-409
Simonson M, Sherwin RW, Anilane JK, Yu WY, Chow BF (1969) Neuromotor development in progeny of underfed mother rats. J Nutr 98:18
Simonson M, Stephan JK, Hanson HM, Chow BF (1971) Open field studies in offspring of underfed mother rats. J Nutr 101:331
Skinner BF (1938) The behavior of organisms: an experimental analysis. Appleton Century, New York, p 6
Smart JL, Dobbing J (1971 a) Vulnerability of developing brain. II. Effects of early nutritional deprivation on reflex ontogeny and development of behavior in the rat. Brain Res 28:85–95
Smart JL, Dobbing J (1971 b) Vulnerability of developing brain. VI. Relative effects of fetal and early postnatal undernutrition on reflex ontogeny and development of behavior in the rat. Brain Res 33:303–314
Sprott RL, Staats J (1979) Behavioral studies using genetically defined mice – a bibliography (July 1976–August 1978). Behav Genet 92:87–102
Spyker JM (1972) Subtle consequences of methylmercury exposure. Teratol 5:267
Spyker JM (1975) Behavioral teratology and toxicology. In: Weiss B, Laties VG (eds) Behavioral toxicology. Plenum Press, NY, p 311–349
Spyker JM, Avery DL (1976) Behavioral toxicology and the developing organism. In: Proceedings, Workshop on behavioral toxicology. DHEW Publication No (NIH) 76–1189. U.S. Dept. Health, Educ and welfare, Washington DC, pp 95–109
Spyker JM, Smithberg M (1971) affects of methylmercury on prenatal and postnatal development in mice. Teratology 4:242–243
Spyker JM, Smithberg M (1972) Effects of methylmercury on prenatal development in mice. Teratology 5:181–190
Spyker JM, Sparber SB, Goldberg AM (1972) Subtle consequences of methylmercury exposure: Behavioral deviations in offspring of treated mothers. Science 177:621–623
Stanton HC (1978) Factors to consider when selecting animal methods for postnatal teratology studies. J Environ Pathol Toxicol 2:201–210
Stehouwer DJ, Campbell BA (1978) Habituation of the forelimb-with drawl response in neonatal rats. J Exp Psychol [Anim Behav] 42:104–119
Stelzner DJ (1971) The normal postnatal development of synaptic end-feet in the lumbosacral spinal cord and of responses in the hindlimb of the albino rat. Exp Neurol 31:337–357
Stott DH (1957) Physical and mental handicaps following a disturbed pregnancy. Lancet I:1006
Sypert GW, Alvord EC (1975) Cerebellar infarction. Arch Neurol 32:357–363

Tachibana T (1979) Effects of early undernutrition on motivation and discrimination learning in rats. Dev Psychobiol 126:539–544
Tamaki Y, Ihouye M (1976) Brightness discrimination learning in a skinner box in prenatally x-irradiated rats. Physiol Behav 16:343–348
Tamaki Y, Shoji R, Takeuchi IK, Murakami U (1976) Facilitatory effect of prenatal x-irradiation on two-way avoidance behavior in rats. Jpn Psychol Res 183:142–146
Thiebot M-H, Soubrie P (1979) Amphetamine-induced circling behavior in rats; effects of unilateral microinjections of GABA and GABA-related drugs into the substantia nigra. Brain Res 167:307–322
Thompson R (1978) A behavioral atlas of the rat brain. Oxford University Press, Oxford New York, pp vii-80
Thompson R, Gates CE, Gross SA (1979) Thalamic regions critical for retention of skilled movements in the rat. Physiol psychol 71:7–21
Thompson RF, Patterson MM, Teyler TJ (1972) The neurophysiology of learning. Annu Rev Psychol 23:73–104
Thompson WR (1957) Influence of prenatal maternal anxiety or emotionality in young rats. Science 125:698
Thompson WR, Olian S (1961) Some effects on offspring behavior of maternal adrenalin injection during pregnancy in three unbred mouse stains. Psychol Rep 8:87
Tonge SR (1973a) Permanent alterations in catecholamine concentrations in dicrete areas brain in the offspring of rats treated with methylamphetamine and chlorpromazine. Br J Pharmacol 4:425
Tonge SR (1973b) Permanent alterations in 5-hydroxyindole concentrations in discrete areas of the rat brain produced by the pre- and neonatal administration of methalamphetamine and chlorpromazine. J Neurochem 20:625
Valle FP, Bols RJ (1976) Age factors in sea differences in open-field activity of rats. Anim Learn Behav 44:457–460
Velayuhan H (1974) Prenatal exposure to drugs: Effect on the development of brain monoamine systems. In: Vernadakis A, Weiner H (eds) Advances in behavioral biology, vol 8. Drugs and the developing brain. Plenum Press, New York, pp 171–198
Vernadakis A, Weiner H (eds) (1974) Advances in behavioral biology, vol 8. Drugs and the developing brain. Plenum Press, New York, pp v-537
Vorhees CV, Brunner RL, McDaniel CR, Butcher RE (1978) The relationship of gestational age to vitamin A induced postnatal dysfunction. Teratology 173:271–276
Vorhees CV, Brunner RL, Butcher RE (1979a) Psychotropic drugs as behavioral teratogens. Science 205:1220–1225
Vorhees CV, Butcher RE, Brunner RL, Sobotka TJ (1979b) A developmental test battery for neurobehavioral toxicity in rats: a preliminary analysis using monosodium glutamate, calcium carrageenan, and hydroxyurea. Toxicol Appl Pharmacol 50:267–282
Wagner JW, Gavoutte B (1963) Relation between myelination and binding of sodium and potassium in rat brain. Proc Soc Exp Biol Med 112:42–46
Walker S, Furchtgott E (1970) Effects of prenatal x-irradiation on the acquisition, extinction, and dicrimination of a classically conditioned response. Radiat Res 42:120–128
Wallace PB, Altman J (1970) Behavioral effects of neonatal irradiation of the cerebellum. I. Qualitative observation in infant and adolescent rats. Dev Psychobiol 2:257–265
Ward JL, Weisz J (1980) Maternal stress alters plasma testosterone in fetal males. Science 207:328–329
Ward R (1980) Some effects of strain differences in the maternal behavior of inbred mice. Dev Psychobiol 132:181–190
Watson JB (1903) Animal education: an experimental study on the psychical development of white rat, correlated with the growth of its nervous system. Contrib Philosophy 4:5–122
Wechkin S, Elden RF, Furchtgott E (1961) Motor performance in the rat as a function of age and prenatal x-irradiation. J Comp Physiol Psychol 54:658–659
Wehmer F, Porter RH, Scales B (1970) Premating and pregnancy stress in rats affects behavior of grand pups. Nature 227:622

Wehner F, Hafez ESE (1975) Psychobiological aspects of fetal and infantile malnutrition. In: Hafez ESE (ed) The mammalian fetus-comparative biology and methodology. Thomas, Springfield, Ill, pp 154–188
Weiss B (1976) Operant techniques in behavioral toxicology. In: Proceedings, Workshop on behavioral toxicology. DHEW Publication No (NIH) 76–1189, U.S. DHEW, Washington DC, pp 49–66
Werboff J, Goodman I, Havlena J, Sikov M (1961) Effects of prenatal x-irradiation on motor performance in the rat. Am J Physiol 201:703–706
Werboff J (1962) Effects of prenatal administration of tranquillizers on maze learning ability. Am Psychol 17:397
Werboff J (1970) Developmental psychopharmacology. In: Clark WG, del Guidice (eds) Principles of psychopharmacology. Academic Press, New York, pp 343–354
Werboff J, Gottlieb JS (1963) Drugs in pregnancy: behavioral teratology. Obstet Gynecol Surv 18:420
Werboff J, Havlena J (1962) Postnatal behavioral effects of tranquillizers administered to the gravid rat. Exp. Neurol 6:263
Werboff J, Havlena J, Sikov MR (1962) Effects of prenatal x-irradiation on activity, emotionality, and maze learning ability in the rat. Radiat Res 16:441–452
Will B, Palland B, Ungever A, Ropartz P (1979) Effects of rearing in different environments on subsequent environmental preference in rats. Dev Psychobiol 12/2:151–160
Wogan GN (1976a) Reproduction, teratology, and human development. In: Nelson N (ed) Human health and the environment: some research needs. DHEW Publication No NIH 77-1277. U.S. D.H.E.W., Washington DC, pp 315–327
Wogan GN (1976b) Behavioral toxicology. In: Nelson N (ed) Human health and the environment: some research needs. DHEW Publication No NIH 77-1277. U.S. D.H.E.W., Washington DC, pp 329–350
Wood H, Rose SPR (1979) Changes in acetylcholinesterase with light exposure, time of day, and motor activity in the rat. Behav Neurol Biol 25:79–89
Yamazaki JN, Bennett LR, McFall RA, Clemente CD (1960) Brain radiation in newborn rats and differential effects of increased age. I. Clinical observations. Neurology (NY) 10:530–536
Yanai J (1979) Strain and sex differences in the rat brain. Acta Anat (Basel) 103: 150–158
Yen-Koo HC, Peterson KW, Balazs T (1978) Conditioned avoidance responses of young mice and offspring of mice treated with neuroleptic or mutagenic agents. J Toxicol Environ Health 4:139–145
Young RB (1964) Effect of prenatal drugs and neonatal stimulation on later behavior. J Comp Physiol Psychol 58:309
Zagon TS, McLaughlin PJ (1978) Perinatal methadone exposure and its influence on the behavioral ontogeny of rats. Pharmacol Biochem Behav 9:665–672
Zamenhof S, van Marthens E, Margolis FL (1968) DNA (cell number) and protein in neonatal brain: Alteration by maternal dietary protein restriction. Science 160:322
Zbinden G (1979) The no-effect level, an old bone of contention in toxicology. Arch Toxicol 43:3–7
Zeman F (1970) Effect of protein deficiency during gestation on postnatal cellular development in the young rat. J Nutr 100:530
Zeman W, King FA (1958) Tumors of the septum pellucidium and adjacent structures with abnormal affective behavior: An anterior midline structure syndrome. J Nerv Ment Dis 127:490–502
Zenick H, Padich R, Tokarek T, Aragon P (1978) Influence of prenatal and postnatal lead exposure as discrimination learning on rats. Pharmacol Biochem Behav 8:347–350
Zimmerman RR, Zimmerman SJ (1972) Responses of protein malnourished rats to novel objects. Percept Mot Skills 35:319

CHAPTER 11

# Behavioral Teratology: A New Frontier in Neurobehavioral Research

D. E. HUTCHINGS

## A. Introduction

Behavioral teratology represents an integration of teratology with experimental psychology, and is primarily concerned with the study of neurobehavioral changes that result from exposure of germ cells, embryos, fetuses, and immature postnatal individuals to a variety of environmental disturbances and events. Like its parent discipline, teratology, these include drugs, industrial chemicals, pesticides, food additives and preservatives, and environmental pollutants, as well as irradiation, stress, infectious agents, and endocrine and metabolic disturbances (WILSON 1973). Its major objective is the description of the behavioral effects induced by these conditions and an understanding of the embryopathic mechanisms by which they are produced. I should emphasize, however, the current state of behavioral teratology as a fledgling discipline; its subject matter remains largely unexplored and uncharted, its methodology has been uneven and occasionally wanting, and its accomplishments strike a tenuous balance between false starts and palpable inroads made by a few pioneering researchers. But despite its immaturity and tentative beginnings, there should be no doubt that it is emerging as a new scientific specialty.

The present chapter is not an exhaustive review of the behavioral teratology literature. Rather, articles have been selected from the animal research literature to elucidate principles as they apply to functional or behavioral manifestations of prenatally administered drugs of use and abuse. Clinical studies are reviewed in order to demonstrate the occurrence of similar behavioral effects in humans.

The notion that the behavior of infants and children can be affected by drugs taken by the mother during pregnancy is by no means new. GOODFRIEND et al. (1956) reviewed articles dating back to 1892 which describe opiate withdrawal in the neonate, and WARNER and ROSETT (1975) cite a medical literature beginning in the early eighteenth century which warns of increased risk of infant death, "puny" children, and mental deficiency associated with alcohol consumption during pregnancy. The term "behavioral teratology" was introduced by WERBOFF and his colleagues when they reported a series of studies, beginning in 1961, dealing with the effects on offspring of psychotropic agents administered to pregnant rats. Unlike teratology, however, this field of study was initially slow to attract many workers, and only in the last few years has begun to emerge as a well-defined research specialty with a firm theoretical identity. In fact, compared with its "parent" discipline, which has flourished vigorously in the past decade or so, behavioral teratology is just beginning to gather some significant momentum. The reasons for this prolonged gestation are complex, but probably stem in part from historical factors.

Historically, behavioral teratology goes back only about 20 years. While much of the early work can be faulted on methodological grounds, one must keep in mind that, at the time, procedural ground rules and organizing theory were lacking. In a series of three studies reported in five articles (WERBOFF and DEMBICKI 1962; WERBOFF et al. 1961 a, b; WERBOFF and HAVLENA 1962; WERBOFF and KESNER 1963) the antidepressants, iproniazid and isocarboxazid, the tranquilizers, reserpine, chlorpromazine, and meprobamate, as well as 5-hydroxytryptophan, and the benzyl analogue of serotonin, 1-benzyl-2-methyl-4-methoxytryptophan, were administered to pregnant rats at various times during pregnancy. In addition to effects on mortality and morbidity, offspring showed differences in maze-learning ability, avoidance conditioning, open-field, and inclined-plane activity, and seizure susceptibility. These impairments pointed to behavioral aspects of prenatal drug safety in humans, but stimulated little further work and attracted only a few new workers to the area (for reviews see JOFFE 1969; YOUNG 1967).

Several problems may have contributed to the apparent lack of interest. The only thing that appeared to be borrowed from the field of teratology was the name; organizing concepts were not. For example, the behavioral studies indicated that a principle of central importance in teratology, the relationship between developmental stage at the time of treatment and the nature of the effects produced in the offspring, had no relationship to the behavioral changes observed. Moreover, the agents employed were not verified teratogens in the strict sense that they could produce malformations in rats or humans. And while the studies assumed that these substances produced biochemical rather than gross morphological alterations in the developing central nervous system (CNS), neither biochemical nor histologic effects were investigated.

Second, the studies were conceived within the context of intelligent curiosity, rather than as experimental tests of specific hypotheses. While such an orientation is both appropriate and understandable as a first step, exploratory studies ultimately must generate testable hypotheses. Each report, however, appeared to end in a kind of cul-de-sac where it languished, generating few suggestions for new directions.

Other studies appeared in the latter part of the 1960s, but most largely failed to replicate the earlier work. The literature progressively became so confused that JOFFE (1969), in his critical review, could conclude only that drugs administered prenatally were capable of altering the behavior of the offspring in the absence of gross structural malformations. From an effort that spanned nearly a decade, no systematic relationship between specific kinds of drugs and specific behavioral effects in the offspring emerged.

In the early 1970s, the quality of the work improved markedly although quantity remained low. The new investigators were considerably more sophisticated about principles of teratology. They began studying agents that were known to interfere specifically with the histogenesis of the fetal CNS; experiments tended to be better controlled, and they often described the neuropathology produced by the agents. Some studies even employed behavioral assessment techniques that permitted speculation as to the implications of the behavioral findings for clinical problems in the human population. Some workers suggested that prenatal drug exposure could produce mental retardation; other emphasized the possibility of more subtle effects, such as impairment of attention and of motivation. Convincing clinical evidence to support these speculations had yet to appear, however. About this time, retrospective clinical reports began appearing in the literature, describing behavioral deviations in infants and children whose mothers had abused alcohol or the opiates, were on methadone maintenance, or had taken the anticonvulsants hydantoin or trimethadione during pregnancy. The effects varied with the drug and ranged from acute neonatal abstinence symptoms to long-term behavioral impairments that included mild to severe mental retardation. Thus, the expectations of the early workers in behavioral teratology expressed 10 years earlier, were finally being realized.

## B. Agents that Cause Gross Structural Malformation and Behavioral Effects

### I. Animal Studies and the Consideration of Critical Periods

With the exception of a few chemical agents that are of large molecular size, biotransformed into inactive metabolites by the placenta, or firmly bound to maternal tissue, most drugs in the maternal circulation readily cross the placenta and enter the embryonic and fetal milieu. Here, they activate one or more embryopathic mechanisms which disrupt the interdependent processes of differentiation (i.e., the appearance of new biochemical and structural properties), growth (i.e., the increase in total mass), and morphogenesis (i.e., the generation of new shape). The embryopathic result may include death, either directly or secondary to malformation, malformation that may or may not be compatible with extrauterine life, growth retardation, and functional alteration that may mediate behavioral effects. The nature of these effects depends on the specificity and toxicity of the agent and, most importantly, on the gestational age or period in development at the time of exposure.

For the sake of discussion, it is convenient to divide prenatal development into three periods: the predifferentiation period, the period of the embryo, and the period of the fetus. The distinction, however, is only conceptual. The conceptus, throughout gestation, is in a continual state of orderly biochemical and structural transition during which new constituents are being formed and spatially rearranged. At any time in the total span of development, these ongoing processes can be subtly deflected, severely perturbated, or abruptly halted, resulting in various embryopathic consequences.

#### 1. Predifferentiation Period

The interval between the fertilization of the oocyte and its implantation in the endometrium is approximately 6 days in both rats and humans; it is referred to as the preimplantation or predifferentiation period. During this time, the ovum, while remaining relatively undifferentiated, undergoes a series of mitotic divisions, changing from a unicellular zygote to a multicellular blastocyst. The blastocyst, suspended in uterine fluid, is actively transported through the fallopian tube to the uterine cavity. Drugs contained in the fluid readily pass into the intercellular spaces of the embryo. Agents that produce malformations later in the development, however, are generally thought to be without teratogenic effect during this early period. It appears that exogenous substances are either toxic to the entire embryo, resulting in its death, or if toxic to alimited number of cells, the "regulative" potentialities of the embryo result in repair with no apparent damage.

Behavioral effects have nonetheless been reported following the administration of drugs during the predifferentiation period in rats (e.g., the studies reported by WERBOFF and HAVLENA 1962). While such early treatment might produce effects by acting directly on the blastocyst, other mechanisms could account for these observations. For example, it has been shown that administration of either phenothiazines (GAURON and ROWLEY 1969) or morphine (FRIEDLER and COCHIN 1972) prior to conception subsequently alters the growth and behavior of the offspring. Even though the drug has presumably cleared from maternal plasma, preconceptional drug exposure alters the maternal environment in some as yet unknown way to modify offspring development. Another possibility is afforded by the socalled ambush effect; agents with a relatively long half-life may be cleared slowly from maternal and/or embryonic fluid. If, for example, such agents are administered during the predifferentiation stage, just prior to organogenesis, they may persist long enough to produce effects at later susceptible periods. Thus, most workers agree that the predifferentiation period is not a susceptible period for teratogenesis. Whether it is similarly refractory for producing behavioral effects awaits further evidence.

## 2. Period of the Embryo

The interval between early germ layer differentiation and the completion of major organ formation (organogenesis) is referred to as the period of the embryo. This phase of development, characterized by the formation of complex, multicellular tissues, and organs of diverse origins and functions, begins soon after implantation and, in humans, continues through approximately the eighth week of gestation. The comparable period in the laboratory rat extends from about day 8 through day 14 of gestation. (The laboratory rat is born around day 22.) During organogenesis, the embryo is maximally susceptible to gross structural malformation if exposed to teratogenic agents. The nature of the defect will depend both on the effect of the agent on embryonic cells and the gestational age at the time of exposure.

Although it is beyond the scope of this chapter to discuss embryopathic mechanisms extensively, an appreciation of how these agents produce structural, and ultimately, behavioral effects derives from a fundamental understanding of such mechanisms. For our purpose here, we might say that to understand the effect of a teratogenic agent is to understand first, what the agent does to embryonic cells (usually, populations of proliferating cells), and second, what developmental processes the cells are carrying out at the time of exposure.

WILSON (1973) has formulated a paradigm of teratogenic action which describes how teratogenic drugs initiate a sequence of pathogenic effects, beginning at the cellular level. Interference with some fundamental aspect of cellular physiology, such as protein synthesis or enzyme activity leads, for example, to cell death or a failure of cellular interaction. WILSON (1973, p. 25) suggests that "... these initially different types of pathogenesis may converge into a relatively narrow channel of abnormal development, for example, one that would lead ultimately to insufficient cells or cell products to carry out morphogenesis or to carry on function at the site of the final defect."

In other words, an agent may have a very specific toxic action at the cellular level. It might, for example kill actively proliferating cells, while sparing those in the resting phase, or only those cells in a particular phase of the cell cycle. In either case, however, populations of cells are killed, and are therefore not available to participate in the development process. The result is a structurally defective embryo.

The nature of the defect will depend on the gestational age of the embryo at the time of exposure, or more specifically, the embryologic processes or events that are correlated with the gestational age of the conceptus. "Critical periods" are recognized for various organs and systems for a given species and refer to the fact that, in general, "particular organs and parts are chemically and morphologically developing at their own paces and according to their own timetables, and each therefore has its characteristic temporal shifts in proneness to damage ..." (KALTER 1968, p. 5). Critical periods for the laboratory rat define a continuum of differential susceptibility that extends from day 8 of gestation through the first several days of postnatal life. A teratogenic agent administered about day 9, for example, will generally give rise to a pattern of gross structural malformations of the brain, spinal cord, eye, and heart. The same treatment administered a few days later, about day 14, will usually produce a very different pattern that includes cleft palate, limb, and digit defects, but none of the defects noted earlier.[1]

With increasing gestational age, there is a corresponding decrease in susceptibility to teratogenesis; agents administered after day 15 or so, as organogenesis becomes complete, do not produce gross defects. They can, however, produce subtle damage in the CNS by interfering with histogenesis.

In summary then, the processes of cell division, differentiation, and migration are of fundamental importance during the prenatal and early postnatal period. And, at different times in development, the dividing cell is carrying out a beautifully integrated and exquisitely timed sequence of events – initially, the creation of specialized cells and tissue underlying organogenesis and later, as these processes continue, the building of the cerebral cortex and the cerebellum, and the "wiring" of their interconnections with other regions of the brain. Until these processes reach their conclusion, they will remain vulnerable to damage caused by drugs.

An obvious constraint in studying behavioral effects produced by teratogenic agents administered during the period of the embryo is that many of the CNS mal-

1 Contrary to older conceptions, suggesting a precise correlation between developmental events at the time of exposure and the specific nature of the malformation, it is now recognized that the critical period for producing a given malformation does not necessarily correspond to the time of rapid organogenesis of its anlage, i.e., the earliest discernible precursor of the structure. Within limits, different agents may produce the same malformation at different gestational ages, sometimes before the appearance of recognizable anlage (e.g., see SHENEFELT 1972). As WILSON (1973, p 123) points out, the notion of critical periods is useful as an approximation of the time of inception of abnormal development, but should not be taken as a definitive scientific principle

formations typically induced (e.g., exencephaly, spina befida) are lethal postnatally. BUTCHER and his colleagues, however, have studied the behavioral effects of two agents teratogenic to the CNS by administering what he called "subteratogenic" doses; that is, dose levels at or just below the teratogenic threshold.

In one study, BUTCHER et al. (1972a) administered 100,000 IU/kg vitamin A on days 9, 10, and 11 of gestation in rats.[2] Learning ability was tested, beginning at 50 days of age by requiring the offspring to learn the escape route from a water-filled multiple T-maze. During five escape trials on each of two successive days, drug-treated offspring made significantly more errors than the control animals. By the third and last test day, however there appeared to be no difference in the number of errors made by either group. Thus, the offspring treated with vitamin A appeared to be impaired in learning the escape task, but with continued training their error rate diminished to the control level.

In a similarly designed study, BUTCHER et al. (1972b) administered 250 mg/kg salicylate on days 9, 10, and 11 of gestation. Offspring were tested as in the first study, except that they were given two additional days of testing during which they were required to learn the backward path through the maze. As in the experiment with vitamin A, the salicylate-treated offspring made significantly more errors than the control animals over the five test days. However, unlike the first experiment, in this study, acquisition data (i.e., error frequency as a function of training) were not provided. Thus, except for the overall finding of more errors, the specific nature of the impairment produced by the salicylate is not clear.

In another study, BUTCHER et al. (1973) investiated the behavioral effects of prenatally administered hydroxyurea. The concern here, however, was not with subteratogenic dose levels, but rather with the specific action of the agent. Hydroxyurea is a potent inhibitor of deoxyribonucleic acid (DNA) synthesis, and when administered during organogenesis in rats, results in cell death in limb buds and the neural tube. At term, however, gross limb malformations are common, while those of the CNS are not. The authors suggested that, despite the absence of gross CNS defects, behavioral impairments might be evident postnatally.

Hydroxyurea in doses of either 375 or 500 mg/kg was administered on day 13 of gestation. Beginning at 30 to 40 days of age, offspring were tested for differences in exploratory and locomotor behavior in an open-field test, followed by escape training as described earlier. Although there were no differences in exploratory behavior among any treated or control group, more than 20% of both dose-level groups displayed an abnormal gait characterized by an outward splaying of the hindlimbs. Compared with the control group, drug-treated offspring made significantly more errors over all training trials on both the forward and the backward path of the maze. There was, however, no clear indication of dose-level effects and acquisition data were not provided.

Acetazolamide, an inhibitor of the enzyme carbonic anhydrase, has an unusual specificity in that the malformation it produces in rats is confined largely to the distal, postaxial parts of the right forelimb and rarely, if ever, includes the CNS. Be-

2 The day of finding sperm is called either day 0 or day 1 of gestation in different studies. So that gestation days refer to the same conceptional age, gestation days have been calculated by designating the day of finding sperm day 1 for all of the studies cited in this chapter

cause of this apparent lack of effect on developing nervous tissue, BUTCHER et al. (1975) investigated whether such an agent could produce behavioral effects. A dose of 500 mg/kg was administered on days 11 and 12 of gestation and offspring tested as described in the open-field and swimming maze. Despite a limp produced by the forelimb defect, drug-treated offspring were no different from control animals in exploratory activity. Similarly, their performance on the maze problem revealed no impairment.

Although confirming studies are needed, these findings suggest the following tentative conclusions: (1) teratogenic agents (such as acetazolamide) that do not produce early CNS pathogenesis or gross CNS malformations do not appear to produce postnatal behavior effects; (2) agents that produce gross malformations of the CNS, such as vitamin A and salicylate, appear to produce behavioral effects when administered at dose levels near or just below the threshold for producing malformations; (3) teratogenic agents (such as hydroxyurea) that produce early pathogenesis in the developing CNS (i.e., cell death), but not gross CNS malformations, may produce a residual functional impairment evident in postnatal behavior. As to the nature of these behavioral effects, the swimming maze used in these studies provides only a preliminary screening technique, indicating either the presence or absence of behavioral differences. Whether these differences are the result of sensory, motivational or perceptual–cognitive deficits awaits a more thorough behavioral analysis.

## 3. Period of the Fetus

Because the embryo becomes increasingly refractory to gross structural malformation as gestational age increases, studies of drug teratogenicity were initially devoted almost exclusively to agents administered during organogenesis. But in 1967, LANGMAN and WELCH initiated studies of the early fetal period and their findings had provocative implications for those concerned with behavioral impairments. They administered an excess of vitamin A, a well-known teratogenic treatment, to mice on two or three successive days during the early fetal period and examined the fetal and neonatal brains at regular intervals up until 10 days of postnatal life. They found that the treatment inhibited DNA synthesis in the neuroepithelial cells of the cerebral cortex. This acted to prolong the cell cycle by appriximately 40%, thus interfering with the differentiation of existing neuroblasts, which resulted in a cerebral cortex with reduced cell density. These findings provided convincing evidence that teratogenic drugs administered later in pregnancy could indeed produce nonlethal brain damage, and encouraged our laboratory to investigate the behavioral correlates.

In our first study (HUTCHINGS et al. 1973), we administered 60,000 IU vitamin A (approximately 230,000 IU/kg) to rats on days 14 and 15 of gestation. Compared with control animals, the vitamin-treated offspring showed a generalized retardation in growth as evidenced by a delayed onset of fur growth and eye opening, and reduced body weight. In adulthood, animals were tested on various operant conditioning tasks in order to asses learning ability. No differences were observed on continuous water reinforcement and on an intermittent reinforcement schedule.

However, differences emerged during the subsequent acquisition of an auditory discrimination. In the presence of the positive cue, S+, in which responding is reinforced, normal subjects typically show elevated rates, while gradually extinguishing their response to the negative cue, S−, in which responding is never reinforced. Both treated and control animals acquired the discrimination during 80 daily training sessions, but the treated group learned more slowly to inhibit their responses to the S− cue. Direct observation suggested a "perseverative" quality, as though treated subjects were not attending as carefully to the onset of the S− signal.

Brain sections from half the treated animals were not obviously different from the control animals, while the remainder showed a diffuse reduction in overall size. However, the amount of brain reduction did not correlate with the discrimination impairment. An auditory impairment in an operant discrimination, similar to that found here, has been reported by other workers, following irradiation in rats at approximately the same gestational age that vitamin A was administered here (FOWLER et al. 1962; PERSINGER 1971), which suggests a critical period for producing the effect.

In a second study, we investigated the effects of 90,000 IU/vitamin A (approximately 280,000 IU/kg) on days 17 and 18 of gestation (HUTCHINGS and GASTON 1974). At this time, the cerebellum is beginning active differentiation, and accordingly we expected motor impairment along with or independent of cognitive deficits. The same control and testing procedures were used as in the previous study.

Unlike animals treated on days 14 and 15, there was no retardation in growth and development. On the operant measures, we found that the treated animals had significantly slower rates of response throughout testing compared with the control group. On the S+, S− discrimination task, they extinguished responding to S− as rapidly as the control animals, and showed no impairment in learning. Although histologic examination showed no reduction in brain size or any obvious abnormality of cellular elements of structures, VACCA and HUTCHINGS (1977) reported in a separate study that the vitamin A treatment interfered with cell proliferation in the developing cerebellum. The major behavioral finding was that the animals treated on days 17 and 18 of gestation failed to acquire a rate of response comparable to that of the control group. The lower rates of the treated animals might have been due to a minor motor disturbance, and, we did observe that some of the 17–18-day-treated animals walked with a peculiar gait. Furthermore, FOWLER et al. (1962), and HICKS and D'AMATO (1966) found that rats irradiated on the same days that vitamin A was administered in our study were more sluggish in their placing reactions, more awkward in their general movements, and did not respond as rapidly as controls in a lever box – observations that nicely parallel our findings. Our study further demonstrates, however, that such an impairment need not be associated with a learning deficit.

The results of the vitamin A work and similar studies using irradiation indicate that there are critical periods during fetogenesis when exposure to teratogenic agents produces a specific kind of behavioral effect. This notion is further corroborated by the more recent work of RODIER et al. (1975) and LANGMAN et al. (1975) with mice. These authors administered 5-azacytidine on either day 15 or day 19 of gestation, or on the third postnatal day. Although its mechanism is unknown, 5-

azacytidine interferes with cell proliferation primarily by killing dividing cells. Treated animals differed from control animals but, a more important finding was that each treated group differed from the other. Animals treated on day 15 had normal locomotor ability the first week of life but persisted in "pivoting", an immature locomotor pattern in which the animal rests on a limp hindlimb and paddles with its forelimbs, thereby producing a spinning in place. Both the day 19 and postnatally treated animals had pronounced intention tremors which disappeared by the third week of life. Animals treated on day 19 displayed normal, if not precocious, motor development, pivoted rarely, and had a well-coordinated gait. By contrast, the postnatal treatment produced animals with an abnormal gait, characterized by splaying hindlimbs and a tendency to pivot. During adulthood, day-15-treated animals were hyperactive, day-19-treated animals hypoactive, while the postnatally treated animals were normally active.

In a separate study, LANGMAN et al. (1975) investigated the morphological effects produced by azacytidine in mice. Treatment on day 15 resulted in an extreme reduction in brain size, particularly in the cerebral cortex. In addition, there was an abnormal layering of the pyramidal cells in the hippocampus and a reduced corpus striatum. Treatment on day 19 produced damage in more restricted brain areas, with dead cells seen mainly in the subependymal layer and external granular layer of the cerebellum. The postnatal treatment killed many proliferating microneurons and microglia in the cerebellum, but did not result in obvious cell deficits in the adult brain. Although they could not explain all of the motor effects in detail, the authors concluded that the deficits produced were quite predictable on the basis of the lesion sites.

The finding of hippocampal damage produced on day 15 and adult hyperactivity is consistent with the inhibitory deficit (given that the hyperactivity attenuates inhibitory control) that we observed in rats for vitamin A administered on days 14 and 15 (HUTCHINGS et al. 1973), and with a similar impairment associated with hippocampal lesions in the adult (ISAACSON 1974). Furthermore, the observation of histologic damage in the cerebellum and adult hypoactivity parallels the cytochemical damage we observed in the same area (VACCA and HUTCHINGS 1977) and the sluggish rates of response for vitamin A administered on days 17 and 18 in rats (HUTCHINGS and GASTON 1974).

These studies indicate that the fetus and neonate, although refractory to gross structural defect, remain vulnerable to more subtle damage, particularly in those areas of the brain that are actively proliferating. Exposure to teratogenic agents either kills the dividing cells outright or slows the rate of proliferation, thereby disrupting subsequent differentiation and migration. Those areas of the brain sustaining cell loss apparently fail to function normally, with resulting behavioral impairment. Although more precise knowledge of the behavioral correlates of the damage awaits further study, the nature of the impairments appears to correspond to the known function of the damaged areas. Whether such effects are produced in humans is not known, but some of the behavioral effects observed (e.g., inhibitory impairment, fine motor dysfunction) in animals bear a striking resemblance to those frequently described for children with so-called minimal brain dysfunction. (For an excellent and thorough review of the chronology of neuron development and the effects of interference during critical periods, see RODIER 1980.)

## II. Human Studies

### 1. The Fetal Alcohol Syndrome

In 1973, JONES et al. described a syndrome of malformation among 11 infants born to chronically alcoholic women. The pattern of defects, which the authors termed the "fetal alcohol syndrome" (FAS) included prenatal and postnatal growth retardation, developmental delay, craniofacial anomalies, and limb defects. The facial dysmorphology in the FAS includes small eye slits (i.e., short palpebral fissures) low nasal bridge, short nose and indistinct or absent groove from the nose to the upper lip, thin, upturned upper lip, a small chin, and flat midface. Other anomalies that have been observed include drooping eyelids, crossed eyes, minor joint anomalies, and hearing defects. A later study indicated a perinatal mortality rate of 17% (JONES et al. 1974) and a study of 30 additional cases (HANSON et al. 1976a) verified the initial diagnosis and provided additional evidence of severe CNS damage, with related intellectual deficits. [For a thorough and critical review of both clinical and animal studies of the FAS, the reader is referred to the following excellent articles: ABEL (1980); STREISSGUTH et al. (1980); and ROSETT and SANDER (1979).]

During the neonatal period, tremulousness, hyperactivity, and irritability have been observed, but their frequency was not initially reported. While these possibly result from alcohol withdrawal, HANSON points out that the tremulousness frequently persists for months to years, while fine motor dysfunction may be permanent.

PIEROG et al. (1977) systematically studied the withdrawal symptoms in six infants showing the dysmorphic features of the FAS. She found an abstinence syndrome very similar to that reported among neonates passively addicted to opiates. Of the six infants, all showed tremors, irritability, increased muscle tone, increased respiratory rate, and hyperacusis. About half the infants showed arching of the back, spontaneous seizure activity, abdominal distention, and vomiting.

STREISSGUTH et al. (1978) studied 20 FAS patients, ranging in age from 9 months to 21 years. IQ scores showed a large variance, ranging from a score of 15 in an 18-month-old infant to 105 in a 9-year-old child. The mean IQ of the entire group was 65, indicating intellectual functioning in the mild to moderately retarded range. The authors further found IQ scores to be correlated with degree of dysmorphogenesis; those with the most severe external features yielded an average IQ of 55, whereas those with less severe features had an average IQ of 82. In addition, many of the children were described as hyperactive as preschoolers, some to the extent that the examiners found them difficult to test. Others with less severe hyperactivity were distractible, had short attention span, and were fidgety.

SHAYWITZ et al. (1980) studied 15 children, ranging in age from 6½ to 18½ years, whose mothers had a history of alcoholism during pregnancy. All had less severe dysmorphic features of the FAS, but demonstrated at least two facial features, with 73% having small palpebral fissures. Standard IQ tests revealed a mean score of 98, with scores ranging from 82 to 113. However, despite the fact that most of the scores fell within the low-average to average range, all of the children had experienced school failure. School records indicated that all had difficulties of short attention span, distractibility, and all but one was described as hyperactive. SHAYWITZ et al. (1980) interpret their findings as corroborating other reports of milder degrees of behavioral impairment frequently found among offspring of alcohol mothers, and suggest that ethanol exerts a continuum of teratogenic effects on the CNS, ranging from learning disabilities and behavioral impairment to mild to severe mental retardation.

JONES and SMITH (1975) described brain findings of an infant with the FAS syndrome who died at 5 days of age. In addition to agenesis of the corpus callosum, there was incomplete development of the cerebral cortex and an abnormal external appearance of the brain, owing to sheets of neuronal and glial cells that had abnormally migrated over the surface of the cerebral hemispheres. Extensive developmental abnormalities resulted from aberration of neuronal migration, and in multiple heterotopias throughout the leptomeninges and cerebral mantle and subependymal regions. The authors suggest that the joint (skeletal) anomalies may be related secondarily to diminished fetal movement associated with the neurologic impairment of the fetus. These observations were corroborated by CLARREN et al. (1978), who studied the neuropathologic findings of four neonates whose mothers consumed large quantities of alcohol during pregnancy. Although two of the infants did not show the external features of the FAS, all showed malformed brains, with hydrocephalus seen in two.

Whether the fetal alcohol syndrome is produced by ethanol directly, one of its metabolites such as acetaldehyde, or an interaction of these with maternal dietary deficiencies is not yet known. It is clear, however, that heavy alcohol consumption during pregnancy produces, among other defects, widespread nervous system embryopathies with mild to severe chronic behavioral impairments.

## 2. The Fetal Hydantoin Syndrome

Although the hydantoins (diphenylhydantoin, mephenhytoin, ethotoin) had been prescribed for the treatment of epilepsy for 40 years, it was not until the early part of the last decade that they came under suspicion as possible teratogens. After HANSON and SMITH (1975) described a pattern of birth defects in five infants prenatally exposed to hydantoin anticonvulsants, HANSON et al. (1976b) carried out a prospective study of 35 children born to 23 women who had been treated with these drugs during pregnancy. They found that four (11%) had sufficient features to be diagnosed as having the fetal hydantion syndrome (FHS). Although there is considerable variability in both the severity and number of defects, the most predominant features include mild to moderate growth deficiency, including reduced brain size, a short nose with anteverted nostrils, a long philtrum and bowed upper lip, and small distal digits with unusually small nails. Three of the four children were administered an IQ test at 7 years of age, and all yielded scores indicating mild to moderate mental retardation. An additional 11 children (31%) each showed several of these dysmorphic features, but not sufficient to warrant a definitive diagnosis of the FHS.

These findings were corroborated in a matched control study of 104 children whose mothers had a convulsive disorder and were treated with hydantoins throughout pregnancy. Moreover, compared with controls, the hydantoin-exposed children had a significantly smaller head circumference at birth, and significantly lower IQ scores at 7 years of age. Because the hydantoins are frequently administered in combination with barbituates, 17 infants born to women with convulsive disorders but treatet only with barbiturates throughout pregnancy were also studied. None of these children showed the dysmorphic pattern similar to the FHS. The authors conclude that the significantly lower IQ scores of the hydantoin-exposed children constitute an area of particular concern.

### 3. The Fetal Trimethadione Syndrome

Since being introduced in 1946, trimethadione and its close congener, paramethadione, have been used to treat childhood petit mal epliepsy. Possibly because of its infrequent use with adults, it was not suspected as a teratogen until GERMAN et al. (1970) described two women who took the drug and had nine pregnancies that resulted in abortion or infants with birth defects. With the discontinued use of the drug, both gave birth to normal children. These observations were corroborated by ZACKAI et al. (1975) who studied three families in which the mothers took trimethadione throughout pregnancy. They described a fetal trimethadione syndrome that included developmental delay, speech difficulty, V-shaped eyebrows, epicanthus, low-set ears with anteriorly folded helix, palatal anomaly, and irregular teeth. Some individuals with the syndrome also show intrauterine growth retardation, short stature, and microcephaly. Of the few cases that have been reported, mild mental retardation is suggested as a component of the syndrome, but additional cases will be required to confirm this possibility.

### 4. Thalidomide

When the teratogenicity of thalidomine was first discovered, the syndrome of malformations was thought to affect limbs, ears, eyes, and viscera, but not the CNS. But, as the children matured, it became increasingly apparent that thalidomide did not spare nervous tissue (STEPHENSON 1976). A review of several studies of intellectual functioning in thalidomide-damaged children by MCFIE and ROBERTSON (1973) indicates that most are within normal range. However, the authors cite one study of 1.5–3.5-year-old affected children that yielded developmental quotients that were below average, with one-third of the subjects scoring in the borderline and mentally retarded categories. In their own study of 56 thalidomide-damaged children 7–10 years old, MCFIE and ROBERTSON (1973) found the mean IQ to fall within or above the normal range. Four subjects, however, were of subnormal or severely subnormal intelligence, which is a much higher proportion than is expected to occur in the general population.

STEPHENSON (1976) reviewed the medical files of a group of 408 thalidomide-damaged children and found 9 ranging in age from 13 to 16 years who had histories suggestive of epilepsy. Further study confirmed 7 with definite epilepsy, yielding a prevalence of 17.2/1,000 compared with 2.42/1,000 for a comparable age group in the general population. In addition, STEPHENSON found the varieties of epilepsy in these children to be unusual. Two had a relatively rare type of severe refractory epilepsy, suggesting widespread brain abnormality. Three had unlocalized or generalized seizures that included episodes of unconsciousness, possibly related to brain stem abnormality. Mental impairment and epilepsy do not occur with the same high frequency as limb reduction among thalidomide-damaged children. Their significantly increased prevalence, however, confirms CNS involvement as an additional component of thalidomide embryopathy in humans.

## C. Agents that Cause Behavioral Effects in the Absence of Gross Structural Malformations

### I. Animal and Human Studies

Several classes of drugs such as tranquilizers, stimulants, hypnotics, and analgesics, while generally not teratogenic in animals or humans, can nevertheless produce intrauterine death, growth retardation, and behavioral deficits. These drugs, unlike the agents already discussed, probably do not selectively kill embryonic cells, but appear rather ot produce functional effects by interfering with neurochemical mechanisms in the developing brain. Their action is poorly understood, but some may act on specific embryonic sites (e.g., synapses) or interfere with the elaboration of neural systems utilizing particular neurotransmitters (e.g., catecholamines) to initiate a sequence of abnormal development. However, early pathogenesis and the final pathway involve biochemical rather than gross morphological effects.

For example, the prenatal administration of reserpine produces a relatively permanent change in brain catecholamine disposition during a critical period in prenatal development in both rat (BARTOLOME et al. 1976) and chick (LYDIARD and SPARBER 1974). In the latter species, the biochemical effect is correlated with a behavioral impairment (SPARBER and SHIDEMAN 1968). The relationship of behavioral effect to gestational age at the time of treatment has yet to be determined for the agents discussed in the following sections. It would appear likely, however, that such a relationship exists and will be demonstrated in future work.

#### 1. Amphetamine

CLARK et al. (1970) administered 1 mg/kg amphetamine sulfate on days 12–15 of gestation in pregnant rats. Compared with a saline-treated control group, the drug-treated offspring showed a significant reduction in locomotor activity at 21 days of age. However, they were not different when tested at younger ages or as late as 60 days of age. Beginning at 33 days of age, offspring were deprived of water and trained to run a T-maze for water reinforcement. Although they did not differ from controls in number of errors, their latency to reach reinforcement was significantly shorter, suggesting heightened activity induced by deprivation.

Because amphetamine affects catecholamine systems in the adult brain, MIDDAUGH et al. (1974) investigated its prenatal administration on brain catecholamines and locomotor activity in the offspring. Amphetamine sulfate (5 mg/kg) was administered daily during the last week of gestation in mice. Some animals were at regular intervals, beginning on the day of birth for determination of brain norepinephrine and dopamine; others were tested behaviorally for activity differences (locomotion, rearing, and grooming) between 13 and 31 days of age, and at

75 days of age. Norepinephrine concentrations in the drug-treated offspring were depressed at birth, rose to control values by day 3, and were elevated at 21 and 30 days of age. Dopamine levels were elevated at 30 days of age; by 75 days of age, neither norepinephrine nor dopamine differed from control concentrations. Significant differences in activity did not clearly emerge until 75 days of age. Not only were the drug-treated offspring more active on total activity scores, but they differed qualitatively as well, their activity was characterized either by increased non-directed locomotion or by greatly reduced locomotion, often coupled with a high frequency of grooming; the relationship of the behavioral differences to the altered catecholamine levels was not clear. Considering that some 570,000 American women of childbearing age are estimated to be using amphetamine-containing diet pills (CHAMBERS and GRIFFEY 1975), additional studies of this agent are certainly indicated.

## 2. Barbiturates

MIDDAUGH et al. (1975a) have emphasized the frequent use of phenobarbital among pregnant women. Some 25% or more use some kind of sedative, often phenobarbital, during the last trimester, many with epilepsy use it throughout pregnancy as an anticonvulsant, and it is sometimes used during late pregnancy as a prophylaxis for neonatal hyperbilirubinemia. Moreover, it is commonly abused among the addict population. A paucity of animal studies of the behavioral effects of prenatal exposure led these authors to carry out the following study.

Three groups of mice were administered either 20, 40, or 80 mg/kg phenobarbital sodium daily during the last week of gestation. The two higher doses have been shown to increase neonatal mortality significantly, and to decrease body weight of surviving offspring (ZEMP and MIDDAUGH 1975). In adulthood, the offspring were placed on a food deprivation schedule and self-trained to lever-press for food reinforcement in operant conditioning chambers. Following this, animals were trained on several fixed-ratio schedules of reinforcement, which required an increasing number of responses for each reinforcement as the training progressed.

There was no difference in the ability of the treated offspring to acquire the lever-press response, compared with saline-injected control animals. On the fixed-ratio schedules, control animals showed the expected increase in response rates with increasingly higher ratio schedules. The treated offspring, however, responded less than controls, and their response decrement became even more pronounced as the schedule demands were increased. The 80 mg/kg dose was less effective in producing the behavioral effect compared with the two lower doses. The authors suggest that this may have been the result of a selection factor due to high neonatal mortality produced by the highest dose. A previous study indicated that phenobarbital-exposed offspring were less responsive to aversive stimuli (MIDDAUGH et al. 1975b). The present study suggested a similar unresponsiveness to appetitive stimuli, leading the authors to postulate that the primary behavioral effects of prenatal phenobarbital exposure is a decreased responsiveness to environmental stimuli.

In the last century, it was recognized that maternal use of narcotics during pregnancy produces withdrawal symptoms in the neonate. Only a decade ago a similar effect was described for barbiturates. DESMOND et al. (1972) reported on 15 infants whose mothers were taking between 60 and 120 mg barbiturates daily, either alone or in combination with anticonvulsants for the treatment of epilepsy throughout pregnancy or only during the last trimester. All of the infants were full-term by weight, had good 1-min Apgar scores, but exhibited a withdrawal syndrome characterized by overactivity, restlessness, disturbed sleep, excessive crying, tremors, hyperflexia, hypertonicity, sneezing, hiccuping, yawning, mouthing movements, hyperacusis, vasomotor instability, hyperphagia, vomiting, and diarrhea. The age of onset of the syndrome was later than that typically seen for heroin and the symptoms in some infants persisted for as long as 6 months. For reasons not clear, symptoms tended to be less severe when the medication included other anticonvulsants. SHAPIRO et al. (1976) reported mental and motor test results at 8 months and 4 years of age of children whose mothers took barbiturates during pregnancy. They found no differences compared with a matched control group. Also, children of epileptic mothers who took barbiturates were no different. The animal work found behavioral effects of prenatal barbiturate exposure that persisted well into adulthood. Whether long-term effects are similarly produced in humans awaits follow-up studies.

## 3. Phencyclidine

Phencyclidine (PCP), most commonly known on the street as "angel dust" but also as "goon", "hog", "the PeaCe Pill", "embalming fluid", and "killer weed", has emerged as one of the most dangerous and widespread drugs of abuse, possibly of epidemic proportion. While still marketed for use as an animal analgesic, its medical use with humans was discontinued following reports of several adverse side effects; severe and persistent postanesthetic hallucinations, agitation, delirium, and disorientation. PCP is manufactured cheaply from chemicals that are easily obtained and its street use became widespread during the early 1970s. Acute use can produce severe and sometimes fatal medical complications, psychotic episodes that may recur, suicidal depression, and acts of violence. Chronic use can lead to both physiologic and psychologic dependence, aggression, and impaired memory. "Bad trips" can include feelings of numbness, paranoia, impending death, anxiety, outbursts of violent behavior, and dissociative reactions. Psychotic symptoms can last from days to weeks and, not infrequently, lead to a diagnosis of acute schizophrenia when patients are seen in the emergency room (STILLMAN and PETERSEN 1979).

In an excellent review of the abuse problem of PCP, STILLMAN and PETERSEN (1979) report findings from the National Institute of Drug Abuse National Survey, the U.S. Drug Abuse Warning Network, and the National Youth Polydrug Study. The figures are indeed alarming: among 12–17-year-old adolescents, users of PCP rose from 3.0% in 1976 to 5.8% in 1977. Similarly, from 1974 to 1976, the number of PCP-related emergencies and deaths increased from 54 to 111. A report from 97 drug abuse treatment programs showed that among 2,750 users below the age of 19, one-third had used PCP, two-thirds of those who had ever tried it were regular users, and its use exceeded that of inhalants, sedatives, cocaine, and opiates. The user of PCP is typically a polydrug abuser and tragically, particularly given the risk of possible organic brain damage, the average age of first use is 14.

Studies of the possible fetal toxicity of PCP are meager. COOPER et al. (1977) administered a single intramuscular dose of PCP to sows just before delivery. He found the plasma concentration of the drug in the piglet to be nearly ten times that of the sow. Moreover, the half-life of the drug was 2–4 h in the sow and 10–20 h in the piglet. MARKS et al. (1980) administered four dose levels of PCP to pregnant mice on days 6–15 of gestation. A significant increase in malformations was found, but only at the highest dose. Because this dose was highly toxic to the dams and no malformations were seen at levels that did not produce excessive maternal toxicity, the authors concluded that PCP is not teratogenic in the mouse. MARBLE et al. (1980) reported that urine samples remain positive for PCP for as long as 7 days postpartum from newborns of mothers with documented PCP use. Such PCP-exposed newborns are described as irritable or hypertonic when handled, lethargic or somnolent when left alone, and may show a vertical nystagmus.

GOLDEN et al. (1980) presented a case report of an infant whose mother used PCP throughout pregnancy. The male infant, born with a dislocated hip, weighed 2,060 g and had a very unusual physical appearance; the face had a triangular shape with a pointed chin and narrow mandibular angle. Visual tracking and head control were poor and nystagmus was observed. Within a few hours after birth, the infant showed increased tone and was extremely jittery; slight auditory or tactile stimulation produced coarse flapping movements of the extremities, but when not stimulated, the infant was floppy and lethargic. During the following weeks, the infant had persistent hypertonicity that suggested cerebral palsy. At 2 months of age, he still had roving eye movements and coarse tremors that were exacerbated by stimulation. Taking into consideration all of the medical findings, the authors suggested that the infant's dysmorphology and cerebral palsy may have resulted from prenatal exposure to PCP. They suggest the establishment of a registry of cases of maternal use of PCP during pregnancy and fetal outcome.

It has been said that PCP is everything we were agraid marijuana would turn out to be, but has not (STILLMAN and PETERSEN 1979). The clinical observations leave little doubt that it is one of the most ravaging drugs of abuse to come on the scene and it may prove equally perilous to the conceptus and newborn. Given its spectacularly high potency in the adult CNS, it is a safe guess that it will not prove benign to the developing CNS. What is needed now are more developmental animal and clinical follow-up studies to determine effects at all levels – structural, functional, and behavioral.

## 4. Opiates

Of the estimated 150,000 opiate-dependent persons in the New York City metropolitan area, approximately 34,000 are women of childbearing age and include some 10,000–12,000 enrolled in methadone maintenance programs. Approximately 3%–5% of the births in New York City municipal hospitals are comprised of infants passively addicted to either heroin or methadone. This places the birthrate of the addicted population at about 3,000 per year in New York City alone (CARR 1975).

Such passively addicted neonates may show signs of acute narcotic withdrawal, characterized by hyperflexia, tremors, irritability, excessive high-pitched crying, and disturbed sleep. For both heroin and methadone, these symptoms usually make their initial appearance within a few days after birth, but for methadone, some infants may not become symptomatic for 2–4 weeks. KANDELL (1977) suggests that fetal storage and prolonged metabolism and excretion of methadone might account for this delayed onset of symptoms. Among a number of heroin-exposed infants studied by WILSON et al. (1973), "subacute" withdrawal, characterized by restlessness, agitation, tremors, and sleep disturbance was found to persist for as long as 3–6 months after birth. Similar symptoms persisting for as long as 12 weeks have been described for infants exposed to methadone (LIPSITZ and BLATMAN 1974), including hyperactivity lasting through 18 months of age (TING et al. 1974).

In order to use a more objective and sensitive measure of neonatal abstinence and detect possible abnormalities of brain dysfunction, some workers have examined the effects of in utero exposure to opiates on sleep patterns. For example, SCHULMAN (1969) found that eight of eight full-term infants born to heroin-addicted mothers showed electroencephalographic (EEG) signs of sleep disturbance similar to those observed among newborns at high risk for CNS impairment. The major effect was a significant decrease in quiet sleep and increase in rapid eye movement (REM) sleep. However, SISSON et al. (1974) reported, in an abstract, that a small group of infants exposed prenatally to either heroin or methadone showed a decrease not only in quiet sleep, but REM sleep as well.

The most thorough and well-controlled sleep study reported to date is that of DINGES et al. (1980) who studied 28 newborns and their mothers enrolled in a methadone treatment program. Unlike some studies of so-called methadone mothers, these authors, through the use of of self-report and frequent random urine tests, closely monitored the mothers for illicit drug use. As a result, it became necessary to divide the mothers, who were receiving an average of 18 mg methadone daily, into three subgroups: (1) a low opiate group that never or only rarely abused heroin; (2) a high opiate group that abused heroin, ranging from daily to once a week; and (3) a polydrug group that frequently abused heroin and other nonopiate psychoactives and drugs of addiction. Compared with an approximately equal number of demographically matched nonaddict control infants, the low and high opiate-exposed groups averaged significantly less quiet sleep and significantly more active REM sleep. Moreover, the effect was dose related; the high dose compared with the low dose produced less quiet sleep and more active REM sleep, and a significantly greater proportion of the high opiate neonates awoke during the recording sessions. These findings agree with those of SCHULMAN (1969), are similar to findings of REM rebound and wakefulness reported for adults undergoing opiate withdrawal, and reflect the increased CNS arousal which characterizes infants undergoing opiate withdrawal.

Similar to both the opiate groups, the polydrug neonates showed significantly less quiet sleep than the controls, but, in contrast, significantly more intermediate sleep. The authors explain that intermediate sleep is not a sleep state as such, but describes a disorganized pattern that does not fit any of the standard sleep parameters. Thus, they conclude that the capacity of the developing CNS to organize psychophysiologic parameters into adaptice states is more severely compromised by polydrug exposure than exposure to opiates alone. A major question raised by findings of neurobehavioral dysfunction in the passively addicted newborn is whether such effects are transitory or possibly associated with long-term sequelae that persist into childhood. Though such longitudinal studies are meager, the few that have reported follow-up findings to the age of 4–6 years, all indicate a range of long-term effects.

WILSON et al. (1979) studied the growth and behavior development of a group of 77 boys and girls, ranging in age from approximately 3–6 years; 22 children whose mothers used heroin during pregnancy were compared with controls. The so-called heroin-exposed group was extremely heterogeneous, however, and included one mother who was drug-free during the last two trimesters, two who substituted morphine, tranquilizers, and sedatives for heroin during the last trimester, and seven polydrug abusers who, along with heroin, used other drugs including codeine, guaiphenesin, barbituates, methadone, and tranquilizers. Unfortunately, urine samples were not analyzed, and drug histories were based solely on self-report, a notoriously unreliable method. Thus, it is not surprising that the severity of neonatal withdrawal in this group correlated poorly with the self-reports of both the quantity and type of drug abused. In addition, half of the heroin-exposed group entered foster care during the newborn period and of these, six were adopted. Thus, compared with the controls, a significantly greater proportion of these children were raised by substitute mothers.

The remaining children comprised three control groups: (1) a "drug environment" group were children of women who lived in the drug culture, i.e., lived an addict or began to abuse drugs subsequent to the birth of the child; (2) a "high risk" group included infants that experienced medical difficulties commonly seen among the addict population, e.e., dysmaturity, intrauterine growth retardation, fetal distress, and disturbed transition; (3) a third group, controlled for socioeconomic factors, were all born following an uneventful pregnancy, uncomplicated delivery and nursery course. For all the control groups, denial of the use of heroin or other psychotropic drugs was based solely on self-report.

Whereas there were no differences between any of the groups with respect to gestational age, both the heroin-exposed and high risk groups had significantly lower birth weights and 1-min Apgar scores. In addition, a greater proportion of the heroin-exposed group were significantly shorter and had a smaller head circumference. There were no mean differences between any of the groups on a measure of IQ and the oberall performance of the heroin-exposed group fell within the normal range. However, they consistently demonstrated poorer performance on several intellectual, perceptual, and behavioral measures compared with controls. They showed deficits in a test of general cognitive abilities and on a test of visual, auditory, and tactile perception, findings which were interpreted by WILSON et al. (1979) as reflecting impaired organizational and perceptual processes, rather than specific sensory deficits. Moreover, the heroin-exposed children were rated by their parents as having greater difficulty in areas of self- and social adjustment which included uncontrollable temper, impulsiveness, poor self-confidence, aggressiveness, and difficulty in making and keeping friends. Although there were no differences between any of the groups on ratings of attention, cooperation, alertness, and measures of play activity, the heroin-exposed group was subjectively rated during the physical examination as significantly more active than the control group. Compared with the heroin-exposed, drug environment, and high-risk groups, the socioeconomic control group was at advantage on several physical and behavioral measures: they were significantly taller, had superior lingustic skills and perceptual abilities, and were rated as significantly less active during the physical examination.

The authors conclude that these findings indicate that chronic exposure to heroin during pregnancy produces significant effects on growth and behavior. Clearly, however, as they point out, these effects cannot be attributed to heroin alone since at least half the mothers admitted to polydrug abuse. Moreover, many of the heroin-exposed infants experienced an unstable parent–child relationship, the effects of which cannot be evaluated. Half of the heroin abusers raised their own infants, and no information with respect to drug use following the birth of their infant is provided. Obviously, such a life-style would unlikely to be associated with a satisfactory mother–infant interaction. And, of those that were either adopted or went to foster homes, there is no way of determining the possible effects of age at separation or the quality and stability of parenting. Regardless of these confounding variables, there is little question, however, that children conceived and raised under the combined intrauterine and postnatal environmental conditions of illicit drug use are at considerable risk for long-term neurobehavioral effects.

Ramer and Lodge (1975) studied 35 infants born to mothers enrolled in a methadone maintenance program. Half of the infants were born to mothers receiving 30–40 mg methadone daily although a few were being maintained at 40–60 mg; urine tests of the infants revealed six positive for heroin as well as methadone. The remaining infants were born to mothers addicted to heroin throughout pregnancy, but who subsequently enrolled in the methadone program. The birth weights of the methadone-exposed infants were within the normal range, whereas the heroin-exposed infants were significantly lighter. Similar to the findings of Dinges et al. (1980), the most severe neonatal abstinence symptoms were seen among infants born to mothers with a history of polydrug abuse, including those abusing heroin while on methadone maintenance.

Lodge (1976), using standard neonatal assessment and developmental scales as well as electrophysiologic measures, studied approximately 24 children from birth to 4 years of age born to mothers enrolled in the methadone maintenance program previously described. These were compared with "normal" controls, but a description of the criteria by which they were chosen is not provided. Infants born to mothers who used heroin during pregnancy were not included in this report. Because the data were derived from both cross-sectional and longitudinal data, Lodge considers these findings as only preliminary. However, to date, Lodge has carried out the most detailed study of methadone-exposed infants and while she is cautious in drawing firm conclusions, at the very least, the findings have considerable heuristic value.

During the neonatal period, the methadone infants scored within the average range on the mental development scale. However, on the behavioral assessment scale, they were rated significantly higher than controls on tonus, activity level, hand–mouth facility, and irritability. They were also rated as showing higher levels of behavioral arousal, increased lability, and more rapid buildup to an aroused state. Moreover, it was found that in general, the performance of the addicted neonates was characterized by an unusually high degree of auditory responsiveness and orientation, but below average visual following and exploration. These effects were reflected on three other measures: (1) lower scores on portions of the behavioral assessment scale that appeared to result from poor attentiveness to visual stimuli and a lack of sustained visual following; (2) low arousal for visual stimulation on an EEG measure; and (3) hypersensitivity to auditory stimulation measured by auditory evoked potential. Similar to the findings of sleep disturbance reported by DINGES et al. (1980), the mothers of the methadone-exposed infants reported that their infants continued to show irritability, excitability, inability to nap, and various sleep irregularities.

As toddlers, the methadone group was described as being highly energetic, active, talkative, and reactive to sensory stimulation, possibly to the extent of being overly distractible. Moreover, their persistence, goal-directedness, and attention span tended to be unusually brief. Nonetheless, in the area of language, an area of particular importance for subsequent intellectual development, the methadone-exposed group showed relative strength; they tended to be above average in naming pictures and objects and precocious in combining words.

STRAUSS et al. (1979) studied 33 children aged 5 years born to mothers who had been enrolled in a methadone maintenance program during their pregnancy. While the dosage received by these mothers is not specified, a previous report indicated that in this clinic, doses in the 6 weeks prior to term rarely exceeded 40 mg/day (STRAUSS et al. 1976), but possible use of illicit drugs during treatment is not mentioned. Compared with an appropriately matched control group of 30 children aged 5 years, the methadone-exposed children did not differ on a standard test of cognitive abilities. During testing, however, the methadone-exposed children were rated by the examiners as significantly more active, energetic, immature, tended to have difficulty in fine motor coordination, and showed more task-irrelevant activity. Moreover, because these children were observed to be no different from controls on a measure of playroom activity, STRAUSS et al. (1979) concluded that their increased activity pattern is found only in structured settings, and suggest that impaired motor inhibition under such circumstances may represent an area of particular vulnerability.

With continuing widespread use of methadone to treat heroin addiction, these clinical reports of both acute neonatal and long-term behavioral effects are disturbing, yet pose a number of interpretive problems. As is apparent from the description of mothers on methadone maintenance, it is difficult to attribute with confidence later sequelae solely to prenatal methadone exposure. Many of the women have poor diets, are heavy smokers, and are currently using amphetamines, barbituates, or alcohol, often in a pattern of polydrug abuse. In addition, the passively addicted neonate is typically administered paregoric, diazepam, chlorpromazine, or phenobarbital, depending on the severity, type, and duration of withdrawal symptoms. Thus, in order to improve our understanding, of both the acute and long-term risk in the human population, several workers have attempted to develop an animal model of prenatal methadone exposure. In our laboratory, we have been carrying out such studies over the past several years with particular emphasis on developmental toxicity and behavioral effects in both the preweanling and adult rat.

Methadone has been found to be teratogenic in the hamster (GEBER and SCHRAMM 1969). However, no evidence of teratogenicity was found in either rabbits or rats (MARKHAM et al. 1971), corroborating similar reports in humans (BLINICK et al. 1973). HUTCHINGS et al. (1976) administered a 5, 10, 15, or 20 mg/kg regimen of methadone to gravid rats in the last 2 weeks of gestation and found a dose-related increase in resorptions and stillbirths, but no teratogenicity. The two intermediate dose levels produced body weights that were reduced at birth, but similar to controls by weaning. Blood levels of methadone were also determined in mothers and litters in the 5, 10, and 15 mg/kg groups sacrificed 24 h before expected parturition. Blood levels were dose related and correspond to those found in human subjects receiving daily maintenance doses of approximately 30, 60, and 100 mg, respectively.

Because of clinical reports of increased lability of state (LODGE 1976) as well as sleep disturbance among opiate-exposed infants (SCHULMAN 1969; SISSON et al. 1974), we examined effects on the rest–activity cycle as well as activity level (HUTCHINGS et al. 1979 a). For this, groups of rats were administered either 10 or 15 mg/kg methadone during the last 2 weeks of gestation and fostered at birth to untreated mothers. Groups of three littermates were tested during an 8-h period on electronic activity monitors at 17, 22, and 30 days of age. Compared with fostered controls, the 10 mg/kg offspring were significantly more active at 17 and 22 days of age and, in addition, were significantly more labile; that is, they showed more frequent shifts from low to high activity. Only an attenuated effect was observed among the 15 mg/kg group.

The activity data of four groups of 22-day-old vehicle controls and 10 mg/kg animals are shown in Fig. 1. From direct observations, we determined that counts of 0 represent periods during which the test group was huddled and sleeping; we refer to these 0 counts as sleep–rest periods. The brief spikes that range from 0–50 were typically produced by periods of waking of one or more of the three animals and repositioning within the group; active exploration by the group produced counts of approximately 50 and above. As shown in Fig. 1 a, b at the outset of the observation period, the control groups showed active exploration for about 30 min, followed by a sleep–rest period. Following this, they tended to show a distinct rhythmicity in their rest–activity cycle. By comparison, the 10 mg/kg groups shown in Fig. 1 c, d revealed striking differences; they remained active throughout virtually the entire 480-min observation period, and their activity pattern was marked by relatively rapid oscillations from low to high levels, with a complete absence of any prolonged sleep–rest periods. By 30 days of age, none of the methadone-treated offspring differed from the controls. The finding of an attenuated effect among the higher dose-level group is not unusual in behavioral teratology studies. MIDDAUGH et al. (1975 a) and HUTCHINGS et al. (1976) have both suggested that dose levels producing a relatively high maternal and offspring mortality may yield survivors that are more resistant to the toxic effects of the drug, and thus not show effects seen among the lower dose-level groups.

ZAGON et al. (1979 a) administered 5 mg/kg methadone to rats during gestation and/or lactation and found that in an activity cage and open-field, methadone-treated rats were less active than controls at 21 days of age, but more active at 45 and 60 days of age. On the other hand, our finding of heightened activity is similar

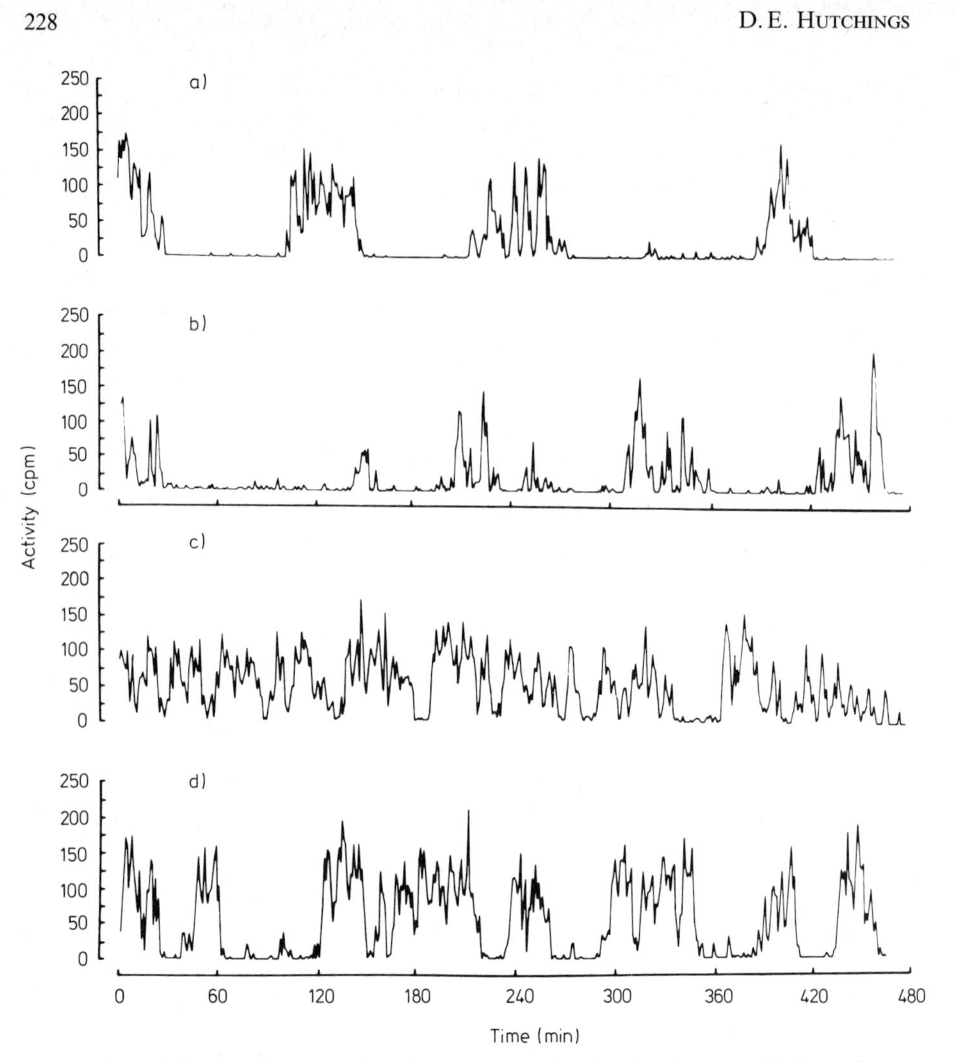


**Fig. 1 a–d.** Activity for offspring of methadone-treated and control rats at 22 days of age. Doses and numbers of rats are as follows! **a** 0 mg/kg, 1 male; 2 females; **b** 0 mg/kg, 1 male, 2 females; **c** 10 mg/kg, 1 male, 2 females; **d** 10 mg/kg, 2 males, 1 female

to the results of SOBRIAN (1977). She exposed rats prenatally to morphine and measured motor activity with electronic activity monitors at 5-day intervals during the first 30 days of life. Compared with controls, the morphine-treated offspring were no different in activity at 5 and 10 days of age. However, from 15 to 25 days of age, the treated offspring showed a sustained period of hyperactivity and, as we found with methadone, their activity level diminished to the level of the controls by 30 days of age.

Although SOBRIAN did not investigate underlying mechanisms, she suggested that prenatal morphine exposure may alter the maturation of the cholinergic–adrenergic or catecholamine systems to produce hyperactivity; methadone could act similarly. It is known that in addition to crossing the placenta, methadone concentrates highly in fetal rat brain (PETERS 1977), and confining exposure only to the prenatal period in the rat produces a significant delay in postnatal brain growth (SLOTKIN et al. 1976; ZAGON and MCLAUGHLIN 1977a) associated with a reduction in brain DNA content measured at 21 days of age (ZAGON and MCLAUGHLIN 1977b).

Alternatively, the heightened activity and increased lability that we found for methadone is analogous to the sleep disturbance and prolonged neonatal abstinence observed among some addicted neonates, and may be related to the persistence of pharmacologically active concentrations of the drug. A study by ROSEN and PIPPENGER (1976) of human neonates suggests that the occurrence of neonatal abstinence is dependent on at least two factors: first, the drug must fall below a critical tissue concentration before symptoms appear and second, once this concentration is reached, the severity of the symptoms are directly related to the rate of its clearance; the more rapid the clearance, the more severe the symptoms.

In order to determine if the behavioral effects that we observed result from the long-term persistence of methadone in offspring tissue, 10 mg/kg methadone was administered as described, with tritiated methadone added on the last 3 days of gestation (LEVITT et al. 1982). In the preliminary study, offspring were killed every 3 days after birth, beginning on day 8 through 20 days of age, and brains and livers were removed. Despite large variability between litters, higher values were found at earlier ages, but most important, tritiated methadone was found both in brain and liver through 20 days of age. These results suggest that after prenatal exposure to methadone, the compound persists in the brain, liver, and perhaps other tissues of the offspring at least until 20 days of age. These findings suggest that the hyperactivity, increased lability of state, and sleep disturbance found at 17 and 22 days of age may be a neonatal abstinence syndrome mediated by the slow clearance of methadone.

Our animal studies have also included the effects of prenatal exposure to methadone on long-term behavioral effects in the adult (HUTCHINGS et al. 1979b). For this, we employed the use of several operant tasks found in our previous work (HUTCHINGS et al. 1973; HUTCHINGS and GASTON 1974) to be sensitive to a variety of behavioral effects produced by vitamin A excess. Rats that had been exposed to a regimen of 10 mg/kg methadone on the last 2 weeks of gestation and fostered at birth to untreated mothers were tested in adulthood. The operant measures included acquisition of a lever-press response for water reinforcement, performance on a variable interval (VI) reinforcement schedule, acquisition and performance of an auditory–visual S+, S− discrimination, and a test of response inhibition using a punishment paradigm.

The operant measures did not reveal any learning or inhibitory deficits associated with prenatal methadone exposure. Treated animals acquired the lever–press response without difficulty, and on the discrimination task, like the controls, extinguished S− responding, maintained short S+ latencies, and acquired long S− latencies. During the punishment phase of testing, the treated animals showed no deficit in inhibiting shock-contingent response, although the methadone-exposed females showed significantly more response suppression compared with both the methadone-exposed and control males. However, among the treated offspring of both sexes, one prominent behavioral effect emerged; even though rapid response rates were not reinforced, the treated animals developed inordinately high rates of responding. During the VI reinforcement phase of testing, methadone-exposed males responded at a rate double that of the controls, and a similar effect was observed for the females during discrimination training. Because we found the treated animals to be no different form controls in a test of home cage activity level (D. E. HUTCHINGS 1979, unpublished work) we characterized this behavioral effect as an impaired ability to modulate task-oriented motor output.

The finding of an increased rate of response in an operant paradigm has also been reported by MIDDAUGH and SIMPSON (1980). The administered either 2.5, 5.0, or 10 mg/kg methadone to mice during the last week of gestation and, at birth, fostered all offspring to untreated mothers. When tested during adulthood, none of the offspring were impaired in the acquisition of the lever-press response. However, on several fixed ratio schedules of reinforcement, the 5 mg/kg group had a significantly higher rate of response compared with vehicle controls. In addition, similar to the increased suppression that we found among the methadone-exposed females during punishment, MIDDAUGH and SIMPSON (1980) found that, in response to the presentation of aversive auditory–visual stimulus, the 5 mg/kg females showed greater suppression of exploratory activity in an open-field experiment.

RECH et al. (1980), administered 5 mg/kg methadone twice daily during gestation and/or lactation and cross-fostered the offspring. Brain monoamines and metabolites were determined at 21 days of age and found to be significantly lower, particularly in limbic regions. At 90 days of age, monoamine levels were normal, but dopamine metabolites were significantly lowever, again, in limbic areas. A group administered methadone during gestation and tested at 90 days of age for acquisition of shuttle box avoidance and during training, was found to acquire the avoidance task faster and show more escapes and intertrial shuttles than controls. The authors suggest that early methadone exposure retards the development of central catecholamine and 5-hydroxytryptamine pathways, possibly producing hyperreactivity to aversive stimuli.

ZAGON et al. (1979 b) administered 5 mg/kg methadone during gestation and/or lactation and, at birth, cross-fostered the offspring. During adulthood, offspring were maze testes for their ability to acquire light–dark discrimination and trained to perform both an active and passive avoidance task. Although there were no differences between any of these groups on passive avoidance, the methadone-exposed animals, compared with vehicle controls, were slower to acquire both the active avoidance task and the light–dark discrimination. However, for this study, only female offspring were tested and the impaired acquisition of active avoidance may have resulted from their hyperreactivity to the aversive stimulus, an effect found by RECH et al. (1980) for both sexes, but only among females by HUTCHINGS et al. (1979 b) and MIDDAUGH and SIMPSON (1980). The finding of impaired learning should be replicated with both male and female offspring, and additional studies should determine whether early methadone exposure produces learning deficits independent of changes in emotionality or hyperreactivity.

In summary, both the clinical and animal studies indicate that prenatal exposure to opiates produces effects that occur in two phases. The acute phase consists of a neonatal abstinence syndrome, characterized by increased CNS arousal. The major behavioral symptoms seen in both humans and animals include hyperactivity, disturbed sleep, and increased lability of state. This early phase can be quite prolonged, lasting from 12 weeks to 6 months in humans and 20–25 days in rats. Although confirming pharmacokinetic studies are needed, it is possible that these persistent symptoms result from the slow clearance of the drug from neonatal tissues. The second phase of the syndrome is less well understood, but the available clinical evidence suggests that exposure to heroin, particularly in a pattern of polydrug abuse, can result in impaired organizational and perceptual abilities, poor self-adjustment, and, in situations requiring motor inhibition, heightened activity. Studies of preschool children exposed prenatally to methadone, reveal no effects on intellectual and cognitive functioning, but do reveal heightened activity or energy level, impulsiveness, brief attention span, and persistence. A finding of impaired motor inhibition while performing a task has been stressed by one worker as an area of particular vulnerability among these children. A strikingly similar effect, characterized as a impaired ability to modulate task-oriented motor activity, has been described for adult rats prenatally exposed to methadone.

## D. Summary

The major concern with drugs administered prenatally has been the risk of structural malformation. It has become increasingly evident, however, that a wide variety of pharmacologic agents can produce a range of effects that includes intrauterine death, growth retardation, and behavioral effects. Several agents that are teratogenic to the developing CNS in animals have been shown to produce learning impairments when administered during embryogenesis at subteratogenic doses; agents not specifically toxic to the CNS appear to be without effect. Further evidence indicates that there are critical periods in fetal development when agents produce histologic and cytochemical damage in specific brain areas. These are associated with behavioral effects, such as inhibitory and motor impairments, which appear to correspond to the known function of the damaged areas. Of the agents known to be teratogenic in humans, alcohol produces the most serious postnatal behavioral consequences. These include delayed development, hyperactivity, fine motor dysfunction, and mental retardation.

Other agents are discussed that do not produce gross structural malformations, but are nevertheless developmentally toxic. These drugs probably do not selectively kill embryonic cells, but appear to produce neurobehavioral effects by interfering with the ontogeny of neurochemical mechanisms. For example, heroin and methadone both produce a neonatal abstinence syndrome in the human neonate, with persistent sleep disturbance and hyperactivity. Studies with young animals have reported similar findings, with behavioral impairments persisting well into adulthood. The actions of these agents are viewed within the conceptual framework of teratology. It is suggested that, through a variety of embryopathic mechanisms, these compounds act on populations of embryonic cells and disrupt their normal pattern of development. An abnormal developmental sequence is initiated, leading to a final common pathway that may include neurobehavioral deficits.

*Acknowledgments.* Preparation of this manuscript was supported by grant DA 02463 from the National Institutes of Health. Portions of the chapter were adapted from HUTCHINGS (1978).

## References

Abel EL (1980) The fetal alcohol syndrome: behavioral teratology. Psychol Bull 87:29–50
Bartolome J, Seidler FJ, Anderson TR, Slotkin TA (1976) Effects of prenatal reserpine administration on development of rat adrenal medulla and central nervous system. J Pharmacol Exp Ther 197:293–302
Blinick G, Jerez E, Wallach RC (1973) Methadone maintenance, pregnancy and progency. JAMA 225:477–479
Butcher RE, Brunner RL, Roth T, Kimmel CA (1972a) A learning impairment associated with maternal hypervitaminosis-A in rats. Life Sci 11:141–145
Butcher RE, Vorhees CV, Kimmel C (1972b) Learning impairment from maternal salicylate treatment in rats. Nature New Biol 236:211–212
Butcher RE, Scott WJ, Kazmaier K, Ritter EJ (1973) Postnatal effects in rats of prenatal treatment with hydroxyurea. Teratology 7:161–165
Butcher RE, Hawver K, Burbacher T, Scott W (1975) Behavioral effects from antenatal exposure to teratogens. In: Ellis NR (ed) Aberrant development in infancy: human and animal studies. L Erlbaum, Hillside NJ, pp 161–167
Carr JN (1975) Drug patterns among drug-addicted mothers: incidence in use, and effects on children. Pediatr Ann 4:65–77
Chambers CD, Griffey MS (1975) Use of legal substances within the general population: the sex and age variables. In: Harbison RD (ed) Perinatal addiction. Spectrum, Holliswood NY, pp 7–19
Clark VH, Gorman D, Vernadakis A (1970) Effects of prenatal administration of psychotropic drugs on behavior of developing rats. Dev Psychobiol 3:225–235
Clarren SK, Alvord EC, Sumi SM, Streissguth AP, Smith DW (1978) Brain malformations related to prenatal exposure to ethanol. J Pediatr 92:64–67
Cooper JE, Cummings AJ, Jones H (1977) The placental transfer of phencyclidine in the pig: plasma levels in the sow and its piglets [Abstr]. J Physiol 267:17P–18P
Desmond MM, Schwanecke RP, Wilson GS, Yasunaga S, Burgdorff I (1972) Maternal barbiturate utilization and neonatal withdrawal symptomatology. J Pediatr 80:190–197
Dinges DF, Davis MM, Glass P (1980) Fetal exposure to narcotics: neonatal sleep as a measure of nervous system disturbance. Sience 209:619–621
Fowler H, Hicks SP, D'Amato CJ, Beach FA (1962) Effects of fetal irradiation on behavior in the albino rat. J Comp Physiol Psychol 55:309–314
Friedler G, Cochin J (1972) Growth retardation in offspring of female rats treated with morphine prior to conception. Science 175:654–656
Gauron EF, Rowley VN (1969) Effects on offspring behavior of mothers' early chronic drug experience. Psychopharmacologia 16:5–15
Geber WF, Schramm LC (1969) Comparative teratogenicity of morphine, heroin and methadone in the hamster [Abstr]. Pharmacology 11:248
German JA, Kowal A, Ehlers KH (1970) Trimethadione and human teratogenesis. Teratology 3:349–362
Golden NL, Sokal RJ, Rubin IL (1980) Angel dust: possible effects on the fetus. Pediatrics 65:18–20
Goodfriend WJ, Shey IA, Klein MD (1956) The effects of maternal narcotics addiction in the newborn. Am J Obstet Gynecol 71:29–36
Hanson JW, Smith DW (1975) The fetal hydantoin syndrome. J Pediatr 87:285
Hanson JW, Jones KL, Smith DW (1976a) Fetal alcohol syndrome: Experience with 41 patients. JAMA 235:1458–1460
Hanson JW, Myrianthopoulos NC, Sedgwick-Harvey MA, Smith DW (1976b) Risks to the offspring of women treated with hydantoin anticonvulsants, with emphasis on the fetal hydantoin syndrome. J Pediatr 89:662–668
Hicks SP, D'Amato CJ (1966) Effects of ionizing radiation on mammalian development. In: Wollam DHM (ed) Advances in teratology. Logos Press, London, pp 195–250
Hutchings DE (1978) Behavioral teratology: embryopathic and behavioral effects of drugs during pregnancy. In: Gottlieb G (ed) Various influences on brain and behavioral development. Academic Press, New York

Hutchings DE, Gaston J (1974) The effects of vitamin A excess administered during the mid-fetal period on learning and development in rat offspring. Dev Psychobiol 7:225–233
Hutchings DE, Gibbon J, Kaufman M (1973) Maternal vitamin A excess during the early fetal period. Effects on learning and development in offspring. Dev Psychobiol 6:445–447
Hutchings DE, Hunt HF, Towey JP, Rosen TS, Gorinson HS (1976) Methadone during pregnancy in the rat: dose level effects on maternal and perinatal mortality and growth in the offspring. J Pharmacol Exp Ther 197:171–179
Hutchings DE, Feraru E, Gorinson HS, Golden RR (1979 a) Effects of prenatal methadone on the rest-activity cycle of the pre-weanling rat. Neurobehav Toxicol 1:33–40
Hutchings DE, Towey JP, Gorinson HS, Hunt HF (1979 b) Methadone during pregnancy: assessment of behavioral effects in the rat offspring. J Pharmacol Exp Ther 208:106–112
Isaacson RL (1974) The limbic system. Plenum Press, New York
Joffe JM (1969) Prenatal determinants of behavior. Pergamon Press, Oxford
Jones KL, Smith DW (1975) The fetal alcohol syndrome. Teratology 12:1–10
Jones KL, Smith DW, Ulleland CW, Streissguth AP (1973) Pattern of malformation in offspring of chronic alcoholic women. Lancet 1:1267–1271
Jones KL, Smith DW, Streissguth AP, Myrianthopoulos NC (1974) Outcome in offspring of chronic alcoholic women. Lancet 1:1076–1078
Kalter H (1968) Teratology of the central nervous system. University of Chicago Press, Chicago
Kandall SR (1977) Late complications in passively addicted infants. In: Rementeria JL (ed) Drug abuse in pregnancy and neonatal effects. CV Mosby, St Louis, pp 116–128
Langman J, Welch GW (1967) Excess vitamin A and development of the cerebral cortex. J Comp Neurol 131:15–26
Langman J, Webster W, Rodier P (1975) Morphological and behavioral abnormalities caused by insults to the CNS in the perinatal period. In: Berry CL, Poswillo DE (eds) Teratology: trends and applications. Springer, Berlin Heidelberg New York, pp 182–200
Levitt M, Hutchings DE, Bodnarenko SR, Leicach LL (1982) Postnatal persistence of methadone following prenatal exposure in the rat. Neurobehav Toxicol Teratol 4:383–385
Lipsitz PJ, Blatman S (1974) Newborn infants of mothers on methadone maintenance. NY State J Med X:994–999
Lodge A (1976) Developmental findings with infants born to mothers on methadone maintenance: a preliminary report. In: NIDA: Symposium on comprehensive health care for addicted families and their children, May 20–21, 1976. pp 79–85
Lydiard RB, Sparber SB (1974) Evidence for a critical period for postnatal elevation of brain tyrosine hydroxylase activity resulting from reserpine administration during embryonic development. J Pharmacol Exp Ther 189:370–379
Marble RD, Thomas RG, Sterling ML (1980) Screening for angel dust in newborns. Pedatrics 66:334
Markham JK, Emmerson JL, Owen NV (1971) Teratogenicity studies of methadone HCL in rats and rabbits. Nature 233:342–343
Marks TA, Worthy WC, Staples RE (1980) Teratogenic potential of phencyclidine in the mouse. Teratology 21:241–246
McFie J, Robertson J (1973) Psychological test results of children with thalidomide deformities. Dev Med Child Neurol 15:719–727
Middaugh LD, Simpson LW (1980) Prenatal maternal methadone effects on pregnant C57BL/6 mice and their offspring. Neurobehav Toxicol 2:307–313
Middaugh LD, Blackwell LA, Santos CA III, Zemp JW (1974) Effects of d-amphetamine sulfate given to pregnant mice on activity and on catecholamines in the brains of offspring. Dev Psychobiol 7:429–438
Middaugh LD, Santos CA III, Zemp JW (1975 a) Effects of phenobarbital given to pregnant mice on behavior of mature offspring. Dev Psychobiol 8:305–313
Middaugh LD, Santos CA III, Zemp JW (1975 b) Phenobarbital during pregnancy alters operant behavior of offspring in C57BL/6J mice. Pharmacol Biochem Behav 3:1137–1139

Persinger MA (1971) Pre- and neonatal exposure to $10^{19}$ Hz and 0.5 Hz electromagnetic fields and delayed conditioned approach behavior. Ph.D. dissertation, University of Manitoba
Peters MA (1977) The effect of maternally administered methadone on brain development in the offspring. J Pharmacol Exp Ther 203:340–346
Pierog S, Chandarasu O, Wexler I (1977) Withdrawal symptoms in infants with the fetal alcohol syndrome. J Pediatr 90:630–633
Ramer CM, Lodge A (1975) Clinical and developmental characteristics of infants of mothers on methadone maintenance. Addict Dis 2:227–234
Rech RH, Lomuscio G, Algeri S (1980) Methadone exposure *in utero:* effects on brain biogenic amines and behavior. Neurobehav Toxicol 2:75–78
Rodier PM (1980) Chronology of neuron development: animal studies and their clinical implications. Child Neurol 22:525–545
Rodier PM, Webster W, Langman J (1975) Morphological and behavioral consequences of chemically induced lesions of the CNS. In: Ellis NR (ed) Aberrant development in infancy: human and animal studies. L Erlbaum, Hillsdale NJ, pp 169–176
Rosen TS, Pippenger CE (1976) Pharmacological observations on the neonatal withdrawal syndrome. J Pediatr 88:1044
Rosett HL, Sander LW (1979) Effects of maternal drinking on neonatal morphology and state regulation. In: Osofsky JD (ed) Handbook of infant development. Wiley, New York, pp 809–836
Schulman CA (1969) Alterations of the sleep cycle in heroin-addicted and "suspect" newborns. Neuropadiatrie 1:89–100
Shapiro S, Hartz SC, Siskind V et al. (1976) Anticonvulsants and parental epilepsy in the development of birth defects. Lancet 1:272–275
Shaywitz SE, Cohen DJ, Shaywitz BA (1980) Behavior and learning difficulties in children of normal intelligence born to alcoholic mothers. J Pediatr 96:978–982
Shenefelt RE (1972) Morphogenesis of malformations in hamsters caused by retinoic acid: relation to dose and stage at treatment. Teratol 5:103–118
Sisson TRC, Wickler M, Tsai P, Rao IP (1974) Effect of narcotic withdrawal on neonatal sleep patterns. Pediatr Res 8:451
Slotkin TA, Law C, Bartolome M (1976) Effects of neonatal or maternal methadone administration on ornithena decarboxylase activity in brain and heart of developing rats. J Pharmacol Exp Ther 199:141–148
Sobrian SK (1977) Prenatal morphine alters behavioral development in the rat. Pharmacol Biochem Behav 7:285–288
Sparber SB, Shideman FE (1968) Prenatal administration of reserpine: effect upon hatching, behavior and brainstem catecholamines of the young chick. Dev Psychobiol 1:236–244
Stephenon JPB (1976) Epilepsy: a neurological complication of thalidomide embryopathy. Dev Med Child Neurol 18:189–197
Stillman R, Petersen RC (1979) The paradox of phencyclidine (PCP) abuse. Ann Intern Med 90:428–429
Strauss ME, Starr RH, Ostrea EM, Chavez CJ, Stryker JC (1976) Behavioral concomitants of prenatal addiction to narcotics. J Pediatr 89:842–846
Strauss ME, Lessen-Firestone JK, Chavez CJ, Stryker JC (1979) Children of methadone-treated women at five years of age. Protracted effects of perinatal drug dependence. Pharmacol Biochem Behav [Suppl] 11:3–6
Streissguth AP, Herman CS, Smith DW (1978) Intelligence, behavior, and dysmorphogenesis in the fetal alcohol syndrome: a report on 20 patients. J Pediatr 92:363–367
Streissguth AP, Landesman-Dwyer S, Martin JC, Smith DW (1980) Teratogenic effects of alcohol in humans and laboratory animals. Science 209:353–361
Ting R, Keller A, Berman P, Finnegan L (1974) Follow-up studies of infants born to methadone-dependent mothers [Abstr]. Pediatr Res 8:346
Vacca L, Hutchings DE (1977) Effect of maternal vitamin A excess on S-100 in neonatal rat cerebellum: a preliminary study. Dev Psychobiol 10:171–176
Warner RH, Rosett HL (1975) The effects of drinking on offspring: an historical survey of the American and British literature. J Stud Alcohol 36:1395–1420

Werboff J, Dembicki EL (1962) Toxic effects of tranquilizers administered to gravid rats. J Neuropsychiatry 4:87–91
Werboff J, Havlena J (1962) Postnatal behavioral effects of tranquilizers administered to the gravid rat. Exp Neurol 6:263–269
Werboff J, Kesner R (1963) Learning deficits of offspring after administration of tranquilizing drugs to the mothers. Nature 197:106–107
Werboff J, Gottlieb JS, Dembicki EL, Havlena J (1961 a) Postnatal effect of antidepressant drugs administered during gestation. Exp Neurol 3:542–555
Werboff J, Gottlieb JS, Havlena J, Word JJ (1961 b) Behavioral effects of prenatal drug administration in the white rat. Pediatrics 27:318–324
Wilson G, Desmond M, Verniaud W (1973) Early development of infants of heroin-addicted mothers. Am J Dis Child 126:457–462
Wilson GS, McCreary R, Kean J, Baxter JC (1979) The development of preschool children of heroin-addicted mothers: a controlled study. Pediatrics 63:135–141
Wilson JG (1973) Environment and birth defects. Academic Press, New York
Young RD (1967) Developmental psychopharmacology: a beginning. Psychol Bull 67:73–86
Zackai EH, Mellman WJ, Neiderer B, Hanson JW (1975) The fetal trimethadione syndrome. J Pediatr 87:280–284
Zagon IS, McLaughlin PJ (1977 a) The effects of different schedules of methadone treatment on rat brain development. Explor Neurol 56:538–552
Zagon IS, McLaughlin PJ (1977 b) Methadone and brain development. Experientia 33:1486
Zagon IS, McLaughlin PJ, Thompson CI (1979 a) Development of motor activity in young rats following perinatal methadone exposure. Pharmacol Biochem Behav 10:743–749
Zagon IS, McLaughlin PJ, Thompson CI (1979 b) Learning ability in adult female rats perinatally exposed to methadone. Pharmacol Biochem Behav 10:889–894
Zemp JW, Middaugh LD (1975) Some effects of prenatal exposure to d-amphetamine sulfate and phenobarbital on developmental neurochemistry and on behavior. Addict Dis 2:307–331

CHAPTER 12

# Abnormal Lung Function Induced by Prenatal Insult

L. M. NEWMAN and E. M. JOHNSON

## A. Introduction

Mammalian susceptibility to teratogenic insult has been of interest and concern for several years. It was apparent as early as the 1940s that the developing embryo was both exposed to and at risk of injury by exogenous agents or conditions (WARKANY 1971). Until recently, expression of developmental abnormalities was thought to be limited to gross structural malformations, and the type of malformations observed were thought to be interrelated with the exact gestational or developmental stage at the time of exposure, as well as with the actual target phase or cell line. Additional evidence suggests, in the case of central nervous system (CNS) and lung evaluation, that the structural level and degree of damage may also dictate the form of expression (HUTCHINGS and GASTON 1974; VORHEES et al. 1978; RODIER 1977; JENSH et al. 1978; NEWMAN and JOHNSON 1980; CHRISTIAN and JOHNSON to be published). A subtle alteration, cellular or biochemical, may not cause a gross structural malformation, yet markedly affect the ability or efficiency by which a particular cell line or organ functions. Two questions arise. First, should a prenatally acquired functional deficit be classified as a teratologic effect; and second, what is the importance of this type of expression? It is our feeling that when a prenatal insult is expressed as a functional deficit with an impact that either threatens the life of an infant or affects the quality of life, it is indeed a teratologic incidence and is as important as any gross structural malformation. Therefore, the primary question becomes "what actual change has occurred and how may that change be manifested?" With this in mind, we have explored the sensitivity of the developing lung.

## B. Lung Development

Proper lung function is critical postnatally for viability and normal growth and development. Survival of the newborn requires that the lung be relatively efficient in the role of gaseous exchange of $O_2$ and $CO_2$, between atmospheric (alveolar) air and the circulating blood, across a tissue barrier immediately at birth. The ability to function is linked to the adequate cellular differentiation and organ development of the embryonic lung buds; first by developing an extensive airway system with a large surface area, matched with an extensive vascular network; and second, by decreasing the tissue mass in relationship to the total air space. These requirements are accomplished by synchronized differentiation of both mesodermal and epithelial components.

**Table 1.** Stages in the histologic development of human and rat lung

| Stage | Rat Time (days) | Human Time (weeks) |
|---|---|---|
| Embryonic | 11–16 | ≦ 6 |
| Pseudoglandular | 17–18 | 7–17 |
| Canalicular | 19–20 | 18–23 |
| Terminal sac | 21 (term) | 24–38 (term) |
| Alveolar | [a] | [b] |

[a] Day 2 postnatal onwards
[b] Term through first decade of life

Histologic ontogeny of lung is quite similar in many mammals, varying greatly, however, in timing and duration from one species to another. In the rat, the respiratory tree is first evidence as an unpaired midline evagination of the pharyngeal floor which has bifurcated to form paired primary bronchi surrounded by dense mesenchyme by day 11 (JOHNSON et al. 1963).[1] Branching of the enlarging respiratory tree is not accompanied by increased epithelial mitotic activity in paired localized sites, but results from interruption of the ordered pattern of collagen fiber deposition and organization (RUDNICK 1933; WESSELS 1970; ALESCIO 1973). TADERERA (1967) observed marked influence of mesoderm on epithelial behavior and failure of mesoderm to undergo normal histogenesis in the absence of epithelium. A reciprocal system appears operative as the epithelium is under control of the mesoderm (ALESCIO and CASSINI 1962; WESSELS 1970) and mesodermal derivatives (WESSELS 1970; ALESCIO 1973). However, in cultures of mouse lung, the epithelial mitotic rate is directly proportional to the quantity of bronchial mesenchyme present (ALESCIO and DI MICHELE 1968).

MORAWETZ (1970) divided the histologic development of lung into three phases for descriptive purposes. Two of these, glandular and canalicular, are prenatal in both rats and humans, and the third or alveolar is postnatal. The term glandular in this staging may prove misleading and we prefer the terminology of *Nomina Embryologica* as discussed by STRANG (1977) wherein five stages are employed. In the rat (specifically the Long-Evans strain in our laboratory), and human (DUNNILL 1962; DAVIES and REID 1970) these are shown in Table 1. It is sufficient to say for this discussion that lung development during the early embryonic phase is comprised primarily of continued or repeated branching of airways. By the end of this period, the histologic picture is one of rather poorly defined epithelial clusters with extremely small lumina, and the adjacent epithelial organizations are separated by abundant mesoderm.

Development of the entire lung is not synchronous, but a gradient of events distributed unevenly throughout the lung's substance. Development tends to proceed

1 The morning on which sperm are found by microscopic examination of a smear of vaginal contents is taken as day 0 of gestation. All citations associated with development events are standardized accordingly in this chapter, provided the authors indicate their method of age designation

both in a craniocaudal and proximodistal pattern. Descriptions for stages and their attainment are related to the major changes, while timing is related to the gestational age at which a predominant portion of the lung is demonstrating a particular structural stage.

The fetal period marks the development of the bronchioles and terminal air spaces. Beginning with the *pseudoglandular* stage (Fig. 1), histologic sections of day 17 and 18 fetal rat lungs typically reveal: (1) circular groups of epithelial cells resembling glandular tissue; (2) tall columnar epithelium with heavily stained and centrally located vesicular nuclei; and (3) large quantities of periodic acid–Schiff positive (PAS+) material, appearing in the basal region of the epithelial cells in histochemical studies with both the light and transmission electron microscopes. Most intracellular organelles are present in moderate numbers. WILLIAMS and MASON (1977) show electron micrographs of intracellular glycogen located in both apical and basal regions of the cells on day 18. However, their mode of counting gestational age is not indicated, and may differ from ours. Additionally, a ±12-h variation in developmental stages within a litter of embryonic or fetal rats is well known.

Changes in epithelial cells become quite evident on day 19: (1) the appearance of the lung becomes *canalicular* (Fig. 2); (2) lining epithelium of developing bronchioles and terminal passages becomes cuboidal, though some columnar cells remain; (3) nuclei are basally located; (4) PAS+ material increases in amount and becomes diffusely scattered throughout the cytoplasm; and (5) the first evidence of two epithelium types, type I and type II alveolar cells, is now seen in developing air spaces. At this stage, the type I alveolar cell is becoming a flattened squamous cell, primarily lining the terminal airway. Increased maturity is associated with condensation of the nucleus, a progressive loss of PAS+ material, and the loss of the numbers of organelles present. Type II cells, in contrast, remain rounded or cuboidal, with the vesicular nucleus basally located. These cells are rich in organelles and often protude into the expanding lumen. PAS+ materials remain and unique granules appear. Strong evidence exists that these granules are the lamellar bodies (O'HARE and SHERIDAN 1970; GIL and REISS 1973), and are believed to be sites of synthesis and storage of the surface active phospholipid, surfactant (e.g., ROONEY et al. 1977).

On day 19 of gestation, lamellar bodies are located in the basal aspects of type II alveolar cells. By day 20, the lamellar bodies have begun to migrate apically while increasing in both size and number. In plastic-embedded 1-μm-thick sections stained in toluidine blue, the accumulating lipid-containing lamellar bodies appear as dark spots (WILLIAMS 1977). By day 20, the PAS+ material has also migrated apically and stains very intensely. This staining subsequently decreases in intensity as lamellar bodies continue to mature and migrate apically. Biochemical determinations indicate that glycogen, which is PAS+, peaks at day 20 and then is rapidly depleted (WILLIAMS and MASON 1977). It is not known whether the glycogen depletion is related to lipid accumulation, except for its temporal connection.

The *terminal sac* period (Fig. 3) is attained by day 21 and represents a continued development of canalicular formation along with the changes already noted in type I and type II cells. This process, which includes connective tissue modifications, continues after birth when true alveoli are formed. In sections of Long-

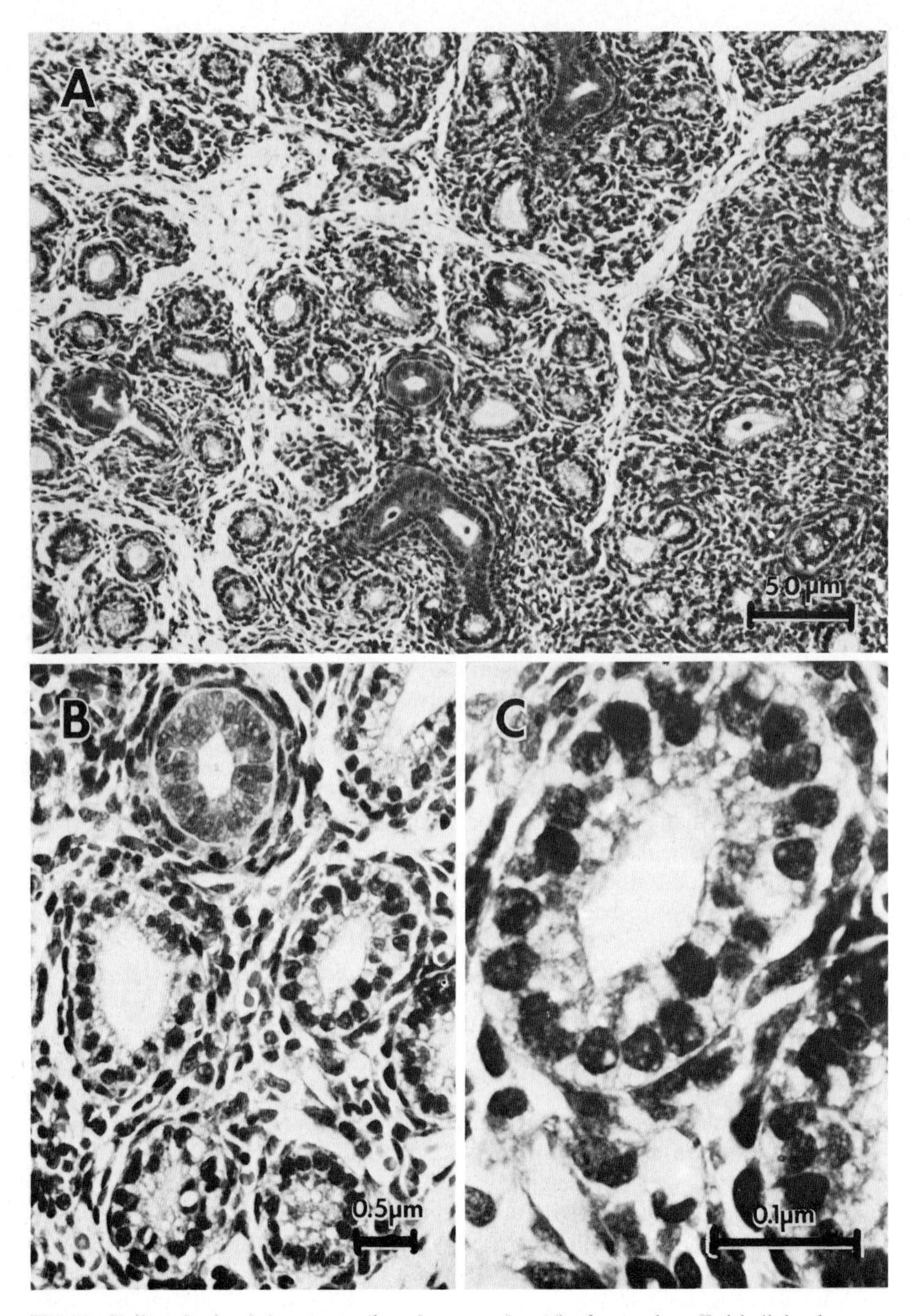


**Fig. 1A–C.** Pseudoglandular stage of rat lung on day 17 of gestation. Epithelial tubes are lined with columnar cells and are surrounded by considerable amounts of mesenchyme. Hematoxylin–eosin stain

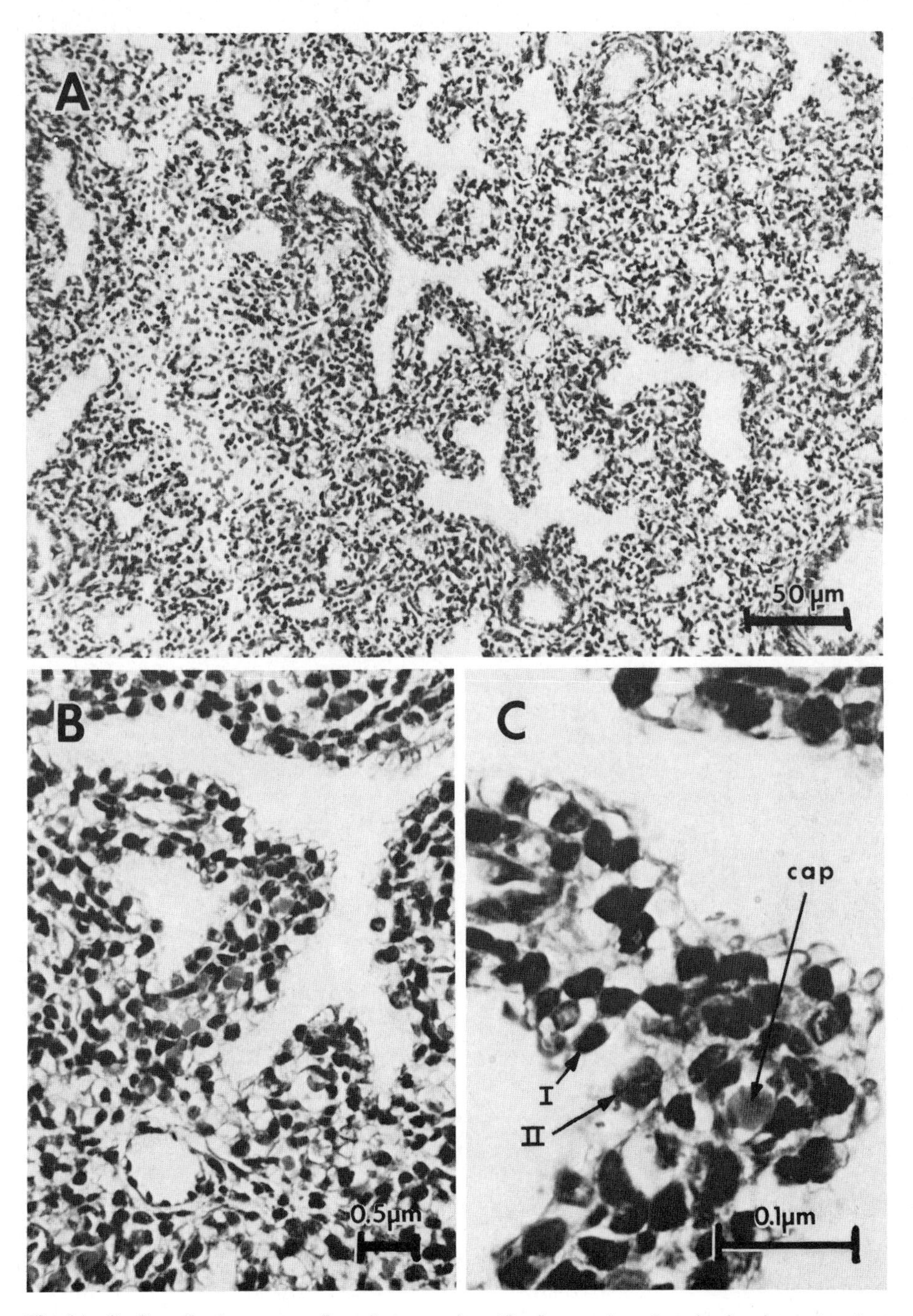


**Fig. 2A–C.** Canalicular stage of rat lung on day 19 of gestation. Luminal volume has increased since day 17. Passages are lined predominantly with cuboidal epithelium. Some cells can be identified as early type I or II pneumocytes, and the capillaries are still surrounded by multiple thickness of connective tissue. Hematoxylin–eosin stain

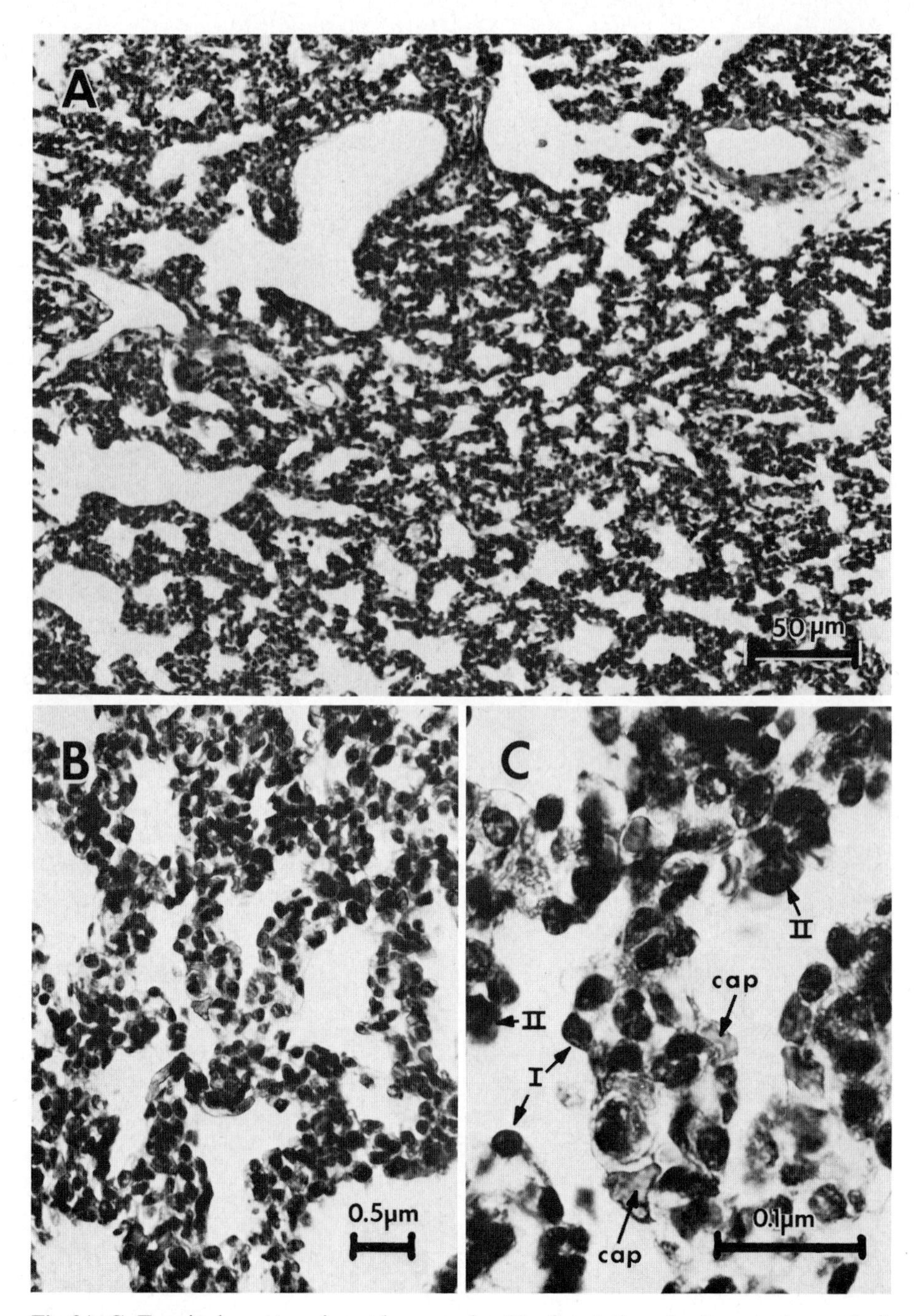


**Fig. 3A–C.** Terminal sac stage in rat lung on day 21 of gestation. Again note the marked increase of luminal area with further maturation of Type I and II cells. Capillaries are now adjacent to the lumina with the air–blood barrier formed by the attenuated cytoplasmic portions of the type I and endothelial cells. Hematoxylin–eosin stain

Evans rat pups collected early on day 21, the lamellar bodies of the type II pneumocytes are plentiful and found both in the apical portion of the cell and within the bronchiolar lumina, ready to be converted into tubular myelin (WEIBEL et al. 1966; MATTHEWS et al. 1981). At least two of our further observations (unpublished) suggest the first significant surfactant release occurs by late day 20: (1) released lamellar bodies and myelin figures were seen in the bronchiolar lumina in Long-Evans rat pup lungs as early as late day 20 (approximately 20.5 days); (2) this same timing (late day 20) compares favorably with the onset of the premature, cesarean-delivered rat pups' ability to exhibit spontaneous breathing, with subsequent survival.

By delivery, the lining epithelium of the entire system has specialized in accordance with the function of the particular region and has the following characteristics. In the upper respiratory tract (trachea, bronchi, and bronchioles), primarily involved with air conduction to the terminal functional units (alevolar ducts and alveoli), we find a tall, pseudostratified columnar ciliated epithelium with numberous goblet cells. As we progress distally, the epithelium becomes simple ciliated columnar, still with many "mucous producing" goblet cells. These become fewer in number and the columnar cells gradually become first cuboidal and ultimately a very thin squamoidal layer as you progress toward the alveoli. Cell type populations are also changing in the small bronchioles now primarily consisting of both ciliated and nonciliated (Clara's) cells with few goblet cells. In the mature terminal regions, the respiratory epithelium has differentiated into the type I and type II pneumocytes. As maturation continues, the ratio of type II to type I pneumocytes tends to decrease (BALIS et al. 1966) as does the ratio of the weight of DNA to dry lung weight (BRUMLEY et al. 1967). The cuboidal type II cells are typically located in the corners of the terminal sac or alveoli. The cytoplasmic extensions of the type I cells are now extensively attenuated, aiding in the formation of a very thin air–blood barrier in conjunction with the underlying capillary endothelial cell, with little or no connective fibers intervening. The cytoplasm of the type I cells, with exception of abundant free ribosomes and micropinocytic vesicles, are sparse in organelles.

The relatively thick septal walls of the newborn have a double capillary loop, with one capillary adjacent to each lumen. The two are separated by a broad band, primarily of interstitial fibroblasts and connective tissue fibers. Later, the thinning out of these walls is probably related to the massive lung growth associated with new alveoli and expansion in general. The newborn infant lung primarily functions with the future respiratory bronchioles and alveolar ducts of the mature lung (referred to as terminal sacs), as most true alveoli are developed postnatally (BURRI et al. 1974; THURLBECK 1975).

Mesodermal derivatives include blood vessels of all sizes, the smooth muscle fibers associated with the large airways (above 1 mm), and connective tissue in general – specifically the collagen, elastin, and reticular fibers providing support. These tissues have been further modified distally to provide the supporting structure, both for the epithelium and for stability of the parenchyma in general, allowing the expansion, with limitations, and recoil required throughout a breath cycle, preventing damage to the thin alveolar walls and/or to the massive capillary bed.

The thick, highly cellular interstitium at birth appears to be made up primarily of large relatively inactive mesenchymal cells (VACCARO and BRODY 1978). In alignment with the massive alveolar development, shortly after birth these cells differentiate into two types of fibroblasts. The first, located in the tips of the new developing septal crests, have similar characteristics to myofibroblasts in that they have intracellular actin-like filaments in the distal cytoplasmic claw-like extensions, and appear to be involved with elastogenesis. Large accumulations of amorphous elastin appear extracellular, adjacent to the claw-like projections. The loaded mitochondria, rough endoplasmic reticulum, Golgi complex, etc. also strongly suggest a role of protein synthesis and secretion for this cell.

The second type of fibroblast, located at the base of developing septae, seems to have a very different, but unknown role. Large stores of lipid material are present, with relatively few organelles (VACCARO and BRODY 1978). Labeling studies noted increased DNA synthesis, with the labeling occurring predominently at the base of new developing septa (KAUFFMAN et al. 1974), suggesting that the lipofibroblasts are new cells rather than senescent, dying cells (VACCARO and BRODY 1978). The fact that the lipid-filled cells have not been observed containing the protein synthesis machinery, strongly suggests these cells are not intermediate forms of the myofibroblast, but an entity of their own. By 3–4 weeks of age, the young rat lung appears similar to the adult. The interstitium is less cellular and the cells are similar in characteristics to the relatively inactive mesenchymal cell at birth (VACCARO and BRODY 1978).

Breathing movements in the human can be recorded as early as 3 months gestation, a process by which pulmonary fluid may be added to the amniotic fluid. These two fluids differ in chemical composition and pulmonary fluid continues to accumulate in normal to slightly excess amounts when the fetal trachea is ligated during gestation (ADAMS et al. 1963 a; CARMEL et al. 1965). Prior to delivery, approximately 26 orders of airway branching have occurred (BOYDEN 1974, 1976) and the luminal spaces and airways are filled with a fluid, rich in surfactant released from the lamellar bodies of the type II cells. Although the source of the pulmonary fluid itself is still undetermined, the chemical composition in lambs suggests a process of serum ultrafiltration with some type of selective secretion or resorption (ADAMS et al. 1963 b).

Delivery is a critical period for the respiratory system. The fetus must adjust rapidly, as the maternal system is no longer providing support, specifically oxygenation, and the infant's environment has changed from a fluid to an air medium. This now requires all of the blood to course through the lungs and that the lungs become filled with air to facilitate rapid transfer of $O_2$ and $CO_2$. The pulmonary fluid is partially removed via the pharynx during the vaginal delivery process. The remaining fluid appears to be absorbed by both alveolar capillaries and peribronchiolar lymphatics, leaving behind a phospholipid film of surfactant coating the saccules (SCARPELLI 1975).

Although the infant must start breathing within a short time after delivery, the total transition from fluid-filled to air-filled lungs is not accomplished in one breath, but takes several days to complete. In comparison with adult lung, the septal walls of the fetus and neonate are relatively thick, and progressively attenuate with repeated inflation–deflation cycles. This process, along with the development of additional alveoli, converts the immature fetal lung to a fully functional and mature lung. Any condition that effects any of the phases of lung development should be examined in terms of its possible impact on function.

## C. Experimental Alteration of Lung

Lung development has been altered at various times of development by different drugs and/or procedures. STANLEY et al. (1975) observed changes in mechanical properties of the lung related to altered molecular structure in connective tissue proteins following exposure of semicarbazide (a lathrogen) in young growing rats (weanlings). Although the lungs ruptured at lower pressures, lung compliance values were within normal limits, as were histologic sections fixed by perfusion at a standard 20 $cmH_2O$ pressure. In contrast, when fixed at 30 $cmH_2O$, dilated terminal air sacs, ruptured alveolar walls, and mathematically, an increased mean linear intercept were easily demonstrated when compared with controls. Biochemical follow-up revealed a decrease in cross-linkage of lung collagen, but unaltered total collagen content. Elastin values were normal.

Owing to the incidence of respiratory distress in newborns (often associated with atelectasis), most prenatal studies have been related in some way to changes in surfactant. This surface active phospholipid lines the terminal passages and alveoli, preventing their total collapse upon expiration by lowering the surface tension of the fluid at the liquid–air interface. A marked increase in surfactant production occurs late in gestation, thus suggesting that respiratory distress, often associated with prematurity, is due to inadequate surfactant (MASON et al. 1977). AVERY and MEAD (1959) showed that extracts of lungs from infants dying of respiratory distress syndrome (RDS) had high surface tension. In contrast, when adult surfactant is placed into the trachea of premature animals prior to the first breath, the surface tension is markedly lowered, as are the opening pressures – lung compliance (ENHORNING et al. 1973) The principal constituent of pulmonary surfactant is dipalmitoyl lecithin (KLAUS et al. 1961). Additional studies now provide evidence that these surface active lipids are stored intracellularly as membrane-bound secretory granules, the lamellar bodies observed in electron microscopy (GIL and REISS 1973). These lamellar bodies are released by the type II cells into the fluid-filled lumina and converted to the surface active tubular myelin (WILLIAMS 1977). As the pulmonary fluid is in constant production, excess is added to the amniotic fluid, either directly by way of the pharynx or indirectly by swallowing and subsequent fetal micturition. Therefore, this surface active material can be detected in: (1) amniotic fluid collected prenatally by amniocentesis (GLUCK et al. 1971); and (2) tracheal washings by means of lung lavage (AVERY and MEAD 1959).

A simple clinical test was devised which depends on the ability of surfactant to generate stable foam in the presence of ethanol (CLEMENTS et al. 1972). Amniotic fluid is mixed with an equal volume of ethanol, then shaken for 15 s. When surfactant is present in sufficient quantity, stable bubbles are generated which form a meniscus around the test tube that persists for 15 min or longer. Bubbles from samples lacking the surface active material are not stable and collapse quickly.

Lecithin (L) and sphingomyelin (S) are two principal lung phospholipids, often utilized in evaluating lung maturity. Until approximately 34 weeks in the human, the L:S ratio is about 1:1 (GLUCK et al. 1972), at about 35–36 weeks, the L:S ratio rises sharply. Similar increases in L:S ratio in the rat also have been reported when lung slices were analyzed directly (FARRELL 1973). The altered ratio (2:1 or greater) is due primarily to marked increase in the amount of lecithin, and is indicative of a mature lung. When pulmonary maturity is achieved, RDS generally does not occur at birth. A quick visual estimation method of the L:S ratio utilizing amniotic fluid on thin layer chromatography plates has been used in assessing the risk of RDS in pregnancies where factors might cause the infant to be delivered prior to adequate lung development (LIPSHAW et al. 1973).

Experimentally, it has been found that hypophysectomy in fetal lambs delays the onset of labor and by giving the fetus adrenocorticotropic hormone (ACTH), premature labor and premature development of lung results (LIGGINS et al. 1967; LIGGINS 1968). Intrauterine decapitation, which destroys the pituitary–adrenal–thyroid axis retards cytodifferentiation of lung and results in large lungs with excess quantities of glycogen (BLACKBURN et al. 1972). LIGGINS ascribed the changes to the induction of lung enzymes by glucocorticoids which altered the architecture of the lung and accelerated the synthesis and secretion of surfactant. It is now known that at least two pathways exist for lecithin synthesis in the fetal lung (FARRELL 1973). The major pathway, termed the choline incorporation pathway, does not become active until late in gestation in many species studied. In the rat, this occurs between days 18 and 19, when lamellar bodies first appear. The hypothesis now exists that corticosteroids induce the enzyme, choline phosphotransferase which enhances lecithin synthesis, surfactant production, and ultimately lung maturation. TORDAY et al. (1981) recently suggested that the observed exogenous glucocoricoid effect, reported by many investigators, mimics the normal spontaneous developmental processes of induction and stimulation of fetal pulmonary surfactant production, with an apparent linkage to induction of cellular differentiation associated with a simultaneous cellular growth inhibition. In the rabbit, there is a marked increase of surfactant and decrease of the lung DNA:protein ratio at 26–28 days gestation, compared with 24–26 and 28–30 days (TORDAY et al. 1981). Excess doses of glucocorticoids markedly accelerate cellular differentiation and may produce hypoplastic lungs as well as total body growth retardation (KAUFFMAN 1977).

Ovine prolactin was injected intramuscularly into rabbit fetuses on the 24th day of gestation. Although the prolactin-treated group showed 40% higher total lung phospholipid content and a 67% higher lung lecithin content, suggesting that prolactin might be a trigger of lung surfactant synthesis in the rabbit fetus (HAMOSH and HAMOSH 1977); VAN PETTEN et al. (1979) found no change in maturation, as evaluated by pressure–volume relationships (lung compliance), suggesting that prolactin does not initiate secretion of sufficient amounts of surfactant to induce physiologic maturation.

Phenobarbital, when administered to pregnant rabbits 7–10 days before delivery, produces pups with fewer lamellar bodies and higher opening pressures than controls (KAROTKIN et al. 1976a). This inhibitory effect was not expected since phenobarbital is a potent enzyme inducer, although it may exert its effect on lung maturation via stimulated hepatic microsomes to oxidize and conjugate endogenous corticosteroids (CONNEY 1967).

Aminophyllin was given to 40 pregnant rabbits, beginning on the 20th gestational day for a period of 7–10 days. The phospholipid content of the lung tissue homogenate from the aminophyllin-treated group was significantly higher than controls, as was the lung compliance slope, derived from pressure–volume curves (KAROTKIN et al. 1976b). Another study, also using rabbits with aminophyllin administration, noted an associated significant increase in lung saturated phosphatidylcholine. Incorporation of choline $^{14}C$ and methionine $^{3}H$ into phosphatidylcholine, was increased (BARRETT et al. 1976). An apparent inverse relation between lecithin and insulin, demonstrated during 34–35 weeks of gestation in the human, tends to support the hypothesis that insulin can inhibit lecithin synthesis (DRAISEY et al. 1977).

Observations concerning the prevalence of RDS as a result of various drug treatments have been reported, thus suggesting that drugs have an effect on development in the human. Prenatal RDS prevention has been achieved using both corticosteroids and bromhexine metabolite VIII, both of which have an inhibitory effect against tissue–fibrinogen–activator (HAAS-DENK et al. 1976). It has been noted that premature infants of heroin-addicted mothers have a lower prevalence RDS than those of nonaddicted mothers (GLASS et al. 1971). Morphine, however, when administered to pregnant rabbits, does not accelerate fetal lung development (ROLOFF et al. 1975).

Effects of maternal nutritional status on lung development have been examined. Low protein (8%) and fat-free diets throughout pregnancy, and 4-day starvation regimes at either 9–13 or 17–21 days gestation, produced small, hypocellular lungs, with transitory low lung lecithin and surface tension activity levels in the rat, as determined by weights and various biochemical assay (FARIDAY 1975). Earlier deprivation periods had no effect at birth. Rat pup lungs, following maternal zinc deficiency, also had reduced surfactant levels, but associated with semicollapsed, histologically hypercellular lungs (VOJNIK and HURLEY 1977).

Postnatal functional respiratory difficulties observed following prenatal cadmium exposure (8.0 mg/kg subcutaneously on days 12–15 of gestation) are apparently related to a delay in number and maturation of the lamellar bodies, and possibly the type II cells (DASTON and GRABOWSKI 1979; DASTON 1981a). The mechanism, in this case, appears to suggest that cadmium acts indirectly by inducing a fetal zinc deficiency (DASTON 1981) such as described by VOJNIK and HURLEY (1977).

Our laboratory has been involved in extensive studies using prenatal administration of excess vitamin A (retinyl acetate 160,000 IU/day on days 15–19 gestation) during the fetal period in the rat. This regime has resulted in many lung changes, both functionally and morphologically (ARMENTI and JOHNSON 1979; NEWMAN and JOHNSON 1980). Spontaneously delivered litters demonstrated a marked increase incidence of stillbirths and neonatal deaths within the first 3 days (Fig. 4). With the fact that terminated pregnancies have no increase in intrauterine deaths, the high stillborn rate suggests difficulty, either during parturition or in the pup's ability to make the transition to the air environment. Late gestational cesarean delivery did not increase postnatal survival, thus suggesting the latter.

Morphologically, although great variation in severity was observed between litters and littermates, and within various regions of the same lung, no experimental

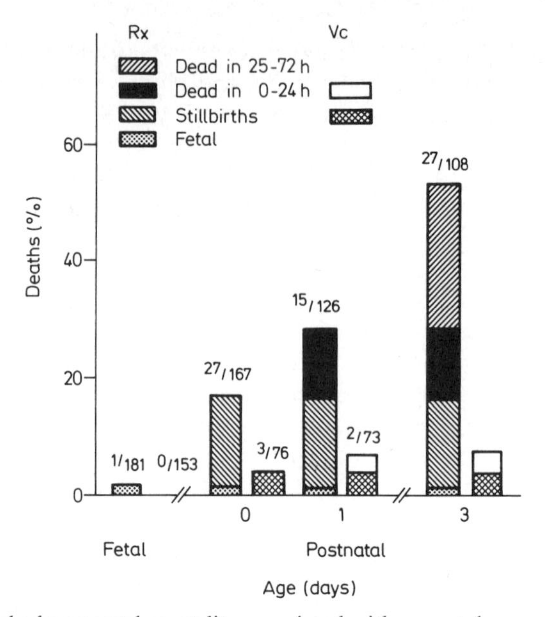


**Fig. 4.** Note the marked postnatal mortality associated with prenatal exposure of excess vitamin A in rat pups compared with controls during the first 72 h. The small numbers over the columns represent the number of dead observed divided by the total number of pups observed for that specific time period. No deaths occurred in the 98 fetal and 63 neonatal normal control pups observed during the same period. *Vc* indicates vehicle controls; *Rx* indicates vitamin-A-exposed pups

**Table 2.** Classification of neonatal lung tissue

| | |
|---|---|
| Grade I | Well-expanded lung with thin septal walls and uniform expansion; most airways demonstrate interconnections (Fig. 5a); functional capability would be expected to be normal |
| Grade II | Well-expanded lung similar to grade I except for thickened septal walls (Fig. 5b and 5c); expansion may ($II_a$) or may not ($II_b$) be uniform; functional capability may be mildly to moderately affected |
| Grade III | Basically, this lung has little or no functional capability; $III_a$ grade lung typically has few open airways with many collapsed alveoli (Fig. 8c), while $III_b$ represents atelectatic lung with rare open lumina (Fig. 8d) |

lung parenchyma appeared totally normal (Figs. 5–9). To aid in evaluating the lungs, a grading system was established on the basis of degree of expansion, thickness of septal walls, and the efficiency with which this would be predicted to function (Table 2). As can be noted in Figs. 5 and 6, the vehicle control (Vc) neonate

**Fig. 5A–C.** Control (*Vc*) neonatal rat lungs (day 2), demonstrating variability in uniformity in septal wall thickness and lung opening in three different animals. Hematoxylin-eosin stain. **A** typical grade I lung with thin septal walls and uniform expansion; **B** grade $II_a$ lung, illustrating uniform expansion and thickened septal walls as are typical for this developmental classification; **C** grade $II_b$ lung, septal walls and expansion are not uniform. See Fig. 6 for higher magnification

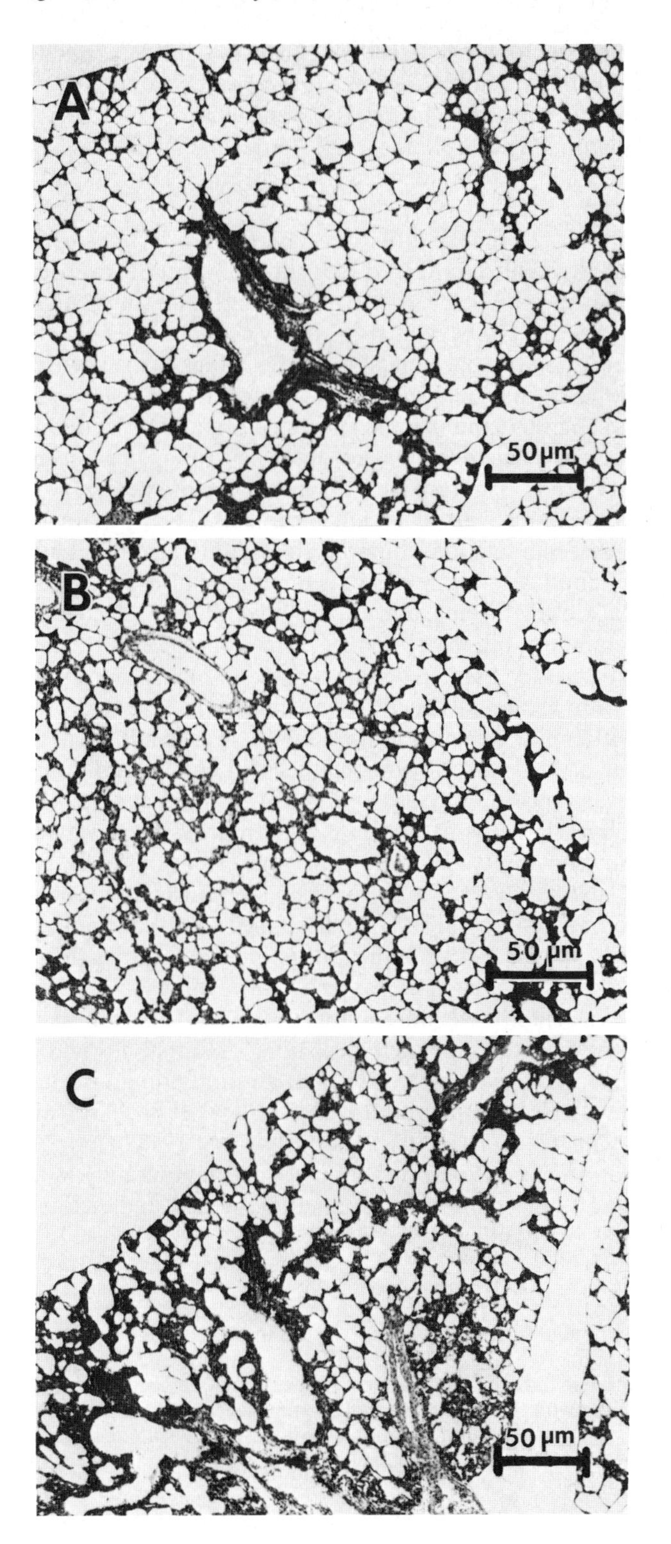
A
50 μm
B
50 μm
C
50 μm

also demonstrates variability in degree of expansion, but to a much less degree in comparison with the vitamin-A-exposed pups (Figs. 7 and 8). When compared with pups from undisturbed pregnancies (normal control, Nc), corn oil appears to have some effect on lung morphology, but this results in minimal impact on function or survival. Figure 7 demonstrates typical examples of regional versus diffuse effects seen in lungs of 2-day-old pups, following the prenatal exposure regime of excess vitamin A. The primary differences are the proportions of lung involved. Many pups' lungs revealed a marked reduction of respiratory surface area, with 25%–50% of the lung parenchyma being of grade III and similar to Figs. 8c and d. These areas do not seem to be related to airway collapse, as expanded airways are observed leading into both open and closed areas (Figs. 9–c). These particular animals would probably have died within a few days. In contrast, pups with grade II lungs similar to Fig. 8b demonstrated projected impaired function, but probably would have survived. Close examination of the general open parenchyma in histologic sections typically demonstrated thickened septal walls 110–120 μm at the thinnest points compared with 60–80 μm in controls. This appears to be largely related to an increase of interstitial components, although epithelial hyperplasia also contributes. Inflation, as already noted, is often nonuniform. Large areas of both partial and total atelectatic lung, and adjacent overdilated lung (compensative emphysema) are common, and may be either diffuse or regional in their distribution. Little or no inflamatory tissue reaction is present. While morphometric studies, evaluating the ratio of luminal space to epithelium of fetal ages day 18–21, revealed no significant difference, an epithelial hyperplasia was identified in terms of an increased number of alveolar cells/$\mu m^2$ epithelial tissue; in addition, an increased mitotic index was noted on days 18 and 19 (MATTHEWS et al. 1981). The overall effect is more epithelial cells packed into a given area, tentatively decreasing the degree of attenuation observed in the cytoplasmic extensions of the type I cell. This may, in turn, cause interference in the diffusion–perfusion of $O_2$ and $CO_2$. Transmission electron microscopy (TEM) studies failed to reveal changes in fetal type I or type II cells, either in developmental timing or structure (MATTHEWS et al. 1981).

Abnormal surfactant levels do not appear to be involved in the expression of excess vitamin A, in spite of the atelectasis noted. Normal morphological parameters of lamellar body development, release, and unfolding into tubular myelin, were observed with electron microscopy (MATTHEWS et al. 1981), and normal reduction of surface tension (ARMENTI and JOHNSON 1978) along with expected changes in L:S ratios measured by thin layer chromatography in amniotic fluid (unpublished data) suggests normal production, release, and quality of surfactant in the fetal lungs of vitamin-A-exposed rat pups.

**Fig. 6A–C.** Higher magnification of similar regions as seen in Fig. 5. (Vehicle control.) Hematoxylin–eosin stain. **A** grade I lung with uniform expansion and thin septal walls; new developing alveoli are identified by the appearance of septal crests (*arrows*); **B** grade $II_a$ uniform expanded lung with thickened septal walls; few developing septal crests are noted (*arrows*); **C** example of grade $II_b$ nonuniform expanded lung with consolidation or collapse areas (*a*) adjacent to open areas (*b*); septal walls are very irregular in thickness, with few septal crests noted

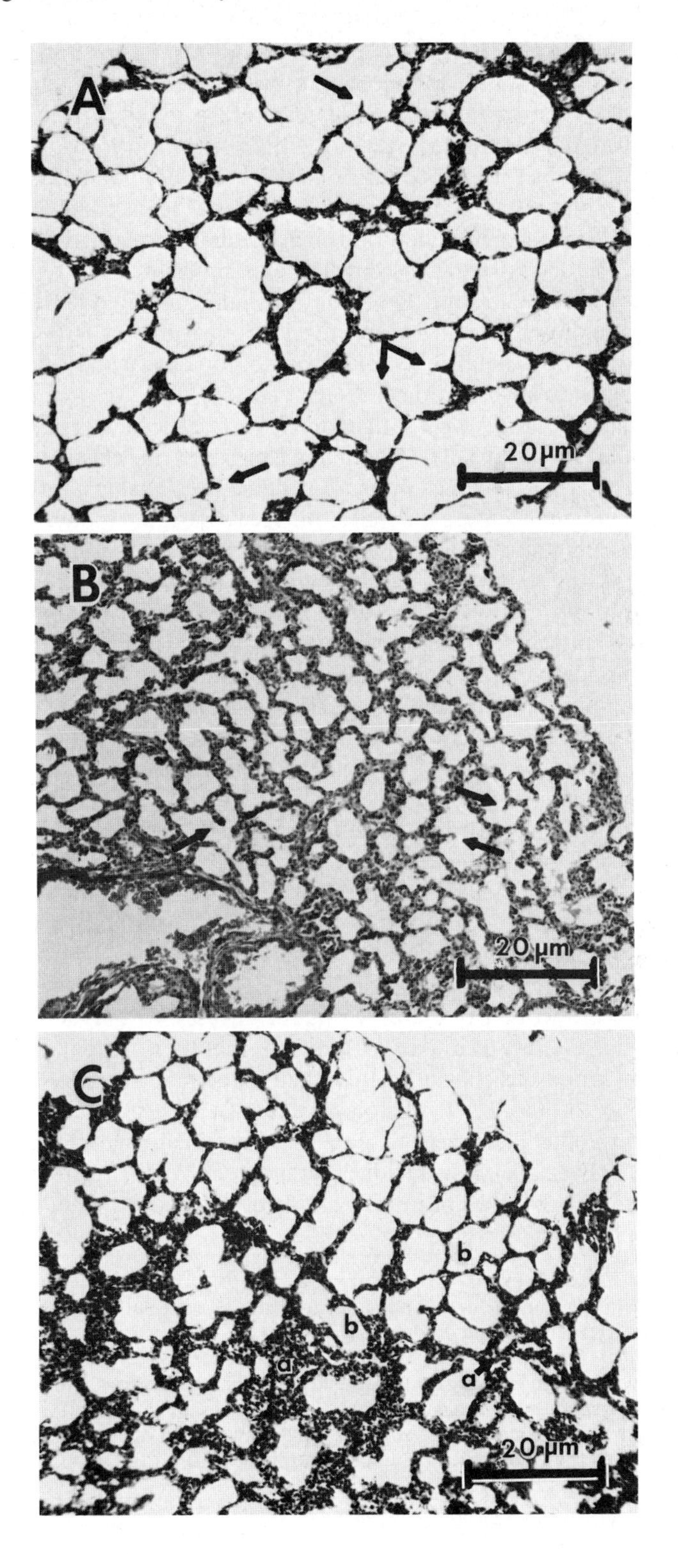
A
20 μm
B
20 μm
C
b
b
a
a
20 μm

As functional parameters, $O_2$ consumption, respiration rate, and lung compliance were studied in the rat neonate (NEWMAN et al. 1978; NEWMAN and JOHNSON 1981). Oxygen consumption and respiratory frequencies were evaluated in similarly treated pups from the day of delivery (day 0) through day 2. On day 0, the $O_2$ uptake values were low but similar to controls (7.4 mg $kg^{-1}$ $min^{-1}$ versus 14.8 ml $kg^{-1}$ $min^{-1}$). On day 1, control pups had increased $O_2$ uptake to 34.3 ml $kg^{-1}$ $min^{-1}$, while experimental pups lagged significantly at 19.7 ml $kg^{-1}$ $min^{-1}$ ($P > 0.05$). The disparity increased on day 2. Similarly, mean respiration rates in treated pups were 58, 81, and 74 respirations/min compared with 72, 111, and 117 in controls on days 0, 1, and 2 respectively. Approximately 50% of the individual pup respiration rates fell below that of controls on days 0 and 1, and 100% by day 2. Few pups lived beyond 4 days of age.

Two types of changes were seen in open chest, static lung compliance air studies (NEWMAN and JOHNSON 1981). Compliance measures the elasticity or recoil ability of the lung tissues in terms of pressure–volume relationships during inflation and deflation. This recoil feature is a reflection of two basic components: first, the tissue components including the amounts, arrangement and structure of elastin and collagen; second, the relationship of surfactant's ability to decrease surface tension on the wet tissue–air interface of the alveoli, thus preventing alveolar collapse. Upon air inflation, both components are in interplay while, if inflated with saline, the surfactant component is eliminated. (Only air inflation results are noted here.) An increase of compliance value implies a stiffer (noncompliant) lung i.e., in fibrosis and a decrease of compliance is a reflection of a more compliant lung, i.e., in emphysema. The inflation limb ($C_{L2-12}$) was significantly increased ($P > 0.02$) in experimental vitamin-A-exposed pups compared with vehicle control pups (Wilcoxon rank sum test). In contrast, the deflation limb ($C_{L12-2}$) mean did not differ, but the frequency distribution revealed an extended curve, suggesting the presence of different subpopulations. This is possibly due to differences in degree of severity of the effect morphologically and/or the uniformity of that effect throughout the lung. With respect to the uniformity factor, lung compliance may not be a good functional parameter for evaluation in the case of excess vitamin A.

Other experimental work, comparing the diffuse effect of blebomycin exposure and the regional effect of radiation, indicates that lung compliance results are not sensitive to conditions that markedly change the percentage of lung involved in ventilation (FINE et al. 1979). Histologic data of our excess vitamin A studies indicate high variability, both in percentage of involvement and diffuse versus regional involvement (Figs. 5, 7). It is obvious that lungs with a diffuse involvement, as seen in Fig. 7c and 8b, would not interfere with basic ventilation; in contrast, regions

→

**Fig. 7A–C.** Vitamin-A-exposed neonatal rat lungs (day 2), demonstrating examples of the typical variability seen in lung expansion in terms of regional and/or diffuse expression. These lungs rarely fit a single grade classification, but often have large regions representing several grades. Hematoxylin–eosin stain. **A** extensive atelectasis incorporating most of the left lower lung (grade III lung); note the adjacent compensative emphysema in the distal portion of the same lobe; **B** a midregion atelectasis (grade III lung) adjacent to relatively normal functioning parenchyma (grade II lung); **C** a typical diffuse expression; note this is quite similar to the poorer vehicle control animals with nonuniform expanded grade $II_b$ lung, i.e., Fig. 5C

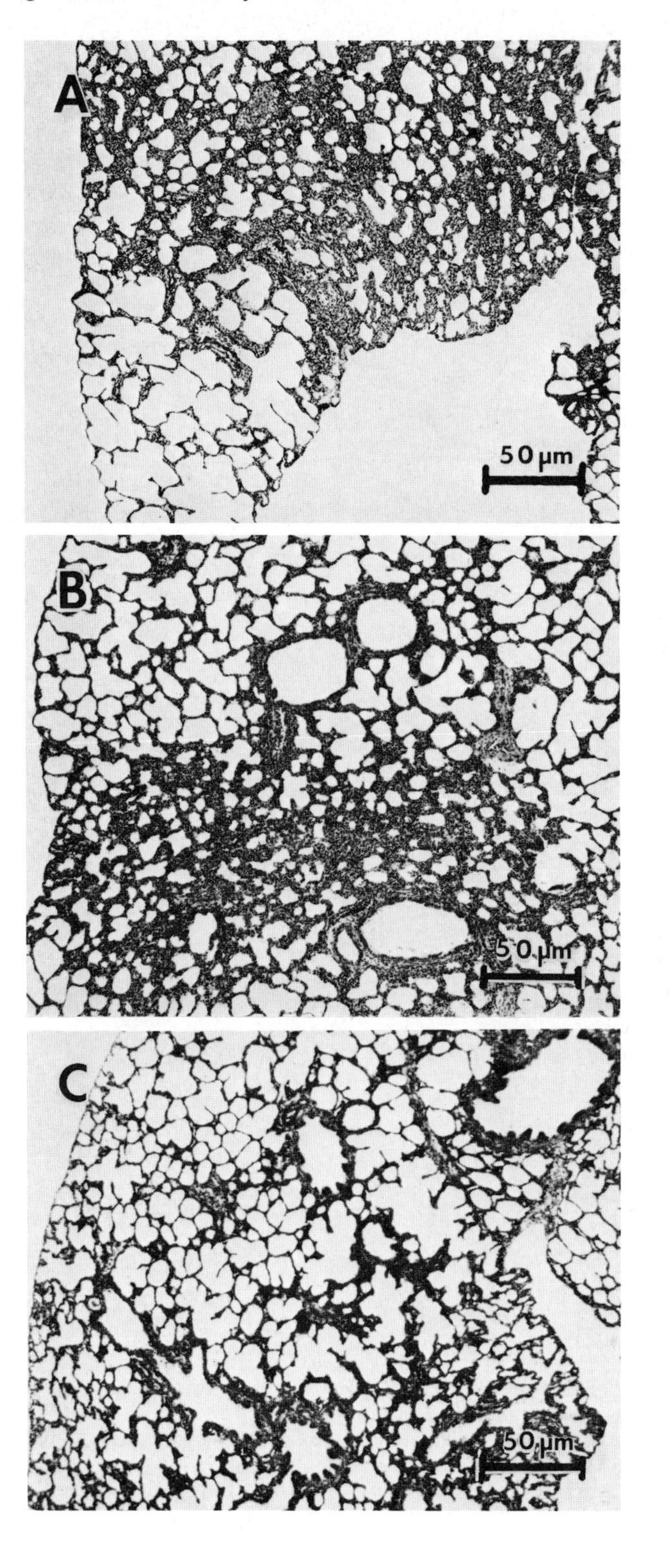
A
50 μm
B
50 μm
C
50 μm

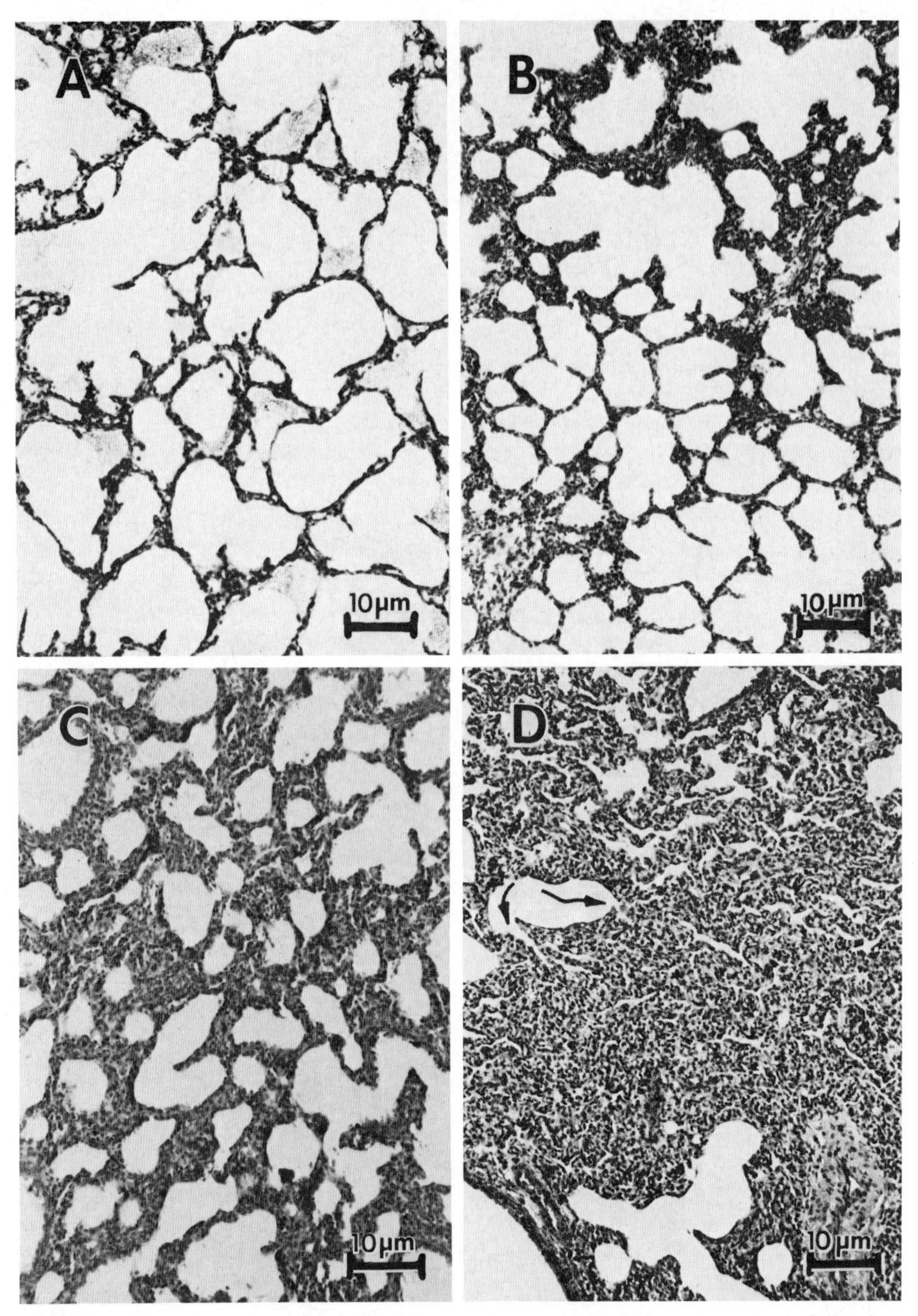


**Fig. 8A–D.** Higher magnification of the degree of variation seen in rat lung tissue following prenatal exposure to excess vitamin A. Selected regions or similar to Fig. 7. Hematoxylin–eosin stain. **A** grade I lung from a region similar to the expanded area of Fig. 7A, except for the slightly thickened septal walls, this tissue could not be distinguished from controls (compare with Fig. 6A); **B** grade $II_b$ expression showing a wide variety of respiratory pathology from Fig. 7C; note there is a mixture of expanded lung, lung with thickened septal walls, and small areas with either consolidation or atelectasis; lung tissue predominantly of this type

of the lung such as those depicted in Figs. 7a, b and 8c, d would have little or no respiratory ventilation. This suggests that, while a diffuse expression in vitamin-A-exposed rat pups would demonstrate a change in total compliance, lungs with large areas of atelectasis may demonstrate normal values if they have somewhat normal parenchyma in the functional areas. Therefore, in terms of compliance, without looking at a specific lung morphologically, it can be said that if lung compliance is abnormal, the lung is affected, but in the case of normal values we may fail to differentiate between normal lungs and those lungs with large atelectatic areas.

## D. Impact and Visibility of Developmental Alterations in Neonatal Population

Respiratory problems account for the largest single cause of neonatal morbidity and mortality in the human. Of these, 90% fall into the category of idiopathic RDS (BIEZENSKI 1976). As eluded to earlier, many chemical exposures or experimental conditions during lung development produce morphological, physiologic, and biochemical changes in the lung. In many respects, the effects seem in various experimental animals are similar to human pulmonary pathologies. Many of these alterations are implicated in the surfactant scheme, some in connective tissue integrity, and others are unknown as of date.

It is difficult, both clinically and experimentally, to identify reliably those individuals with compromised respiratory function. Individuals with severely effected lungs are easily identified as the condition is often life-threatening. In contrast, those with more subtle damage may have changes in functional efficiency, growth development, or susceptibility to various diseases. The identification of this latter group is difficult because "normal" values are themselves quite variable. This is well demonstrated by the typically broad range of physiologic values derived from untreated individuals. This problem is compounded in experimental animal studies where data from several observations are pooled and averaged for the presentation of results. Pooled data tend to mask the appearance of subtle effects in highly variable populations. If the standard deviation (SD) is large, the frequency distribution curve should be closely examined. Irregularly shaped, extended, or skewed curves tend to suggest the presence of inhomogenous populations. It is apparent that a need exists to establish criteria and methods to identify subpopulations within a given population.

Comparison of experimental animals with controls is difficult because of the broad range of variation encountered, regardless of which lung parameter one chooses to examine. We find that all normal rat lungs have at least some negative features. For instance, when we examine the microscopic appearance of a partic-

would most likely demonstrate a moderate detrimental effect on functional capabilities. Poor regions of the lung are usually a mixture of grade II tissue depicted in Figs. 8C and D, and would have little if any functional capability (see Fig. 7A and B for low magnification); **C** typical grade $III_a$ lung; although some airways are seen, much of the area appears collapsed; **D** an atelectetic lung area with rare open lumina (grade $III_b$ lung); note the slit-like airways, some leading out to larger open airways (*arrow*)

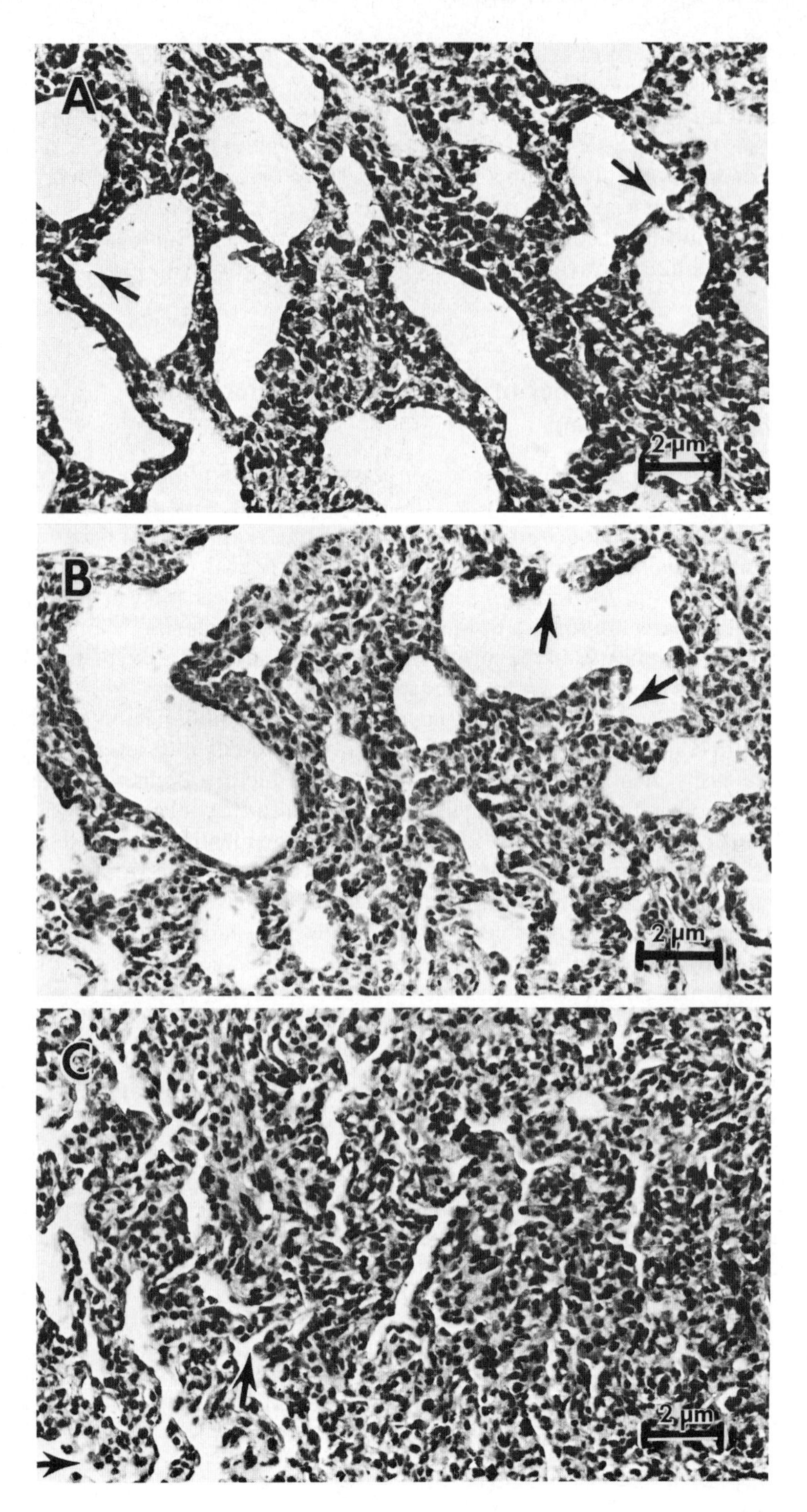
A
2 μm
B
2 μm
C
2 μm

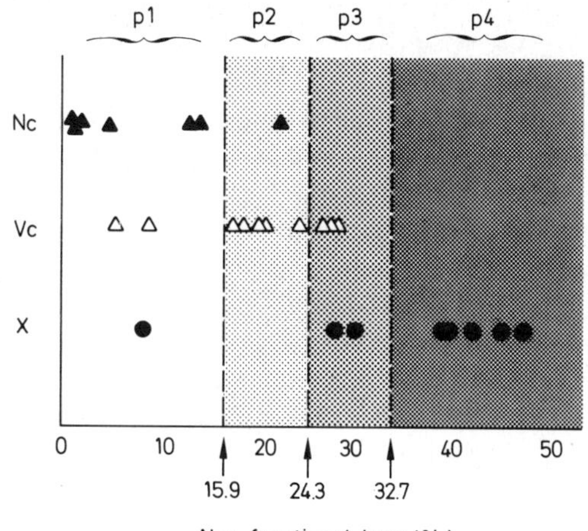


**Fig. 10.** Distribution of a given population (control or experiment) into subpopulations according to the percentage of grade III lung seen in a representative midhilar coronal histologic section of the entire lung. Normal limits (p 1) are dictated by the maximum acceptable percentage of grade III lung and are the mean +1 SD of values seen in normal control animals. Each subsequent SD increment sets the boundaries for each subpopulation, and thus for increasing severity of expression. *Full triangles* undisturbed control (*Nc*); *open triangles* vehicle control (*Vc*); *full circles* vitamin-A-exposed (*X*). See text for further explanation. Note most vitamin-A-exposed pups fall either between 2 and 3 SD (p 3) or beyond 3 SD (p 4)

ular normal control lung, some area will be found to be grade III according to the criteria presented in Table 2. As an example, to set a baseline, all available rat lungs were examined and the average percentage of grade III lung tissue in normal control lungs determined. This average value plus 1 SD was arbitrarily taken as the outside value for normal limits. All individual pup lung values were then compared with this base value and determined as falling within or outside normal limits. Abnormal pups were further subdivided into subpopulations on the basis of subsequent SD increments. Figure 10 demonstrates a scattergram utilizing this process of sorting individuals into subpopulations on the basis of histologic evaluation of their lungs. The percentage of lung parenchyma categorized as grade III, for instance, allows each pup to be evaluated and ranked as an individual in regard to severity of effect. If the value: (1) falls within the acceptable range (p 1) – the pup is classified as unaffected; (2) falls between 1 and 2 SD (p 2) – the pup is classified as mildly affected; (3) falls between 2 and 3 SD (p 3) – moderately affected; and (4) falling beyond 3 SD (p 4) – severely affected. This sorting and ranking method is also applicable in physiologic studies. Individual pups demonstrating subtle changes in either lung morphology or function can be effectively identified (manuscript in preparation).

**Fig. 9A–C.** Higher magnification of grade III lung regions similar to Fig. 8C and D, demonstrating connections between expanded airways and the slit-like openings in collapsed lung (*arrows*); Fig. 8A–C are progressively more severely affected; hematoxylin–eosin stain

## E. Conclusion

Although most neonatal laboratory animals are small and have organ systems which are extremely difficult to evaluate functionally, the importance of testing is unquestionable. Structure–function studies clearly indicate that teratogens (agents or conditions), applied any time up through early postnatal development, adversely alter development of the lung. This can be expressed as a functional deficiency in addition to the commonly acknowledged gross structural malformations. Though decrements of functional ability may be more subtle than gross abnormalities, their potential impact on normal growth, function and/or susceptibility to later pulmonary diseases may be considerable. As demonstrated by treatment with excess vitamin A (acetate), fetal stages are subject to abnormal development and a "teratogenic zone" must be considered as extending beyond the first third of pregnancy.

The extent to which such hidden decrements in attaining development of full genetic functional potential occur in the general population is unknown. Experiments to date would seem to imply that, as regards the lung, there could be significant factors markedly influencing the quality of postnatal life. These subtle effects perhaps also lead to confounding and unrecognized variables affecting functional capabilities of other organ systems.

*Acknowledgments.* The authors extend special thanks to ALBERT CADOGAN for his excellent technical assistance and to DEBRA LUNDGREN for her preparation of the manuscript.

## References

Adams FH, Fujiwara T, Rowshan L (1963a) The nature and origin of the fluid in the fetal lamb lung. J Pediatr 63:881–888
Adams FH, Moss AJ, Fagen L (1963b) The tracheal fluid in the fetal lamb. Biol Neonate 5:151–158
Alescio T (1973) Effect of a proline analogue acetidine-2-carboxylic acid on the morphogenesis *in vitro* of mouse embryonic lung. J Embryol Exp Morphol 29:439–451
Alescio T, Cassini A (1962) Induction *in vitro* of tracheal buds by pulmonary mesenchyme grafted on tracheal epithelium. J Exp Zool 150:83–94
Alescio T, di Michele M (1968) Relationship of epithelial growth to mitotic rate in mouse embryonic lung developing *in vitro*. J Embryol Exp Morphol 19:227–237
Armenti VT, Johnson EM (1978) Effects of retinyl acetate on fetal lung maturation in the rat [Abstr]. Teratology 17:46A
Armenti VT, Johnson EM (1979) Effects of maternal hypervitaminosis A on perinatal rat lung histology. Biol Neonate 36:305–310
Avery ME, Mead J (1959) Surface properties in relation to atelectasis and hyaline membrane disease. Am J Dis Child 97:517–523
Balis JU, Delivori M, Conen PE (1966) Maturation of postnatal human lung and idiopathetic respiratory distress syndrome. Lab Invest 15:530–546
Barrett CT, Sevanian A, Lavin N, Kaplan SA (1976) Role of adenosine 3′,5′ Monophosphate in maturation of fetal lungs. Pediatr Res 10:621–625
Biezenski JJ (1976) Pulmonary surfactant amniotic fluid lipids. Obstet Gynecol Annu 5:71–102
Blackburn WR, Travers H, Potter DM (1972) The role of pituitary-adrenalthyroid axes in lung differentiation I. Studies of the cytology and physical properties of anencephalic fetal rat lung. Lab Invest 26:306–318

Boyden EA (1974) The mode of origin of pulmonary acini and respiratory bronchioles in the fetal lung. Am J Anat 141:317–328
Boyden EA (1976) The development of the lung in the pig-tail monkey (*Macaca nemestrina*, L). Anat Rec 186:15–38
Brumley GW, Chernick V, Hodson WA, Normand C, Fenner A, Avery ME (1967) Correlations of mechanical stability, morphology, pulmonary surfactant, and phospholipid content in developing lamb lung. J Clin Invest 46:863–873
Burri PH, Dbaly J, Weibel ER (1974) The postnatal growth of the rat lung I. Morphometry. Anat Rec 178:711–730
Carmel JA, Friedman F, Adams FH (1965) Fetal tracheal ligation and lung development. Am J Dis Child 109:452–456
Christian MS, Johnson EM (to be published) Postnatal functional teratology resulting from fetal insult I. Alteration of gastrointestinal physiology. J Environ Pathol Toxicol
Clements JA, Platzker ACG, Tierney DF et al. (1972) Assessment of the risk of the respiratory-distress syndrome by a rapid test for surfactant in amniotic fluid. N Engl J Med 286:1077–1081
Conney AH (1967) Pharmacological implications of microsomal enzyme induction. Pharmacol Rev 19:317–366
Daston GP (1981 a) Effects of cadmium on the prenatal ultrastructural maturation of rat alveolar epithelium. Teratology 23:75–84
Daston GP (1981 b) Effects of maternal cadmium exposure on fetal lung maturation: relation to fetal zinc levels [Abstr]. Teratology 23:32A
Daston GP, Grabowski CT (1979) Toxic effects of cadmium on the developing rat lung I. Altered pulmonary surfactant and the induction of respiratory distress syndrome. J Toxicol Environ Health 5:973–983
Davies G, Reid L (1970) Growth of the alveoli and pulmonary arteries in childhood. Thorax 25:669–681
Draisey TF, Gagneja GL, Thibert RJ (1977) Pulmonary surfactant and amniotic fluid insulin. Obstet Gynecol 50:197–199
Dunnill MS (1962) Postnatal growth of the lung. Thorax 17:329–333
Enhörning G, Grossman G, Robertson B (1973) Tracheal deposition of surfactant before the first breath. Am Rev Respir Dis 107:921–927
Fariday EE (1975) Effect of maternal malnutrition on surface activity of fetal lungs in rats. J Appl Physiol 39:535–540
Farrell PM (1973) Regulation of pulmonary lecithin synthesis. In: Villee CA; Villie DB, Zuckerman J (eds) Respiratory distress syndrome. Academic Press, New York, pp 271–293
Fine R, McCullough B, Collins JF, Johanson WG Jr (1979) Lung elasticity in regional and diffuse pulmonary fibrosis. J Appl Physiol 47:138–144
Gil J, Reiss OK (1973) Isolation and characterization of lamellar bodies and tubular myelin from rat lung homogenates. J Cell Biol 58:152–171
Glass L, Rajegowda BK, Evans HE (1971) Absence of respiratory distress syndrome in premature infants of heroin-addicted mothers. Lancet 2:685–686
Gluck L, Kulovich MV, Burer RC Jr, Brenner PH, Anderson GG, Spellacy WN (1971) Diagnosis of the respiratory distress syndrome by amniocentesis. Am J Obstet Gynecol 109:440–445
Gluck L, Kulovich MV, Eidelman AI, Cordero L, Khazin AF (1972) Biochemical development of surface activity in mammalian lung IV. Pulmonary lecithin synthesis in the human fetus and newborn and etiology of the respiratory distress syndrome. Pediatr Res 6:81–99
Haas-Denk S, Krieglsteiner P, Wreidt-Lübbe I, Erhardt W, Münnich W, Blümel G (1976) Tissue-plasminogen-activators of maternal and fetal rat lungs after application of betamethasone or bromhexine-metabolite VIII. Z Geburtshilfe Perinatol 180:398–403
Hamosh M, Hamosh P (1977) The effect of prolactin on the lecithin content of fetal rabbit lung. J Clin Invest 59:1002–1005
Hutchings DE, Gaston J (1974) The effects of vitamin A excess administered during the midfetal period on learning and development in rat offspring. Dev Psychobiol 7:225–233

Jensh RP, Ludlow J, Weinberg I, Vogel WH, Rudder T, Brent RL (1978) Studies concerning the postnatal effects of protracted low dose prenatal 915 MHz microwave radiation [Abstr]. Teratology 17:21A
Johnson EM, Nelson MM, Monie IW (1963) Effects of transitory pteroylglutamic acid (PGA) deficiency on embryonic and placental development in the rat. Anat Rec 146:215–224
Karotkin EH, Kido M, Cashore WJ et al. (1976a) Acceleration of fetal lung maturation by aminophyllin in pregnant rabbits. Pediatr Res 10:722–724
Karotkin EH, Kido M, Redding RA et al. (1976b) The inhibition of pulmonary maturation in the fetal rabbit by maternal treatment with phenobarbital. Am J Obstet Gynecol 124:529–531
Kauffman SL (1977) Acceleration of canalicular development in lungs of fetal mice exposed transplacentally to dexamethasone. Lab Invest 36:395–401
Kauffman SL, Burri PH, Weibel ER (1974) The postnatal growth of the rat lung II. Autoradiograph. Anat Rec 180:63–76
Klaus MH, Clements JA, Havel RJ (1961) Composition of surface-active material isolated from beef lungs. Proc Natl Acad Sci USA 47:1858–1859
Liggins GC (1968) Premature parturition after infusion of corticotropin or cortisol into fetal lambs. J Endocrinol 42:323–329
Liggins GC, Kennedy PC, Holm LW (1967) Failure of initiation of parturition after electrocoagulation of the pituitary of the fetal lamb. Am J Obstet Gynecol 98:1080–1086
Lipshaw LA, Weinberg JH, Sherman AI, Foa F, Foa P (1973) A rapid method for measuring the lecithin-sphingomyelin ratio in the amniotic fluid. Obstet Gynecol 42:93–98
Mason RJ, Dobbs LG, Greenleaf RD, Williams MC (1977) Alveolar type II cells. Fed Proc 36:2697–2702
Matthews LM, Johnson EM, Newman LM (1981) Introduction of late gestational teratogenesis in rat lung by hypervitaminosis A. Teratology 23:253–258
Morawetz F (1970) Zur Entwicklung der menschlichen Lunge. Pneumonologie 143:136–138
Newman LM, Johnson EM (1980) Characterization of morphological and physiological abnormalities following fetal hypervitaminosis A exposure in the rat [Abstr]. Teratology 21:58A
Newman LM, Johnson EM (1981) Effect of fetal exposure to hypervitaminosis A on lung compliance in the neonatal rat [Abstr]. Teratology 23:54A
Newman LM, Johnson EM, Armenti VT (1978) Effect of prenatal vitamin A on neonatal respiratory frequency and $O_2$ consumption in the long-Evans' rat [Abstr]. Teratology 17:44A
O'Hare KH, Sheridan MN (1970) Electron microscopic observations on the morphogenesis of the albino rat lung, with special reference to pulmonary epithelial cells. Am J Anat 127:181–206
Rodier PM (1977) Correlations between postnatally-induced alterations in CNS cell population and postnatal functions. Teratology 16:235–246
Roloff DW, Howatt WF, Kanto WP, Borer RC (1975) Morphine administration to pregnant rabbits: effect on fetal growth and lung development. Addict Dis 2:369–379
Rooney SA, Nardone LL, Shapiro DL, Motoyama EK, Gobran L, Zachringer N (1977) The phospholipids of rabbit type II alveolar epithelial cells: comparison with lung lavage, lung tissue, alveolar macrophages and a human alveolar tumor cell line. Lipids 12:438–442
Rudnick D (1933) Developmental capacities of the chick lung in chorioallantoic grafts. J Exp Zool 66:135–154
Scarpelli EM (1975) Perinatal respiration. In: Scarpelli EM (ed) Pulmonary physiology of the fetus, newborn, and child. Lea & Febiger, Philadelphia, pp 117–139
Stanley NN, Alper R, Cunningham EL, Cherniack NS, Kafalider NA (1975) Effects of a molecular change in collagen on lung structure and mechanical function. J Clin Invest 55:1195–1201
Strang LB (1977) Growth and development of the lung: fetal and postnatal. Annu Rev Physiol 39:253–276
Taderera JV (1967) Control of lung differentiation *in vitro*. Dev Biol 16:489–512

Thurlbeck WM (1975) Postnatal growth and development of the lung. Am Rev Respir Dis 111:803–844
Torday JS, Zinman HM, Nielsen HC (1981) Reciprocal relationship between fetal lung cell proliferation and functional differentiation in vivo, 6/I [Abstr]. Fed Proc 40:557
Vaccaro C, Brody JS (1978) Ultrastructure of developing alveoli I. The role of the interstitial fibroblast. Anat Rec 192:467–480
Van Petten GR, Bridges R (1979) The effects of prolactin on pulmonary maturation in the fetal rabbit. Am J Obstet Gynecol 134:711–714
Vojnik C, Hurley LS (1977) Abnormal prenatal lung development resulting from maternal zinc deficiency in rats. J Nutr 107:862–872
Vorhees CV, Brunner RL, McDaniel CR, Butcher RE (1978) The relationship of gestational age to vitamin A induced postnatal dysfunction. Teratology 17:271–276
Warkany J (1971) Congenital malformations. Year Book, Chicago
Weibel ER, Kistler GS, Tondury G (1966) A stereologic electron microscope study of "tubular myelin figures" in alveolar fluids of rat lungs. Z Zellforsch Mikrosk Anat 69:418–427
Wessels NK (1970) Mammalian lung development. Interactions in formation and morphogenesis of tracheal buds. J Exp Zool 175:455–466
Williams MC (1977) Conversion of lamellar body membranes into tubular myelin in alveoli of fetal rat lungs. J Cell Biol 72:260–277
Williams MC, Mason RJ (1977) Development of the type II cell in the fetal rat lung. Am Rev Respir Dis 115:37–47

CHAPTER 13

# Postnatal Alterations of Gastrointestinal Physiology, Hematology, Clinical Chemistry, and Other Non-CNS Parameters

M. S. CHRISTIAN

## A. Introduction

Although interest in teratology has existed since prehistoric times, scientific studies of the subject are restricted to the last century. Initially, it was assumed that mammalian conceptuses were protected from external influences by the maternal organism, and early experiments were restricted to studies of amphibian and avian development (WARKANY 1965). HALE'S (1933, 1935, 1937) demonstration of the relationship of vitamin A deficiency and teratogenicity in pigs, disproved the theoretical nonsusceptibility of mammalian conceptuses to external influences and initiated investigation of mammalian teratogenic risk (WILSON and WARKANY 1964). In the 1960s, as a direct result of the thalidomide tragedy (LENZ 1961; MCBRIDE 1961), scientific and regulatory interest was restimulated, with subsequent expansion of research efforts associating morphological changes with first trimester teratogenic insult (WILSON and FRASER 1977).

Until recently, many investigators assumed that susceptibility to morphological change resulting from teratogenic insult vanished at completion of organogenesis (KALTER 1968; WILSON 1973). It is now evident that teratogenic insult during the fetal period may produce changes of different types. Clinical examples of human fetal susceptibility include modification of infant thyroid function by naturally occurring thiourea-like substances, enzyme induction by barbiturates, growth retardation associated with maternal smoking (LOWE 1974), and depression of the immune system associated with maternal alcohol consumption (MONJAN and MANDELL 1980).

Within the past decade, it has been clearly demonstrated that the developing central nervous system (CNS) is susceptible to teratogenic insult during the fetal period. Postnatal functional impairment subsequent to prenatal insult of the CNS has been reported (BUTCHER et al. 1973; INOUYE et al. 1972; KHERA and NERA 1971; SPYKER and SMITHBERG 1972; VACCA and HUTCHINGS 1977). Correlation of neonatal functional deficits and observed alteration of CNS histogenesis sometimes occurs (PETIT and ISAACSON 1976; RODIER 1977). Selection of appropriate methods for detection of behavioral deficits and the relative importance of these findings currently comprises an area of intense debate (BUELKE-SAM and KIMMEL 1979; BUTCHER 1976; COMMITTEE on POSTNATAL EVALUATION of ANIMALS SUBJECTED to INSULT DURING DEVELOPMENT 1976; GRANT 1976; KIMMEL 1976; RODIER 1976). The theory of a pure "behavioral teratogen" has even been proposed (VORHEES et al. 1979), although this has been discounted by others (JOHNSON et al. 1980).

Altered development of organ systems other than the CNS was demonstrated about 20 years ago (JOHNSON 1964), but only recently have acceptance and recognition of functional alterations resulting from prenatal insult occurred. Most of the early reports of functional changes have two limitations. First, the evaluation was of a single organ system, and second, only one test agent was used. Fetal insult has been reported to delay maturation of the lung (ARMENTI et al. 1977; JOHNSON and ARMENTI 1978; NEWMAN et al. 1978), liver, spleen, heart, testis, ovary (JOHNSON 1964), and adrenals (EGUCHI et al. 1976). Alteration of hemopoiesis (AMORTIGUI et al. 1976; HOFFMAN and CAMPBELL 1977), derangement of carbohydrate metabolism (DEMEYER et al. 1972; SNELL 1977), liver enzyme system (LUCIER 1976), hematocrits and plasma electrolytes (CHERNOFF and GRABOWSKI 1971), increased heart: body weight ratio (GRABOWSKI 1976), altered heart rate (GRABOWSKI and TURNSTALL 1971), and partial or total sterility (MUKHERJEE et al. 1975) have been reported as secondary to teratogenic insult of the fetus.

This chapter will review some of these reported postnatal sequelae of fetal insult, and describe a series of possible screening tests for postnatal gastrointestinal teratogenic effects and effects on multiple systems in the same animals exposed to different agents during the fetal period (CHRISTIAN 1979; CHRISTIAN and JOHNSON 1978, 1979a, b; CHRISTIAN and JOHNSON to be published).

## B. Functional Teratology of the Gastrointestinal Tract

### I. Gastrointestinal Congenital Malformations

The gastrointestinal tract is an organ system which demonstrates significant development during the fetal period (HAMILTON and MOSSMAN 1972). In a review of congenital gastrointestinal malformations, HEINONEN et al. (1977) reported an incidence of 6/1,000, based on 346 malformations in 301 children of a total population of 50,282. Pyloric stenosis was the most common malformation, occurring in 32% of the children presenting gastrointestinal tract anomalies. Umbilical hernia occurred in 17%, Hirschsprung's disease in 4.3%, tracheoesophageal fistula in 3.7% and various types of atresia in 2%–3% of the children with malformations. Pyloric stenosis occurred four times more frequently in whites than in blacks, with the gastrointestinal tract malformation rates 7.4, 5.0, and 3.8/1,000 in whites, blacks, and hispanics, respectively. Gastrointestinal tract malformations were much more frequent in children of low birth weight, and approximately 50% more frequent in males.

Variables positively associated with gastrointestinal tract malformations and with a statistically significant relative risk greater than 3/1,000 included: single umbilical artery (8.8/1,000), birth weight less than 1,500 g (5.4/1,000) and hydramnios (4.7/1,000). Also statistically significant and positively associated with gastrointestinal tract malformations were hemorrhagic shock (2.6/1,000), convulsive disorder (2.5/1,000), Rh incompatibility (2.2/1,000), maternal age of 40 years or more (2.0/1,000), malformation in a family member (1.9/1,000), abruptio placentae (1.8/1,000), male sex (1.6/1,000), and white ethnic group (1.4/1,000) (HEINONEN et al. 1977).

Several gastrointestinal tract malformations have been associated with abnormal development of the intramural plexuses. For example, the pathology producing esophageal achalasia, in which the pharyngeal swallowing reflex and action of the pharyngoesophageal sphinter are normal, but peristalsis is absent, is agenesis of the myenteric plexuses (DAVENPORT 1977). Infants with hypertrophic pyloric stenosis have a similar number of myenteric plexuses per unit area as normal infants, but the plexuses in the abnormal infant are primarily comprised of undifferentiated ganglia (FRIESEN et al. 1956).

Hirschsprung's disease, congenital megacolon, which is four times more frequent in male infants, also has abnormal myenteric plexuses as the causal pathology (EHRENPREIS 1971). Many cases of idiopathic megacolon have a similar histopathology (BODIAN et al. 1949). Classically, Hirschsprung's disease is defined by the absence of ganglia in the narrow distal segment of the rectosigmoid (WHITEHOUSE and KERNOHAN 1948). EHRENPREIS (1971) expanded the classification of megacolon with abnormal ganglia to include: (1) absent, as in Hirschsprung's disease with aganglionosis or hypoganglionosis; (2) degenerated or reduced, as in Chagas' disease and as a complication of anorectal surgery; and (3) immature, a developmental phenomenon sometimes associated with temporary intestinal obstruction in fetuses and premature infants.

The piebald-lethal mouse demonstrates a congenital malformation similar to human Hirschsprung's disease. In mice expressing the recessive trait, the rectal segment is hypoganglionic or aganglionic, and the colon is grossly distended with impacted feces (BRANN and WOOD 1976). These examples of pathology in the human and animal model demonstrate that mature intramural plexuses must be present for intestinal propulsion to occur.

## II. Normal Anatomy, Development, and Physiology of the Gastrointestinal Tract

The nerve layer in the stomach of the human fetus segments into plexuses at approximately 16 weeks gestation. However, mature ganglia are not observed until 2–4 weeks after full-term birth, and not until 4–8 weeks after birth are mature ganglia present in every plexus (FRIESEN et al. 1956). Similar postnatal increase in absolute cell number and size is reported in the rat (GABELLA 1971), indicating that this species is an appropriate model system for study.

Coordinated peristaltic propulsion requires an adequate number of functional intramural plexuses (FEHER and VAJDA 1972; VIZI 1976; WOOD 1976). Five intramural plexuses composed of individually distinct cells can be distinguished: (1) subserous; (2) myenteric (Auerbach's); (3) deep muscular; (4) internal; and (5) submucous (Meissner's). The two major divisions, the myenteric and the submucous, are present in the muscle layers and submucosa, respectively. Terminal fibers of these two plexuses probably give rise to the other three (DAVENPORT 1977; GUNN 1968; IKEDA 1957; IRWIN 1931; SCHOFIELD 1968; WOOD 1975).

Regional differences in motility are believed to reflect a gradient in intrinsic innervation of the gastrointestinal tract (BENNETT 1974). Postganglionic sympathetic and pregnaglionic parasympathetic fibers comprise a large portion of the plexuses. Branches of the plexuses synapse with other plexuses, the circular and longitudinal muscle layers, the muscularis mucosae, the gland cells of the mucosa, endocrine cells, and muscular tissue within the mucosa.

Reflex arcs are formed by cells in the submucous plexus, which have dendrites acting as receptor organs in the mucosa, and muscle layers and axons synapsing with cells in either the submucous or myenteric plexuses. This vast network of ganglia interconnecting with ganglia also interconnects with efferent sympathetic and parasympathetic fibers, the various muscle tissues, and the mucosal secretory and endocrine cells (DAVENPORT 1977; SZURSZEWSKI 1976). It is probable that the intramural plexuses not only coordinate peristalsis, but in addition mediate secretory and endocrine activity of the mucosa and participate in feedback mechanisms.

## III. Physiologic Teratology of the Gastrointestinal Tract

The emphasis of the following research (CHRISTIAN 1979) on investigation of possible alteration of gastrointestinal function was based on the theory that many of the functional disorders related to abnormal number and/or maturation of the intramural plexuses may be secondary to teratogenic insult. The elements of the intramural plexuses originate from neural crest cells and migrate to their final destination (WESTON 1970). Intramural neural elements have been observed in the small intestine of 12-mm human fetuses at approximately week 6 of gestation (KUBOZOE et al. 1969), and in rabbits on day 12 of gestation (DAIKOKU et al. 1975). It was demonstrated that, in the rat, the intramural plexuses are not present in the fetal gastrointestinal tract on days 14 or 15 of gestation, are possibly present on day 16, and are definitely present on day 17 of gestation (CHRISTIAN 1979). The full complement of mature ganglia is not present until some time after birth.

Initial interest in experimental delay of proliferation and maturation of the ganglia was on the assumption that such a delay might provide an animal model for evaluation of human gastrointestinal pathology and reveal this pathology to be a functional teratogenic effect. It was also assumed that inhibited neural crest cell migration was a means by which development of the inramural plexuses could be delayed. As ablation techniques were not used, specific sensitivities of various developing organ systems to a teratogen would be expected to result in alteration of concurrently developing systems. It was expected that experimental delay of cell proliferation in the fetus might possibly result in functional defects in the gastrointestinal tract and in other systems which develop during fetal and early postnatal life.

## IV. Test Agents

Four known teratogens which reduce cell proliferation were tested in rats. Three of the agents have been used for chemotherapy; the fourth is a different type of agent, a nutritional requirement. Agents tested were:

1. Actinomycin D, a teratogen (JORDAN and WILSON 1970; TUCHMANN-DUPLESSIS and MERCIER-PAROT 1960) which interferes with RNA transcription by binding to guanine and inhibiting DNA-dependent RNA polymerase (REICH 1963; STOCK 1966; WAKSMAN CONFERENCE on ACTINOMYCINS 1974).
2. Hydroxyurea, a teratogen (CHAUBE and MURPHY 1966; SCOTT et al. 1971) which interferes with DNA synthesis by inhibiting ribonucleoside diphosphate re-

ductase, the enzyme which catalyzes the reductive conversion of ribonucleotides to deoxyribonucleotides (AGRAWAL and SARTORELLI 1975; KRAKOFF 1975; YARBRO 1968).

3. Methotrexate, a teratogen (BERRY 1971; JORDAN et al. 1977; KHERA 1976; MILUNSKY et al. 1968; SKALKO and GOLD 1974; WILSON 1970) which inhibits DNA synthesis by inactivating dihydrofolate reductase and thus prevents the conversion of dihydrofolic acid to tetrahydrofolic acid, a cofactor of thymidine synthetase (BERTINO 1975; HANDSCHUMACHER and WELCH 1960; HITCHINGS and BURCHALL 1965; JOHNS and BERTINO 1973).

4. Vitamin A (retinyl acetate), a teratogen (COHLAN 1954; KALTER and WARKANY 1961) which may act be reducing the rate of mitosis and the subsequent proliferative rate in surviving cells (MARIN-PADILLA 1966).

Actinomycin D is reported to have a tissue half-life of 26–47 h in the rat (GALBRAITH and MELLETT 1975) and has been observed in fetal tissues, indicating that placental transfer occurs (BARANOV et al. 1968; JORDAN and WILSON 1970). Hydroxyurea has a short half-life of approximately 85 min in rat embryos (WILSON et al. 1975). Methotrexate persists in mammalian tissues; and in mice has been detected months after administration (CHARACHE et al. 1960). Although its metabolism is different in mice and rats, as the excretion of methotrexate is slower in the rat, it may be assumed that the drug also produces long-term effects in the rat (ZAHARKO and OLIVERIO 1970). It is evident that it reaches the fetus, because methotrexate can be used in studies of transient inhibition of DNA synthesis in the rat, and its effect can be rapidly reversed by administration of calcium folinate (BERRY 1971). Vitamin A (retinyl acetate) is a fat-soluble vitamin which persists in tissues, particularly liver, and enters enterohepatic circulation. Only 25%–35% of a dose is excreted within 24 h (ROBERTS and DELUCA 1967; ZACHMAN et al. 1966).

Hydroxyurea has a relatively short half-life and was therefore administered twice each day at 8-h intervals. The other agents, with longer half-lives, were administered once each day of treatment. Saline (0.9%) was administered to control rats once each day of treatment. The teratogens were administered intraperitoneally at 10 ml/kg to rats on days 15–17 (chemotherapeutic agents) via gavage, or days 15–19 (vitamin A) of gestation. Dosages administered were 10 ml/kg$^{-1}$/day$^{-1}$, 0.05–0.1 mg/kg$^{-1}$/day$^{-1}$, 250 mg/kg twice a day, and 0.25–1.0 mg/kg$^{-1}$/day$^{-1}$ 0.9% saline, actinomycin D, hydroxyurea, and methotrexate, respectively. Corn oil was given at 1.0 ml/kg and vitamin A at 250,000–1,000,000 U.S.P. units/kg$^{-1}$/day$^{-1}$. It was assumed that continual exposure to these agents, beginning on day 15 of gestation and continuing through days 17 or 19 of gestation, would result in decreased cell proliferation at a time just prior to and during genesis of the intramural plexuses in the rat.

## V. Observations

### 1. Anatomic

Only a subjective examination of a few treated rats was performed because a meaningful statistical analysis of the absolute number of intramural plexuses would require a large number of animals, special staining techniques, and a great length of time, and because absolute number and maturity of the ganglia are co-determinants of coordinated gastrointestinal function. In a methotrexate-treated male rat, there appeared to be a reduced number of intramural plexuses in the stomach and small intestine. This subjective alteration was not observed in the methotrexate-treated female rat, nor in the male and female rats administered either actinomycin D or hydroxyurea.

Although it was not possible to determine an anatomic basis for the observations, altered postnatal gastrointestinal physiology was found in teratogen-exposed rats. In postnatal functional evaluations of various segments of the gastrointestinal tract, rats exposed during the fetal period to teratogens performed differently from control rats. Postnatal evaluations studied were rectal emptying, transit time, food consumption and utilization, and gastric emptying (CHRISTIAN and JOHNSON 1978a, 1979a, b to be published). Because only a few rats were administered vitamin A, these results are not tabulated; however, results appeared similar to those observed for rats administered the three chemotherapeutic agents, and are discussed when differences were observed.

## 2. Rectal Emptying

The rectal emptying assay is a modification of a pharmacologic test used to detect antidiarrheal agents (VON SCHOTTEK 1967). It evaluates the time required to expel an inserted bead from the rectum. Results of this test may reflect innervation and integrity of feedback mechanisms in the colon and anal sphincter, ability of the anal sphincter to remain contracted, sensitivity of the tissues, internal pressures, ileal outflow, propulsive movements in the colon, and coordination and sequencing of defecation (DAVENPORT 1977).

Rectal emptying was altered in rats in all teratogen-treated groups (Fig. 1). Rats exposed to teratogens during the fetal period emptied beads more rapidly than control rats. Sex-related differences in response were apparent in the teratogen-treated groups. Male rats were generally more affected than female rats. Rectal emptying was more rapid in rats in both control and teratogen-exposed rats when a rod was used to insert the bead 1 cm into the colon than when the bead was inserted without using a rod (Fig. 2). Although the differences were not significant at $P<0.05$, whether or not a rod was used to insert the bead, the response was more rapid when a rod was used. This variation possibly indicates that the additional stress inherent in the method contributed to the observed difference in performance of teratogen-exposed and control rats.

## 3. Transit Time

Transit time is a standard physiologic evaluation. In these studies it measured the duration of time from intubation of rats with an opaque X-ray medium until this medium was observed in fecal material. Transit time in rat intestine, using charcoal in feed, has been reported as 6–32 h (SIKOV et al. 1969). In these studies, all rats had opaque medium in feces within 24 h after intubation. Transit time was more rapid in teratogen-exposed rats than in 0.9% saline control rats (Fig. 3). As in the previous assay, a sex-related difference in response was observed. Although transit times were similar in male and female control rats, teratogen-treated male rats had shorter transit times than teratogen-treated female rats.

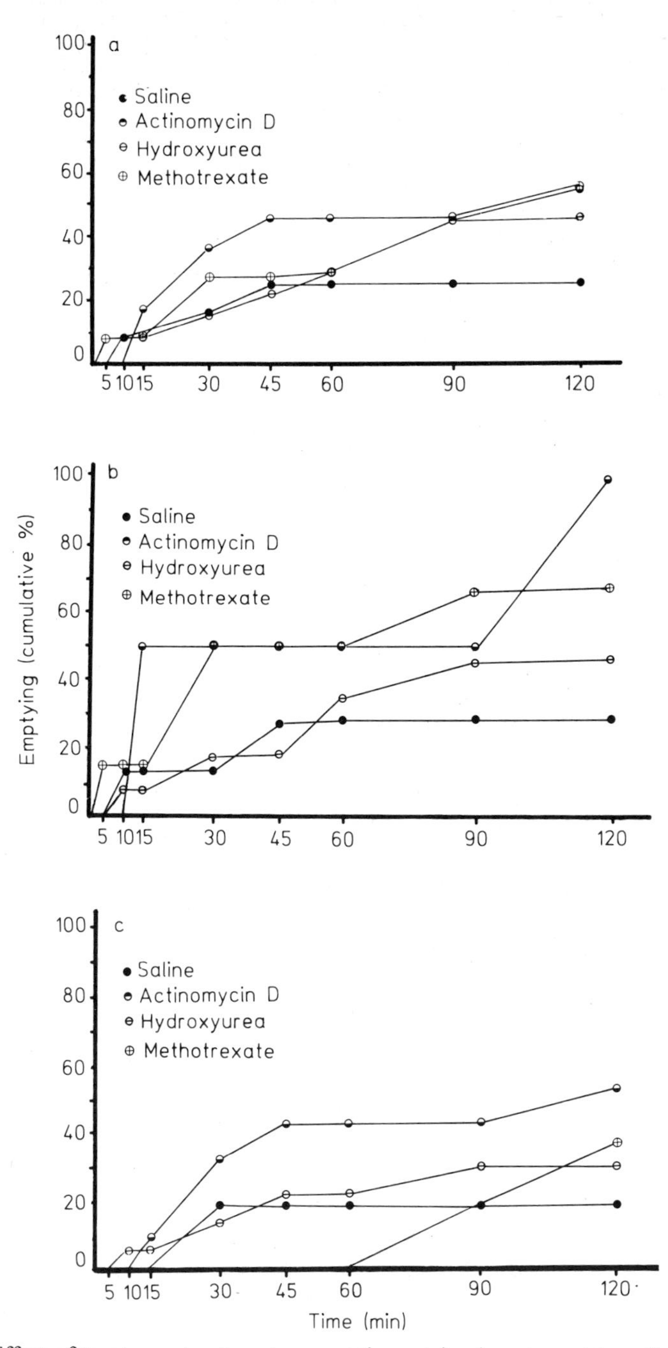


**Fig. 1 a–c.** Effect of teratogen treatment on rectal emptying in rats, rod insertion method. **a** combined sexes; **b** males; **c** females

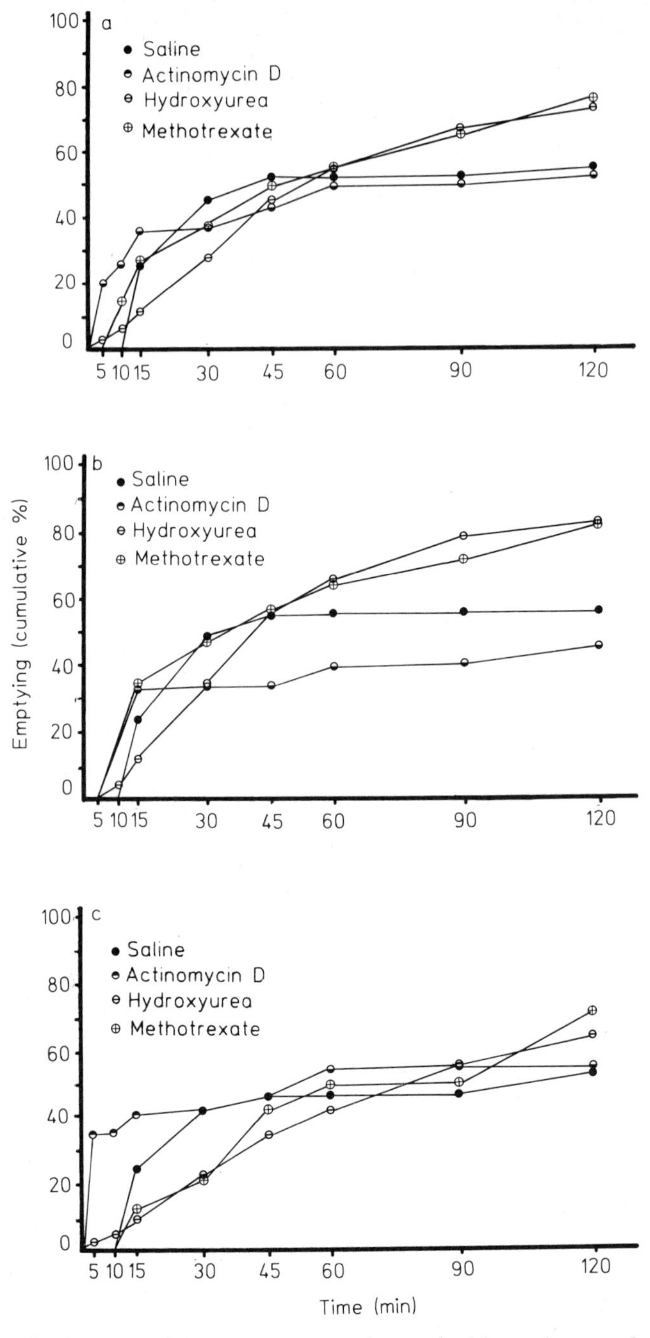


**Fig. 2 a–c.** As Fig. 1, except that teratogens were inserted without the use of a rod

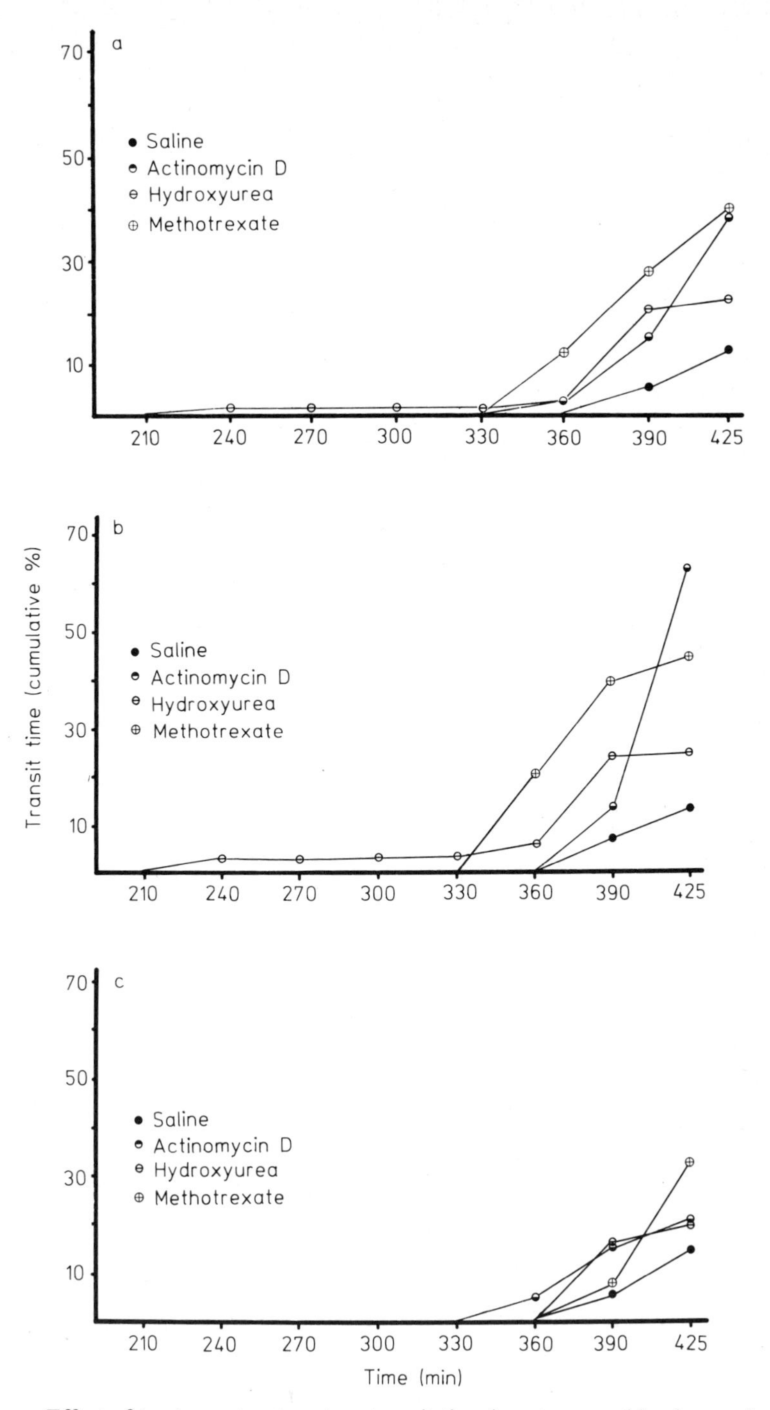


**Fig. 3 a–c.** Effect of teratogen treatment on transit time in rats. **a** combined sexes; **b** males; **c** females

Transit time and rectal emptying are subject to similar types of alteration. Passage time of the intubated medium from the stomach to the anus may be altered at any sphincter; propulsion through the various segments of the small and large intestine may differ with retention in one area and could possibly be compensated for by more rapid transit in another. Factors reported to alter normal gastrointestinal function include osmotic pressure (HUNT and PATHAK 1960), fasting (DOLUISIO et al. 1969; ORR and BENET 1975; YOUNG and LANDSBERG 1977), diet (FORD 1977; HUNT et al. 1975), age (SIGNER and FRIDRICH 1975), ingested volume (HUNT and MACDONALD 1954), and drugs (BRIDGES et al. 1976). The absolute cause of the observed alteration in this assay cannot be determined. Two possible mechanisms are increased peristaltic activity and incontinence of sphincters, both of which can be related to the multiple factors previously mentioned.

### 4. Food Consumption and Utilization

Among basic requirements of all living systems are food consumption and food utilization. In general, the amount of a specified diet consumed correlates with the change in body weight observed in an animal during the interval evaluated. In these studies, food was available to the rats ad libitum. There was an indication that the presumed correlation of food consumed and body weight gained was somewhat impaired in rats in teratogen-exposed groups. A sex-related difference in response was apparent, but the response varied in rats treated with different teratogens. Female rats given chemotherapeutic agents during the fetal period were more affected than male rats. Male rats treated with vitamin A were more affected than female rats.

### 5. Gastric Emptying

The gastric emptying assay is a modification of a test for pharmacologic activity of an agent (JACOBY and BRODIE 1967). The assay measures the rapidity with which a fixed number of pellets intubated using a constant volume of distilled water is expelled from the stomach. It does not measure the factors which can contribute to the speed with which the pellets are emptied from the stomach. In these studies (Fig. 4), gastric emptying was decreased in rats exposed to teratogens. Sex-related differences in response were present. The control male and female rats differed in response with more rapid gastric emptying in control female than in control male rats. The observations in male rats were more variable than in female rats, and the direction of alteration differed with each of the chemotherapeutic agents evaluated.

Gastric emptying is dependent not only on coordinated peristalsis, but also on integrity of the sphincters, intraabdominal pressure, muscle tone, afferent impulses from the mouth and esophagus, blood glucose levels, the diet ingested, and feedback from receptors in the duodenum. The speed at which the stomach empties is primarily regulated by chemical and physical properties of chyme in the duodenum. Three pathways are involved in regulating gastric motility: (1) reflex mechanisms whose afferent and efferent fibers are in sympathetic and parasympathetic nerves; (2) reflexes not involving higher centers, but operating through intrinsic plexuses or the celiac plexus; and (3) blood-borne hormones liberated from the intestinal mucosa in response to chemical properties of chyme (DAVENPORT 1977; SCHOFIELD 1968).

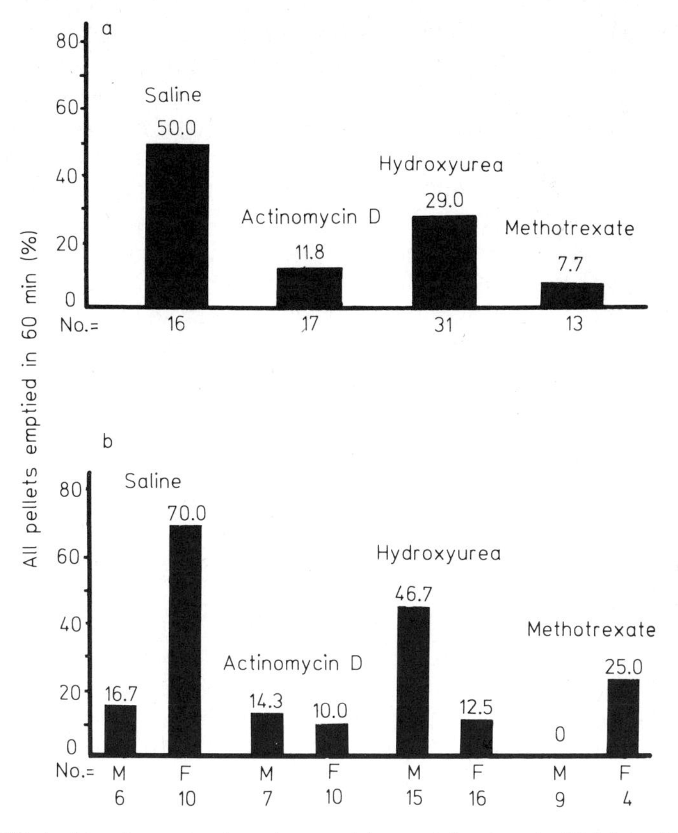


**Fig. 4 a, b.** Effect of teratogen treatment on gastric emptying in rats. Heights of bars show the percentage of rats which emptied all pellets in a 60-min period. **a** combined sexes; **b** separate sexes

## VI. Discussion of Observed Physiologic Changes

Alteration observed in assays of gastrointestinal function in teratogen-treated rats may be the result of multiple factors. Decreased and increased motility in the teratogen-exposed rats, as compared with 0.9% saline controls, may reflect variation in response to the stress of the assay, as well as inherent changes in gastrointestinal function. It is reasonable to presume that teratogenic insult during the fetal period may have altered the function of the gastrointestinal tract, not only via possible inhibition of development of the intramural plexuses, but also by altered development of the mucosa itself, with secondary changes in cell kinetics and the response of these cells to stimuli.

Cellular migration of intestinal epithelia is extremely slow in rats less than 2 weeks old, as compared with that in adult rats (Koldovsky et al. 1966). The mucosa of the gastrointestinal tract changes dramatically during the fetal period (Kammeraad 1942). Epithelial cellular migration time was observed to be even longer in the fetal rat than in the 2-week-old rat, with parietal and zymogen cells not identifiable until late in the fetal period (Yeomans and Trier 1976).

The cell dynamics of the intestinal epithelium can be altered by starvation, protein depletion, and refeeding (CLARKE 1975; HAGEMANN and STRAGAND 1977; HOPPER et al. 1968). Cell dynamics in these tissues are also regulated by internal feedback mechanisms (GALJAARD et al. 1972). The observed alteration of gastrointestinal physiology has extensive implications. Not only was food utilization changed, but also the length of time available for digestion of the ingested food. Nutritional status can affect longevity, fertility (BERG 1960), and the onset of disease (BERG and SIMMS 1960a, b). Excess or deprivation of specific diet requirements can influence spontaneous tumor prevalence (ROSS and BRAS 1973).

The absorption, not only of food, but of pharmacologic agents (JACOBY and BRODIE 1967) and environmental toxins is dependent upon gastrointestinal physiology. Individual differences in the rate of gastric emptying (HEADING et al. 1973) and cell response to pharmacologic agents ingested (JOLLY and FLETCHER 1977) can alter not only the pharmacologic dose of any agent administered orally, but also the toxic dose. Decreased integrity of gastrointestinal function and feedback mechanism can result in altered response to other external influences, such as radiation (QUASTLER et al. 1959).

It is not unexpected that the observed sex-related differences in gastrointestinal physiologic response to teratogenic agents occurred. Two examples of sex-related differences in rats are: (1) normal postnatal CNS development, in which the male rat develops more slowly than the female (GREGORY 1975); and (2) "catch-up growth" after perinatal retardation due to large litter size, in which the skull in female rats appears to compensate completely, but remains stunted in male rats (WILLIAMS and HUGHES 1978). The observed sex-related difference in the incidence of gastrointestinal malformation in humans, previously cited, conforms to these experimental results. The fact that all rats were not equally affected may reflect not only pharmacokinetics of the test agents evaluated and genetic complement of the fetus, but also circadian periodicity of fetal growth (BARR 1973) and circadian modification of teratogenesis (CLAYTON et al. 1975).

## C. Other Non-CNS Functional Alterations

In order to examine the generality of functional alterations produced by fetal teratogenic exposure, in addition to effects on gastrointestinal physiology, CHRISTIAN and JOHNSON (1979b) evaluated a battery of non-CNS parameters evaluated in a limited number of the same rats. Many of these tests have been used in the past for diagnosis of disease states, and were selected because of their known ability to indicate pathology (Table 1).

Few references citing hematology, clinical chemistry, or urinalysis profiles in neonatal rats are published. Recent technical advances and the development of microtechniques for analysis of blood samples have eliminated the major difficulty, obtaining sufficient volumes of blood for examination. Because of the paucity of data, and the variation in rat strains and laboratory techniques, data from the limited number of animals evaluated in the CHRISTIAN and JOHNSON studies cannot be directly compared with published reviews. Neither should they be considered as absolute findings, but rather as indicators of possible functional changes which

**Table 1.** Tests for diagnosis of disease

| Evaluations | Methods | |
|---|---|---|
| Hematocrit (%) | Coulter counter (Model ZBI-6) or Spun-International microcapillary centrifuge and reader | |
| Hemoglobin (g/dl) | Coulter hemoglobinometer | |
| RBCs × $10^6/mm^3$ | Coulter counter (Model ZBI-6) | |
| WBCs × $10^3/mm^3$ | Coulter counter (Model ZBI-6) | |
| Mean corpuscular volume ($\mu m^3$) | Coulter counter (Model ZBI-6) | |
| Differential (%) | Stained blood smear (manual count) | |
| Nucleated RBCs/100 WBCs | Stained blood smear (manual count) | |
| Albumin (g/dl) | Bromocresol green | Union Carbide Centrifi Chem 400 |
| Blood urea nitrogen (mg/dl) | Modified urease | Union Carbide Centrifi Chem 400 |
| Creatinine (mg/dl) | Modified Jaffee | Union Carbide Centrifi Chem 400 |
| Glucose (mg/dl) | Kornberg (hexokinase) | Union Carbide Centrifi Chem 400 |
| Serum glutamic oxalacetic Transaminase (IU/L) | Modified Karmen | Union Carbide Centrifi Chem 400 |
| Serum glutamic pyruvic Transaminase (IU/l) | Modified Wroblewski | Union Carbide Centrifi Chem 400 |
| Total protein (g-%) | Chaney (Biuret) | Union Carbide Centrifi Chem 400 |
| Urinalysis: | | |
| Blood | Bili-Labstix (NDC 0193–2813–21) | |
| Bilirubin | Bili-Labstix (NDC 0193–2813–21) | |
| Ketone | Bili-Labstix (NDC 0193–2813–21) | |
| Glucose | Bili-Labstix (NDC 0193–2813–21) | |
| Protein | Bili-Labstix (NDC 0193–2813–21) | |
| pH | Bili-Labstix (NDC 0193–2813–21) | |
| Heart and respiration rates | Stethoscope and auditory count | |
| Estrous cycling, mating, fertility | Microscopic evaluation of smears of vaginal cytology | |
| Histopathology | Microscopic evaluation | |

require further evaluation. Blood and urine samples from saline control, corn oil control, and teratogen-treated pups in these studies were collected and evaluated at the same time points, using the same techniques. The older data can be considered for similarity of normal values and trends. These preliminary reports should be considered as indicators of parameters which should be further evaluated.

## I. Hematology

Published data in white rats indicate that there are developmental changes in hemopoiesis. Hemoglobin levels peak at approximately 4–6 months and then slightly decrease. Red blood cells (RBCs) rapidly increase in number during the first month after birth to a maximum level at approximately 6 months. Mean corpuscular volume, and the number of nucleated RBCs/100 white blood cells (WBCs) decrease with age. WBCs gradually increase in number with age and are subject to variation reflecting sampling technique; the number is higher in samples from blood obtained by tail snip than in blood obtained by cardiac or orbital sinus puncture techniques. The neutrophil:lymphocyte ratio is greatest in young rats (DAVIDSOHN and

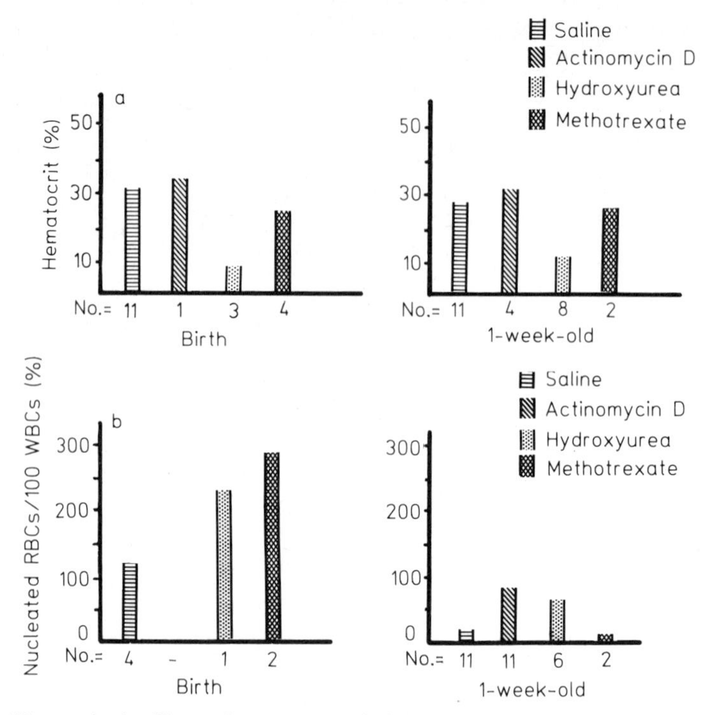


**Fig. 5 a, b.** Hematologic effects of teratogens administered to rats. **a** hematocrit; **b** nucleated red blood cells/100 white blood cells

Henry 1962; Schalm et al. 1975). Hematology values can be markedly altered by fasting and/or water deprivation, particularly in young rats, with hemoconcentration as the result (Apostolou et al. 1976).

Control rats in these studies generally conformed to the expected hemopoietic developmental pattern. However, transient anemia in hydroxyurea-treated rats, characterized by decreased hematocrit, and increased incidence of nucleated RBCs in hydroxyurea- and methotrexate-treated rats, may have indicated delayed maturation or some other developmental change (Fig. 5). Increased neonatal hemoglobin level has been reported in rats exposed to carbon dioxide throughout gestation and early postnatal life (Hoffman and Campbell 1977). The carbon dioxide-exposed rats also had slightly increased heart weight and heart:body weight ratio. Hydroxyurea-exposed rats in this study had a decreased hematocrit level. These data, in which teratogenic exposure was limited to the fetal period, indicate that prolonged exposure is not required for hemopoietic changes to occur, and that the cardiovascular system is another target organ for functional alteration.

## II. Clinical Chemistry

Even fewer published evaluations of clinical chemistry than of hematology parameters in neonates exist. Blood glucose levels have been reported to decrease from day 17 to day 19 of gestation and subsequently rise toward adult levels just before

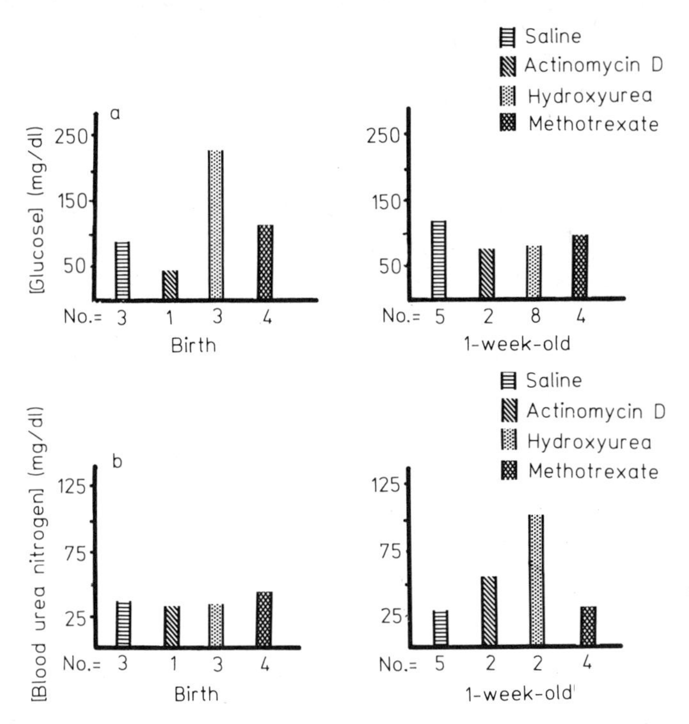


**Fig. 6 a, b.** Effects of teratogens on clinical chemistry in rats. **a** glucose; **b** blood urea nitrogen

birth (WATTS et al. 1976). Glycogen deposition in the liver is initiated at day 17 of gestation and increases through day 19 (AVDALOVIC et al. 1970; DAWKINS 1963). Subtle changes in rat perinatal carbohydrate metabolism were observed at birth in rats exposed to methylmercuric chloride on day 6 of gestation. Impaired glycogen mobilization, with resultant hypoglycemia, was observed and postulated as a contributing factor to neurologic disturbances present in the animals at later times (SNELL 1977; SNELL et al. 1977). DEMEYER et al. (1972) reported hypoglycemia secondary to exposure to actinomycin D during the fetal period in the rat. In these studies, by CHRISTIAN and JOHNSON (1979 b) glucose level in rats exposed in utero to actinomycin D was slightly depressed at birth and at 1 week of age. In rats exposed in utero to hydroxyurea, glucose level was elevated at 1 week of age (Fig. 6 a).

Altered development of liver enzyme systems secondary to fetal insult in the rat has been reported (LUCIER 1976). Not previously reported were transient increases in blood urea nitrogen (BUN) levels in hydroxyurea-treated rats in evaluations performed on serum from 1-week-old rats (Fig. 6 b). This transient increase in BUN level may indicate liver and/or kidney pathology. Also not previously reported was the alteration of serum glutamic pyruvic transaminase (SGPT) levels in 5-week-old, teratogen-exposed rats. Both increased and decreased serum enzyme levels were observed, possibly indicating liver pathology (DAVIDSOHN and HENRY 1962; SCHALM et al. 1975).

## III. Urinalysis

Relatively few urinalysis studies of newborn animals or humans are published. In newborn infants, a transient proteinurea occurs (RHODES et al. 1962). A similar high urine protein level was observed in all control and teratogen-treated neonatal rats. Glucose also is frequently observed in urine from newborn infants, and was occasionally present in urine from teratogen-treated rats. Not expected was the increase in occult blood in urine from corn oil control and teratogen-treated rats (Fig. 7). This increase may have been secondary to the minor trauma of urine collection and possibly indicate increased sensitivity to the procedure. Bilirubin, ketone bodies, protein, and urine pH were slightly increased in urine from rats exposed to some of the teratogens. The incidence of ketone bodies and pH may have reflected undiagnosed metabolic changes, while the presence of bilirubin may indicate kidney functional deficiency (DAVIDSOHN and HENRY 1962; KARK et al. 1963). A series of postnatal functional evaluations of renal development in rats has been reported (MCCORMACK et al. 1980). These include organic ion transport capacity, inulin and PAH clearance, BUN, and maximal urine osmolality. These tests have not yet demonstrated functional teratogenic change.

## IV. Reproduction

Neonatal hypothyroidism has been proposed as a cause of impaired brain development in rats with concomitant delay in puberty, and first estrus, and prolonged estrous cycles (BAKKE et al. 1976). Altered sexual behavior in adult male rats has been associated with maternal stress during gestation (MASTERPASQUA et al. 1976). Vitamin $B_{12}$ deficiency can produce reduced testicular maturation and size (JOHNSON 1964). In mice, reduced fertility or total sterility have been reported as secondary to teratogenic effect on RNA synthesis in fetal ova (MUKHERJEE et al. 1975).

In these studies, delayed vaginal opening was observed in rats exposed during the fetal period to hydroxyurea and methotrexate. Male rats treated with vitamin A had decreased mating performance. Examination of smears of vaginal contents of inseminated female rats revealed an apparent increase in abnormal spermatozoa from male rats treated with vitamin A. A methotrexate-treated male rat was observed to have immature testes. Fertility was decreased in rats in all teratogen-treated groups (Fig. 8). Decreased fertility was possibly the result of altered RNA synthesis in fetal ova, but not necessarily via this mode, since not all of the agents tested have been demonstrated to interfere with RNA synthesis.

## V. Cardiovascular

GRABOWSKI and TURNSTALL (1977) developed a technique for recording fetal electrocardiograms at 20 days of gestation and have demonstrated functional alteration secondary to embryonic teratogenic insult. Although a simple technique for evaluating heart rate was not developed in these studies, there was an indication that the normal cardiovascular pattern was altered by teratogen exposure of the fetus.

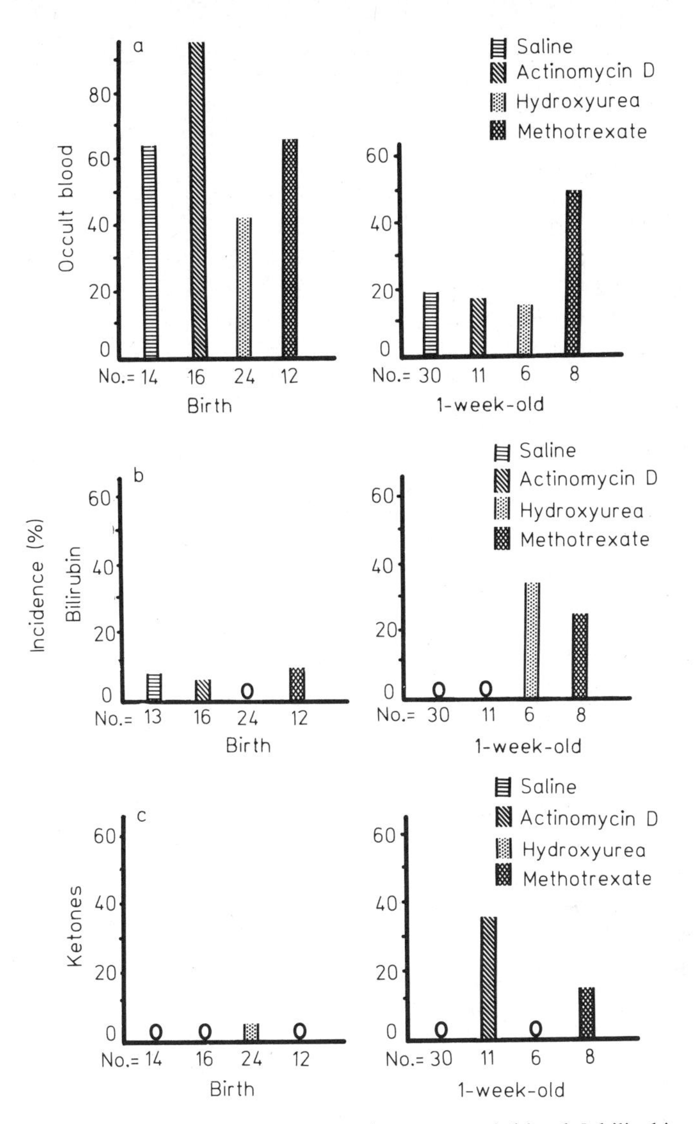


**Fig. 7 a–c.** Urinalysis studies of teratogen-treated rats. **a** occult blood; **b** bilirubin; **c** ketones

## VI. Organ Weights

Organ weight evaluations are not considered extremely valuable in toxicity tests because of inherent variation in body weights in growth-retarded animals (SCHARER 1977). Various methods of adjusting data for growth changes are suggested (SHIRLEY 1977; STEVENS 1977). The fact that body weight changes during treatment are used to separate toxic from physiologic admustments may, in fact, indicate that organ weight changes are actually good tests of the physiologic capacity of an animal to adjust under stress.

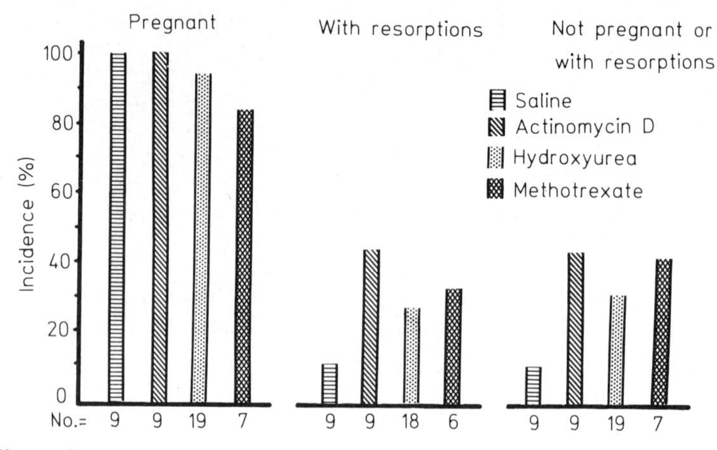


**Fig. 8.** Effects of teratogen treatment on mating and fertility in 68-day-old rats

### VII. Histopathology

Despite observed alteration of hematology, clinical chemistry, and urinalysis profiles, which would indicate heart, liver, and kidney pathology, no specific histopathology of these organs was observed in tissues from a few experimental animals. Absence of histopathology may reflect the small population evaluated and/or the early state of the pathology. However, the organ: body weight ratio of these tissues was altered, and it is believed that appropriate functional tests would probably reveal that, under stress conditions, overt pathology would result.

### VIII. Immunology

Although no evaluation of alteration of the immune system was performed in the CHRISTIAN and JOHNSON (1979a, b) work, recent work by BARNETT et al. (1980) has indicated alteration of postnatal immunocompetence in mice exposed in utero to carbofuran or diazinon.

## D. Summary and Conclusion

Postnatal functional evaluations are not presently included in the standard battery of tests used to determine teratogenic effect (*Food and Drug Administration* 1966; *Environmental Protection Agency* 1978, 1979). However, functional tests may demonstrate alterations not apparent in a strict morphological evaluation. Appreciation of the potential toxic effects of fetal exposure to foreign agents and conditions, and the possible long-term effects of this exposure, requires that animal models be developed to aid in evaluationg risks. Fetal target organ systems need to be determined, and the normal and altered development of these systems evaluated, so that predictive tests may be devised and used as guides to determine the potential hazards of fetal exposure.

The CHRISTIAN and JOHNSON (1979a, b) studies of multiple organ systems, excluding the CNS, demonstrated that changes in postnatal gastrointestinal function in rats can be produced by exposure of these rats to different types of teratogens during the fetal period. Limited studies of changes in hemopoiesis, glucose, BUN, and SGPT values, urinalysis profile, sexual maturation, and fertility were observed in the same rats which had been exposed to teratogens during the fetal period, and which had altered gastrointestinal function. There was also an indication of changes in heart and respiration rates, and development of the liver, kidney, and thymus in these rats. All of these changes may indicate altered development secondary to fetal insult.

These data demonstrate that functional teratogenic changes associated with insult during the fetal period are not restricted to the CNS, but can include multiple systems, and that relatively simple physiologic tests can be used to reveal additional underlying mechanisms for "behavioral changes" which have been presumed to reflect only CNS alteration.

## References

Agrawal KC, Sartorelli AC (1975) -(N)-heterocyclic carboxaldehyde thiosemicarbazones. In: Sartorelli AC, Johns DG (eds) Antineoplastic and immunosuppressive agents. II. Springer, Berlin Heidelberg New York, pp 793–807

Amortegui AJ, Feinberg SS, Figallo EM (1976) Postnatal effects of chemically induced intrauterine growth retardation on some hematological values in the rat. Biol Neonate 29:216–221

Apostolou A, Saidt L, Brown WR (1976) Effect of overnight fasting of young rats on water consumption, body weight, blood sampling and blood composition. I. Lab Anim Sci 26:959–960

Armenti VT, Masters E, Cliver A, Johnson EM (1977) Effects of teratogenic insult on fetal lung maturation. Teratology 15:30A

Avdalovic N, Rukavina D, Eberhardt P (1970) Hormonal aspects of glycogen accumulation in fetal and neonatal rat liver. Proc Soc Exp Biol Med 134:943–946

Bakke JL, Lawrence NL, Robinson S, Bennett J (1976) Lifelong alterations in endocrine function resulting from brief perinatal hypothyroidism in the rat. J Lab Clin Med 88:3–13

Baranov VS, Weismann BL, Nikitina SS, Repina GV, Repina VS (1968) Differentialinhibition of serum protein synthesis in mammalian embryos by actinomycin-D in various stages of liver development (in Russian). Biochimie 33:1174–1182

Barnett JB, Spyker-Cranmer JM, Avery DL, Hoberman AM (1980) Immunocompetence over the lifespan of mice exposed in utero to carbofuran or diazinon: 1. Changes in serum immunoglobin concentrations. J Environ Pathol Toxicol 4:53–63

Barr M Jr (1973) Prenatal growth of Wistar rats: circadian periodicity of fetal growth late in gestation. Teratology 7:283–288

Bennett A (1974) Relation between gut motility and innervation in man. Digestion 11:392–396

Berg BN (1960) Nutrition and longevity in the rat. I. Food intake in relation to size, health and fertility. J Nutr 71:242–254

Berg BN, Simms HS (1960 a) Nutrition and longevity in the rat. II. Longevity and onset of disease with different levels of food intake. J Nutr 71:255–263

Berg BN, Simms HS (1960 b) Nutrition and longevity in the rat. III. Food restriction beyond 800 days. J Nutr 74:23–32

Berry CL (1971) Transient inhibition of DNA synthesis by methotrexate, in the rat embryo and foetus. J Embryol Exp Morphol 26:469–474

Bertino JR (1975) Folate antagonists. In: Sartorelli AC, Johns DG (eds) Antineoplastic and immunosuppressive agents. II. Springer, Berlin Heidelberg New York, pp 468–483

Bodian M, Stephens FD, Ward BCH (1949) Hirschsprung's disease and idiopathic megacolon. Lancet 256:6–11

Brann L, Wood JD (1976) Motility of the large intestine in piebald-lethal mice. Dig Dis 21:633–640
Bridges JW, Dent JG, Johnson P (1976) The effects of some pharmacologically active amines on the rate of gastric emptying in rats. Life Sci 18:97–108
Buelke-Sam J, Kimmel CA (1979) Development and standardization of screening methods for behavioral teratology. Teratology 20:17–30
Butcher RE (1976) Behavioral testing as a method for assessing risk. Environ Health Perspect 18:75–78
Butcher RE, Scott WJ, Kazmaier K, Ritter EJ (1973) Postnatal effects in rats of prenatal treatment with hydroxyurea. Teratology 7:161–166
Charache S, Condit PT, Humphreys SR (1960) Studies on the folic acid vitamins. VI. The persistence of amethopterin in mammalian tissues. Cancer 13:236–240
Chaube S, Murphy ML (1966) The effects of hydroxyurea and related compounds on the rat fetus. Cancer Res 26:1448–1457
Chernoff N, Grabowski CT (1971) Responses of the fetus to maternal injections of adrenalin and vasopressin. Br J Pharmacol 43:270–278
Christian MS (1979) Postnatal functional teratology resulting from fetal insult. Ph.D. dissertation, Thomas Jefferson University
Christian MS, Johnson EM (1978) Prenatal alteration of postnatal gastrointestinal function. Teratology 17:44a
Christian MS, Johnson EM (1979a) Functional teratology of the gastrointestinal tract resulting from fetal insult in the rat. 18th annual meeting, society of toxicology [Abstr 237, A119]. Academic Press, New York
Christian MS, Johnson EM (1979b) Postnatal alteration of non-CNS physiology evaluated in rats treated with teratogens during the fetal period. Teratology 19:23A
Christian MS, Johnson EM (to be published) Postnatal functional teratology resulting from fetal insult. 1. Alteration in gastrointestinal physiology. J Environ Pathol Toxicol
Clarke RM (1975) The time-course of changes in mucosal architecture and epithelial cell production and cell shedding in the small intestine of the rat fed after fasting. J Anat 120:321–327
Clayton DL, McMullen AW, Barnett CC (1975) Circadian modification of drug-induced teratogenesis in rat fetuses. Chronobiologia 2:210–217
Cohlan SQ (1954) Congenital anomalies in the rat produced by the excessive intake of vitamin A during pregnancy. Pediatrics 13:556–569
Committee on Postnatal Evaluation of Animals Subjected to Insult during Development (1976) Document – Including sample behavioral test battery. National Institute of Environmental Health Sciences, Research Triangle
Daikoku S, Ikeuchi C, Miki S (1975) Electronmicroscopic studies on developing intramural ganglia of the small intestine in human and rabbit fetuses. Acta Anat (Basel) 91:429–454
Davenport HW (1977) Physiology of the digestive tract, 4th edn. Year Book, Chicago
Davidsohn I, Henry JB (1962) Clinical diagnosis by laboratory methods, 14th edn. WB Saunders, Philadelphia
Dawkins MJR (1963) Glycogen synthesis and breakdown in fetal and newborn rat liver. Ann NY Acad Sci 111:203–211
DeMeyer R, Verellen G, Gerard P (1972) Study of carbohydrate metabolism in the newborn rat as a tool for evaluating effects of drugs administered during pregnancy. In: Klingberg MA, Abramovici A, Chemke J (eds) Advances in experimental medicine and biology, vol 27. Drugs and fetal development. Plenum Press, New York, pp 83–96
Doluisio JT, Tan GH, Billups NF, Diamond L (1969) Drug absorption II: effect of fasting on intestinal drug absorption. J Pharm Sci 58:1200–1202
Eguchi Y, Arishima K, Morikawa Y, Hashimoto Y (1976) Changes in the weight of the adrenal glands and in the concentration of plasma corticosterone in perinatal rats after prenatal treatment with estradiol benzoate. J Endocrinol 69:427–531
Ehrenpreis T (1971) Hirschsprung's disease. Dig Dis 16:1032–1052
Environmental Protection Agency (August 22, 1978) Pesticide programs, proposed guidelines for registering pesticides in the US; hazard evaluation: humans and domestic animals. Federal Register, Part II, 43(163):163.83-3 Teratogenicity studies; 163.83-4 Reproduction study

Environmental Protection Agency (July 26, 1979) Proposed health effects test standards for toxic substances control act test rules and proposed good laboratory practice standards for health effects. Federal Register, Part IV, 44(145): Subpart F-Teratogenic/Reproductive Health Effects: 772/116-1 General; 772.116-2 Teratogenic effects test standards; 772.116-3 Reproductive effects test standards

Fehér E, Vajda J (1972) Cell types in the nerve plexus of the small intestine. Acta Morphol Acad Sci Hung 20:13–25

Food and Drug Administration (1966) Guidelines for reproduction studies for safety evaluation of drugs for human use. FDA Washington DC

Ford DJ (1977) Influence of diet pellet hardness and particle size on food utilization by mice, rats and hamsters. Lab Anim 11:241–246

Friesen SR, Boley JO, Miller DR (1956) The myenteric plexus of pylorus: its early normal development and its changes in hypertrophic pyloric stenosis. Surgery 39:21–29

Gabella G (1971) Neuron size and number in the myenteric plexus of the newborn and adult rat. J Anat 109:81–95

Galbraith WM, Mellett LB (1975) Tissue disposition of 3H-Actinomycin-D (NSC-3053) in the rat, monkey and dog. Cancer Chemother Rep Part 1 59:1061–1069

Galjaard H, van der Meer-Fieggen W, Giesen J (1972) Feedback control by functional villus cells on cell proliferation and maturation in intestinal epithelium. Exp Cell Res 73:197–207

Grabowski CT (1976) Postnatal effects on rats of prenatal exposure to carbon monoxide [Abstr]. Teratology 13:23A

Grabowski CT, Turnstall AC (1977) An electrocardiographic study of rat fetuses treated with Trypan blue [Abstr]. Teratology 15:32A

Grant LD (1976) Research strategies for behavioral teratology studies. Environ Health Perspect 18:85–94

Gregory E (1975) Comparison of postnatal CNS development between male and female rats. Brain Res 99:152–156

Gunn M (1968) Histological and histochemical observations on the myenteric and submucous plexuses of mammals. J Anat 102:223–239

Hagemann RF, Stragand JJ (1977) Fasting and refeeding: cell kinetic response of jejunum, ileum and colon. Cell Tissue Kinet 10:3–14

Hale F (1933) Pigs born without eyeballs. J Hered 24:105–106

Hale F (1935) The relation of vitamin A to anophthalmos in pigs. Am J Ophthamol 18:1087–1093

Hale F (1937) The relation of maternal vitamin A deficiency to microphthalmia in pigs. Tex J Med 33:228–232

Hamilton WJ, Mossman HW (1972) In: Hamilton WJ, Mossman HW (eds) Human embryology, 4th edn. Williams and Wilkins, Baltimore, pp 291–376

Handschumacher RE, Welch AD (1960) Agents which influence nucleic acid metabolism. In: Chargoff E, Davidson JN (eds) The nucleic acids, vol 3. Academic Press, New York, pp 453–526

Heading RC, Nimmo J, Prescott LF, Tothill P (1973) The dependence of paracetamol absorption on the rate of gastric emptying. Br J Pharmacol 47:415–421

Heinonen OP, Slone S, Shapiro S (1977) Malformations of the gastrointestinal tract. In: Kaufman DW (ed) Birth defects and drugs in pregnancy. Publishing Sciences Group, Littleton, pp 163–175

Hitchings GH, Burchall JJ (1965) Inhibition of folate biosynthesis and function as a basis for chemotherapy. In: Ford FF (ed) Advances in enzymology. Interscience, New York, pp 417–468

Hoffman DJ, Campbell KI (1977) Postnatal toxicity of carbon monoxide after pre- and postnatal exposure. Toxicology Lett 1:147–150

Hopper AF, Wannemacher RW Jr, McGovern RA (1968) Cell population changes in the intestinal epithelium of the rat following starvation and protein-depletion. Proc Soc Exp Biol Med 128:695–698

Hunt JN, MacDonald I (1954) The influence of volume on gastric emptying. J Physiol 126:459–474

Hunt JN, Pathak JD (1960) The osmotic effects of some simple molecules and ions on gastric emptying. J Physiol 154:254–269
Hunt JN, Cash R, Newland P (1975) Energy density of food, gastric emptying and obesity. Lancet 905–906
Ikeda T (1957) An histological study of the submucous nerve plexus of the alimentary canal with special reference to the three types of nerve plexus. J Comp Neurol 107:43–56
Inouye M, Hoshino K, Murakami U (1972) Effect of methylmercuric chloride on embryonic and fetal development in rats and mice. Annu Rep Res Inst Environ Med Nagoya Univ (Engl Ed) 19:69–74
Irwin DA (1931) The anatomy of Auerbach's plexus. Am J Anat 49:141–166
Jacoby HI, Brodie DA (1967) Gastrointestinal actions of metoclopramide. Gastroenterol 52:676–684
Johns DG, Bertino JR (1973) Folate antagonists. In: Holland JF, Frei E (eds) Cancer medicine. Lea and Febiger, Philadelphia, pp 739–754
Johnson EM (1964) A histologic study of postnatal vitamin $B_{12}$ deficiency in the rat. Am J Pathol 44:73–83
Johnson EM, Armenti VT (1978) Postnatal effects of prenatal insult on lung development in the rat. Anat Rec 190:432–433
Johnson EM, Staples RE, Hoar RM (1980) Behavioral teratogens-unfortunate terminology. Neurobehav Toxicol 2:IV
Jolly LE Jr, Fletcher HP (1977) The effect of repeated oral dosing of methotrexate on its intestinal absorption in the rat. Toxicol Appl Pharmacol 39:23–32
Jordan RL, Wilson JG (1970) Radioautographic study of RNA synthesis in normal and actinomycin D treated rat embryos. Anat Rec 168:549–564
Jordan RL, Wilson JG, Schumacher HJ (1977) Embryotoxicity of the folate antagonist methotrexate in rats and rabbits. Teratology 15:73–79
Kalter H (1968) Teratology of the central nervous system. University of Chicago Press, Chicago pp 5–6
Kalter H, Warkany J (1961) Experimental production of congenital malformations in strains of inbred mice by maternal treatment with hypervitaminosis A. Am J Pathol 38:1–21
Kark RM, Lawrence JR, Muehrcke RC, Pirani CL, Pollak VE, Silva H (1963) A primer of urinalysis. Harper and Row, New York
Kammeraad A (1942) The development of the gastro-intestinal tract of the rat. 1. Histogenesis of the epithelium of the stomach, small intestine and pancreas. J Morphol 70:323–351
Khera KS (1976) Teratogenicity studies with methotrexate, aminopterin and acetylsalicylic acid in domestic cats. Teratology 14:21–28
Khera KS, Nera EA (1971) Maternal exposure to methyl mercury and postnatal cerebellar development in mice [Abstr]. Teratology 4:233
Kimmel CA (1976) Behavioral teratology: overview. Environ Health Perspect 18:73
Koldovsky O, Sunshine P, Kretchmer N (1966) Cellular migration of intestinal epithelia in suckling and weaned rats. Nature 212:1389–1390
Krakoff IH (1975) Clinical and pharmacologic effects of hydroxyurea. In: Sartorelli AC, Johns DG (eds) Antineoplastic and immunosuppressive agents. Springer, Berlin Heidelberg New York, pp 789–792
Kubozoe T, Daikoku S, Takita S (1969) Electron-microscopic observations on Auerbach's plexus in a 12 mm human embryo. J Neuro-Visc Relat 31:291–307
Lenz W (1961) Kindliche Mißbildungen nach Medikamenteinnahme während der Gravidität? Deutsch Med Wochenschr 86:2555–2556
Lowe CU (1974) Pediatric aspects: from the embryo through adolescence: special susceptibility and exposure. Pediatr 53:779–782
Lucier GW (1976) Perinatal development of conjugative enzyme systems. Environ Health Perspect 18:25–34
Marin-Padilla M (1966) Mesodermal alterations induced by hypervitaminosis A. J Embryol Exp Morphol 15:261–269

Masterpasqua F, Chapman RH, Lore RK (1976) The effects of prenatal psychological stress on the sexual behavior and reactivity of male rats. Dev Psycholbiol 9:403–411
McBride WG (1961) Thalidomide and congenital abnormalities. Lancet 2:1358
McCormack KM, Abuelgasim A, Sanger VL, Hook JB (1980) Postnatal morphology and functional capacity of the kidney following prenatal treatment with dinoseb in rats. J Toxicol Environ Health 6:633–643
Milunsky A, Graef JW, Gaynor MF (1968) Methotrexate-induced congenital malformations. J Pediatr 72:790–795
Monjan AA, Mandell W (1980) Fetal alcohol and immunity: depression of mitogen-induced lymphocyte blastogenesis. Teratology 21:4A
Mukherjee AB, Chan M, Waite R, Metzger MI, Yaffee SJ (1975) Inhibition of RNA synthesis by acetyl salicylate and actinomycin-D during early development in the mouse. Pediatr Res 9:652–657
Newman L, Johnson EM, Armenti VT (1978) Effect of prenatal vitamin A on neonatal respiratory frequency and $O_2$ consumption in the Long-Evans rat [Abstr]. Teratology 17:44A
Orr JM, Benet LZ (1975) The effect of fasting on the rate of intestinal drug absorption in rats: preliminary study. Dig Dis 20:858–865
Petit TL, Isaacson RL (1976) Anatomical and behavioral effects of colchicine administration to rats late in utero. Dev Psychobiol 9:119–129
Quastler H, Bensted JPM, Chir B, Lamerton LF, Simpson SM (1959) II. Adaptation to continuous irradiation: observations on the rat intestine. Br J Radiol 32:501–512
Reich E (1963) Biochemistry of actinomycins. Cancer Res 23:1428–1441
Rhodes PG, Hammel CL, Bermen LB (1962) Urinary constituents of the newborn infant. J Pediatr 60:18–23
Roberts AB, DeLuca HF (1967) Pathways of retinol and retinoic acid metabolism in the rat. Biochem J 102:600–605
Rodier PM (1976) Critical periods for behavioral anomalies in mice. Environ Health Perspect 18:79–83
Rodier PM (1977) Correlations between prenatally-induced alterations in CNS cell populations and postnatal function. Teratology 16:235–246
Ross MH, Bras G (1973) Influence of protein under- and overnutrition on spontaneous tumor prevalence in the rat. J Nutr 103:944–963
Schalm OW, Jain OC, Carroll EJ (1975) Veterinary hematology, 3rd Edn. Lea and Febiger, Philadelphia
Schärer K (1977) The effect of chronic underfeeding on organ weights of rats. How to interpret organ weight changes in cases of marked growth retardation in toxicity tests? Toxicology 7:45–56
Schofield GC (1968) Anatomy of muscular and neural tissues in the alimentary canal. In: Schofield GC (ed) Handbook of physiology. vol IV/6. American Physiology Society, Washington DC, pp 1579–1627
Scott WJ, Ritter EJ, Wilson JG (1971) DNA synthesis inhibition and cell death associated with hydroxyurea teratogenesis in rat embryos. Dev Biol 26:306–315
Shirley E (1977) The analysis of organ weight data. Toxicology 8:13–22
Signer E, Fridrich R (1975) Gastric emptying in newborns and young infants. Acta Paediatr Scand 64:525–530
Sikov MR, Thomas JM, Mahlum DD (1969) Growth 33:57–68
Skalko RG, Gold MP (1974) Teratogenicity of methotrexate in mice. Teratology 9:159–164
Snell K (1977) Effect of prenatal exposure to methylmercury on perinatal carbohydrate metabolism in the rat [Abstr]. International congress on toxicology, March 30–April 2, 1977, p 13
Snell K, Ashby SL, Barton SJ (1977) Disturbances of perinatal carbohydrate metabolism in rats exposed to methylmercury in utero. Toxicology 8:277–283
Spyker JM, Smithberg M (1972) Effects of methylmercury on prenatal development in mice. Teratology 5:181–187
Stevens MT (1977) An alternative method for the evaluation of organ weight experiments. Toxicology 7:275–281

Stock JA (1966) Antitumor antibiotics. II. The actinomycins. In: Schnitzer RJ, Hawkins F (eds) Experimental chemotherapy, vol 4. Academic Press, New York, p 243–267

Szurszewski JH (1976) Neural and hormonal determinants of gastric antral motility. In: Bülbring E, Shuba MF (eds) Physiology of smooth muscle. Raven Press, New York, pp 379–383

Tuchmann-Duplessis H, Mercier-Parot L (1960) The teratogenic action of the antibiotic actinomycin D. In: Wolstenholme GEW, O'Connor CM (eds) Ciba Foundation Symposium on Congenital Malformations. Little, Brown, Boston, pp 115–133

Vacca L, Hutchings DE (1977) Effect of maternal vitamin A excess on S-100 in neonatal rat cerebellum: a preliminary study. Dev Psychobiol 10:171–176

Vizi ES (1976) The role of α-adrenoceptors situated in Auerbach's plexus in the inhibition of gastrointestinal motility. In: Bülbring E, Shuba MF (eds) Physiology of smooth muscle. Raven Press, New York, pp 357–367

Von Schottek W (1967) Der Glaskugeltest – eine orientierende Methode zur Prüfung des Einflusses von Pharmaka auf die Dickdarmperistaltik der Ratte. Arzneim Forsch 17:649–650

Vorhees CV, Brunner RL, Butcher RE (1979) Psychotropic drugs as behavioral teratogens. Science 205:1220–1225

Waksman Conference on Actinomycins (1974) Their potential for cancer chemotherapy. Cancer Chemother Rep 58:1–123

Warkany J (1965) Development of mammalian teratology. In: Wilson JG, Warkany J (eds) Teratology principles and techniques. University of Chicago Press, Chicago, pp 1–20

Watts C, Gain K, Sandin PL (1976) Glucose homeostasis in the developing rat. Biol Neonate 30:88–94

Weston JA (1970) The migration and differentiation of neural crest cells. In: Abercrombie M, Brachet J, King TJ (eds) Advances in morphogenesis. Academic Press, New York, pp 41–114

Whitehouse FR, Kernohan JW (1948) Myenteric plexus in congenital megacolon. Arch Intern Med 82:75–111

Williams JPG, Hughes PCR (1978) Catch-up growth in the rat skull after retardation during the suckling period. J Embryol Exp Morphol 45:229–235

Wilson JG (1970) Embryotoxicity of the folic antagonist methotrexate [Abstr]. Anat Rec 166:398

Wilson JG (1973) Environment and birth defects. Academic Press, New York

Wilson JG, Fraser FC (eds) (1977) Handbook of teratology, vols 1–4. Plenum Press, New York

Wilson JG, Warkany J (1964) Teratology principles and techniques. University of Chicago Press, Chicago

Wilson JG, Scott WJ, Ritter EJ, Fradkin R (1975) Comparative distribution and embryotoxicity of hydroxyurea in pregnant rats and Rhesus monkeys. Teratology 11:169–178

Wood JD (1975) Neurophysiology of Auerbach's plexus and control of intestinal motility. Physiol Rev 55:307–324

Wood JD (1976) Neuronal interactions within ganglia of Auerbach's plexus of the small intestine. In: Bülbring E, Shuba MF (eds) Physiology of smooth muscle. Raven Press, New York, pp 321–329

Yarbro JW (1968) Further studies on the mechanism of action of hydroxyurea. Cancer Res 28:1082–1087

Yeomans ND, Trier JS (1976) Epithelial cell proliferation and migration in the developing rat gastric mucosa. Dev Biol 53:206–216

Young JB, Landsberg L (1977) Suppression of sympathetic nervous system during fasting. Science 196:1473–1475

Zachman RD, Dunagin PE Jr, Olson JA (1966) Formation and enterohepatic circulation of metabolites of retinol and retinoic acid in bile duct-cannulated rats. J Lipid Res 7:3–9

Zaharko DS, Oliverio VT (1970) Short communications. Reinvestigation of methotrexate metabolism in rodents. Biochem Pharmacol 19:2923–2925

# In Vitro Screens of Teratogenic Potential

CHAPTER 14

# Detection of Teratogens Using Cells in Culture

J. H. GREENBERG

## A. Introduction

Chemical teratogens are toxic substances which cause structural or functional abnormalities during the development of the fetus. Teratogenesis is dependent on the fetal environment, and maternal–fetal interactions, genetic factors affecting drug metabolism, tissue repair, and nutrition may determine whether or not a substance will be teratogenic for a particular fetus. Tests for teratogenicity in animals (COLLINS 1978), particularly in those species whose metabolism resembles that of humans, are the most relevant procedures for assessing human risk. Current tests in animals, however, are time consuming and likely to become more complex as testing is extended into the postnatal period to detect functional and behavioral defects. Rapid in vitro systems therefore may be useful in preliminary screening of chemicals, making it possible to assign priorities for subsequent testing in animals. In addition, in vitro methods in conjunction with animal testing are valuable for identifying the proximate teratogen and for understanding the mechanism of action of a teratogen, both of which are of great importance in estimating hazards to humans.

In vitro methods have been used extensively to assess toxicity (for a review, see DAWSON 1972) and carcinogenicity (for a review, see AMES 1979) of a wide variety of compounds. Toxicity tests generally measure alterations in cell number, morphology, or some biochemical parameter. Carcinogenicity tests using cultured eukaryotic cells measure neoplastic transformation, chromosomal changes such as sister chromatid exchange, or the ability of cells to undergo DNA repair. In addition, bacteria are employed to assess genetic alterations based on the correlation between mutagenicity and carcinogenicity of compounds.

Testing of teratogenicity in vitro requires analysis of a variety of parameters in addition to cell death and mutagenicity. Systems for detecting teratogens in vitro should be selected with regard to their relevance as models for normal developmental processes, such as cell proliferation, migration, differentiation, and cellular interactions. Whole embryo cultures and organ cultures as test systems are discussed in Chaps. 15 and 16. This chapter will consider in vitro systems using isolated cells. Table 1 summarizes potential systems, as well as two systems which are currently being investigated, to assess teratogenicity of compounds.

## B. Differentiating Cells in Culture to Detect Teratogens

Various populations of cultured embryonic cells, under appropriate conditions, differentiate into chondrocytes, melanocytes, muscle cells, neurons, and cells of other phenotypes. Teratogens have been shown to cause changes in the differentiation of certain types of cells in culture. For example, 5-bromo-2′-deoxyuridine inhibits chondrogenesis (LEVITT and DORFMAN 1972), melanogenesis (GARCIA et al. 1979), and myogenesis (BISCHOFF and HOLTZER 1970). Vitamin A analogs inhibit chondrogenesis (HASSELL et al. 1978) and alter the differentiation of cultured mouse epidermal cells (YUSPA and HARRIS 1974). Diazepam (BANDMAN et al. 1978) and dimethylsulfoxide (BLAU and EPSTEIN 1979; MIRANDA et al. 1978) both inhibit myogenesis. These results suggested that differentiating cells in culture might provide a suitable system for detecting teratogens.

Therefore, we recently tested a group of teratogenic and nonteratogenic compounds to determine whether there is a correlation between teratogenicity of a compound in vivo and its effect on growth or differentiation of embryonic cells in culture (WILK et al. 1980). Two cell types, neural crest and limb mesenchymal cells, were chosen since they represent differentiating systems at two stages of development. Cranial neural crest cells from chick embryos of $1^1/_2$ days of incubation are multipotential, and in culture differentiate within 6 days into melanocytes in the presence of fetal bovine serum or calf serum and into neuron-like cells in the presence of horse serum (GREENBERG and SCHRIER 1977). Limb bud mesenchymal cells from 4-day-old chick embryos differentiate into chondrocytes within 4 days when plated at high cell density (UMANSKY 1966). Neural crest and limb mesenchymal cells might be expected to detect teratogens which affect cell–substrate interactions, mitosis, response to inductive or permissive factors, synthesis of specialized gene products, and elaboration of an extracellular matrix.

Primary cultures of neural crest cells were established from outgrowths of explanted cranial neural tubes from chick embryos of stage 9 (HAMBURGER and HAMILTON 1951), as described previously (GREENBERG and SCHRIER 1977). After 2 days of culture in Eagle's minimal essential medium (MEM) containing 2% chick embryo extract, 5% horse serum, and antibiotics, the neural tubes were removed and the remaining monolayer of neural crest cells was dissociated from the dish. The cell suspension was adjusted to $4–7 \times 10^5$ cells/ml culture medium. Replicate cultures (usually 20–50) were prepared by placing 15-μl drops of the cell suspension in the center of 35-mm culture dishes. Since previous experiments demonstrated that the type of serum present in the medium during the first 2 days of culture does not affect subsequent differentiation (GREENBERG and SCHRIER 1977), it was possible to use the same cell population to assess differentiation into both neurons and melanocytes. Therefore, after the subcultured cells attached to the substrate, 2 ml medium containing either 5% horse serum or fetal bovine serum were added to the cultures. Compounds to be tested were added 1 day later. Cultures were examined daily for 1 week by phase contrast microscopy to assess growth and differentiation. In some cases, cultures were assayed on day 7 for choline acetyltransferase activity (GREENBERG and SCHRIER 1977) or for melanin synthesis (GREENBERG and OLIVER 1980).

Primary cultures of limb bud mesenchymal cells were prepared by dissociating cells from prechondrogenic chick limb buds (stage 23–24), as described previously (UMANSKY 1966; GOETINCK et al. 1974; HASSELL et al. 1978). Cell suspensions were adjusted to $2 \times 10^7$ cells/ml MEM containing 10% fetal bovine serum, and 20-μl drops were plated on 35-mm culture dishes. After 3 h, cells attached and 2 ml me-

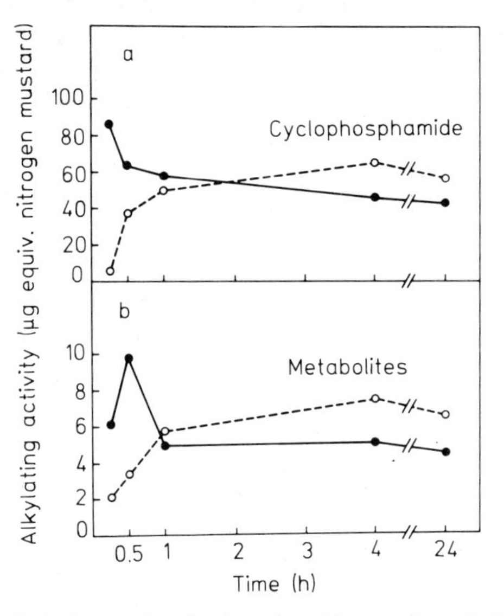


**Fig. 1a, b.** Time course for release of cyclophosphamide **a** and total alkylating metabolites **b** after incubation of cyclophosphamide (100 μg/ml) with S9 mix inside a dialysis bag. Cyclophosphamide, which has no alkylating activity, was hydrolyzed in acid prior to reaction with 4-(p-nitrobenzyl)pyridine. The values at each time point represent an individual determination of alkylating activity found inside the dialysis bag (*closed circles*) or in the medium (*open circles*) of a single dish. WILK et al. (1980)

dium were added. Compounds to be tested were added after 1 day and sometimes again after 3 days. Cultures were examined daily by phase contrast microscopy for 4 days. The accumulation of sulfated proteoglycans, which is a measure of cartilage formation, was determined by alcian blue staining (HASSELL et al. 1978). Proteoglycans were extracted from the stained cultures with 4 *M* guanidinium hydrochloride, and absorbance at 600 nm was determined to quantitate their levels.

Concentrations of drugs tested in the culture were in the range of blood levels that have been associated with malformations in cases where these values were known. When serum levels of teratogens were unknown, at least three series of concentrations were used: 500, 250, and 125 μg/ml; 100, 50, 25, and 10 μg/ml; or 1, 0.5, and 0.1 μg/ml. Some compounds require metabolic activation before they can exert their effect. Therefore test compounds were incubated with the postmitochondrial supernatant fraction (S9) of liver microsomes of phenobarbital-treated rats plus a NADPH-generating system (AMES 1973). Because the S9 mixture added directly to the medium is toxic to cells, it was combined with the test compound in autoclaved dialysis bags (6 × 25 mm; MADLE and OBE 1977), which were placed into the cultures. A single dialysis bag containing the S9 fraction (0.04 ml), 5 m*M* NADP, 10 m*M* glucose-6-phosphate, 8 m*M* $MgCl_2$ (0.05 ml), and the test compound or vehicle control (0.01–0.05 ml) was incubated with the cells for 4 h. During this time, the compound and its metabolites diffused into the medium, as shown in Fig. 1 for cyclophosphamide.

Of 14 compounds with proven teratogenic effects in vivo, 13 induced readily detectable morphological alterations in the neural crest cultures which differentiate

**Table 1.** In vitro systems which may detect teratogens

| |
|---|
| Differentiating cells |
| Neural crest |
| Limb mesenchyme |
| Fusing myoblasts |
| Teratocarcinoma or embryonal carcinoma |
| Erythroleukemia cells |
| Cell-cell and cell-substrate interactions |
| Reaggregation of dissociated cells |
| Synapse formation |
| Adhesion to lectin-coated surfaces |
| Attachment to collagen |
| Migratory activity |
| Chemotaxis |
| Phagokinetic tracks |

into pigmented and neuron-like cells, and in the limb mesenchyme cultures which differentiate into chondrocytes (Table 2). In contrast, nonteratogenic compounds had no effect on the growth or differentiation of these cultures. The effects of the teratogens on the cultured cells included detachment from the substrate, decreased cell proliferation, abnormal morphology, and inhibition of differentiation into the expected phenotypes. The effects of the teratogens were dose dependent, and in the cases of phosphoramide mustard, diphenylhydantoin, β-aminopropionitrile, norchlorcyclizine, and acetylsalicylic acid, the cells were affected at concentrations similar to the maternal blood levels associated with malformed embryos. 5-Bromo-2′-deoxyuridine and retinoic acid, in contrast, appeared to be active at lower concentrations than in vivo, presumably due to maternal effects which reduce access of the drug to the embryo. The only teratogen which was without effect on the cultured cells was thalidomide, possibly due to insolubility or lack of activation by the liver microsomal system. To overcome these problems, a recent approach has been to treat animals known to be sensitive to a compound (for example, rhesus monkeys for thalidomide) and to add serum obtained before and after treatment to cultures of differentiating cells. Serum from some monkeys treated with thalidomide decreases the chondrogenesis of limb mesenchymal cells (L. DENCKER and E. HORIGAN, personal communication 1980).

With the exception of the cyclophosphamide metabolites, the teratogenic compounds tested are not considered to be general inhibitors of DNA or protein synthesis. Cultured differentiating cells are therefore sensitive to teratogens which specifically alter tissue development, as well as to those which exert a general toxic effect. In addition, since the teratogens produced similar effects on neural crest and limb mesenchymal cells, it is likely that differentiating cells may detect compounds which act generally on developmental processes, as well as those whose teratogenic effect is specific for the particular cell type. However, it might be useful to examine the effects of teratogens on other embryonic cells in which special processes occur during differentiation. For example, fusion of myoblasts to form myotubes in-

**Table 2.** Teratogenic effects of drugs on differentiating neural crest and limb mesenchymal cells in culture (WILK et al. 1980)

| Compound | Concentration[a] (μg/ml) | Neural crest[b] | Limb mesenchyme chondrogenesis[c] (% of control) |
|---|---|---|---|
| *Teratogens* | | | |
| β-Aminopropionitrile | 125 | Cell vacuoles (transient) | 60 |
| 5-Bromo-2′-deoxyuridine | 1 | Prevents differentiation[e] | 0 |
| Phosphoramide mustard | 5 | 50% cells detached | 20 |
| +S9 | 5[d] | Not tested | 50 |
| Nornitrogen mustard | 10 | Not tested | 50 |
| Norchlorcyclizine | 10 | Not tested | 40 |
| Retinoic acid | 0.1 | Alters melanocyte morphology[e] | 5 |
| | 0.3 | Alters neuronal morphology[e] | |
| Retinyl acetate | 1 | Alters melanocyte morphology; no effect on neuronal morphology | 80 |
| | 3 | Not tested | 10 |
| Diphenylhydantoin | 50 | 25% cells detached | 40 |
| +S9 | 50[d] | Not tested | 80 |
| Thalidomide | 500 | No effect | 100 |
| +S9 | 500[d] | No effect | 100 |
| Acetylsalicyclic acid | 250 | No effect | 80 |
| 6-Diazo-5-oxo-L-norleucine | 5 | Cells detached | Not tested |
| Diazepam | 50 | Cells detached | Not tested |
| *Nonteratogens* | | | |
| Cyclophosphamide | 50 | No effect | 100 |
| +S9 | 50[d] | Cells detached | 0 |
| Carboxycyclophosphamide | 50 | No effect | 100 |
| +S9 | 50[d] | Not tested | 100 |
| Glutethimide | 500 | No effect | 100 |
| +S9 | 500[d] | No effect | 100 |
| Isoniazid | 500 | No effect | 100 |
| +S9 | 500[d] | No effect | 100 |
| Bendectin (doxylamine succinate + pyridoxine-HCl) | 250 | No effect | Not tested |
| +S9 | 50 | No effect | Not tested |

[a] Concentrations given are lowest effective concentration, or for compounds without effect, the highest concentration tested. All compounds tested were added to neural crest cultures on day 3: 5-Bromo-2′-deoxyuridine, cyclophosphamide, nornitrogen mustard, phosphoramide mustard, retinoic acid, and retinyl acetate were added to mesenchyme cultures on day 1. Other compounds were added to mesenchyme cultures on both days 1 and 3

[b] Unless indicated, effects were similar for cells cultured under conditions where neurons and melanocytes differentiate

[c] Alcian blue staining of matrix proteoglycans was used to quantitate chondrogenesis

[d] Concentration in medium assuming that 50% of the original compound, or its metabolites, placed into the dialysis bag is accessible to the cells (see Fig. 1)

[e] Decreased melanin synthesis and choline acetyltransferase activity were observed (GREENBERG et al. 1980)

volves recognition of specific sites on the plasma membrane. Failure of myoblasts to fuse might detect teratogens which affect those or other cellular interactions.

The use of embryonic cells limits somewhat the number of replicates that can be assayed at one time. Although a differentiating cell line such as neuroblastoma, teratocarcinoma, or erythroleukemia would provide more cells, these lines are malignant, and may not react to teratogens as do normal embryonic cells. However, embryonal carcinoma cells have recently been used as a screening system for teratogenicity of benzo[*a*]pyrene metabolites (FILLER 1980). Nonmalignant but nondifferentiating cell types such as fibroblasts would also provide greater numbers of cells, but such cultures would probably only detect substances which are toxic, and not those which affect specific functions of developing cells.

## C. In Vitro Cell Interactions

During development, cells interact specifically with other cells and matrix components, and it might be expected therefore that compounds which interfere with these interactions might be teratogenic. MOSCONA and co-workers have shown that dissociated embryonic cells will aggregate in vitro, forming characteristic homotypic and heterotypic associations (for a review, see MOSCONA and HAUSMAN 1977). These interactions are energy dependent and appear to be mediated by tissue-specific macromolecules (LILIEN 1968; HAUSMAN and MOSCONA 1975). Systematic studies have not been performed to determine whether teratogens interfere with reaggregation of embryonic cells, although inhibitors of DNA, RNA, or protein synthesis block reaggregation of trypsin-treated cells (MOSCONA and HAUSMAN 1977).

Recently, BRAUN et al. (1979) suggested that tumor cells, which are available in large quantities and which interact with lectin-coated surfaces, might mimic the more complex embryonic interactions that occur during development. Accordingly, they measured the effect of a large number of teratogenic and nonteratogenic agents on the attachment of tumor cells to plastic disks coated with concanavalin-A. Ascitic mouse ovarian tumor cells labeled in vivo with thymidine $^3H$ were preincubated with the test compound for 30 min at 37 °C and then exposed to the coated disks. After 20 min at room temperature, the disks were washed and counted for radioactivity. Of the teratogens tested, 31 of 39 (79%) inhibited attachment (Table 3). Of the nonteratogenic agents tested, 14 of 16 (88%) did not inhibit attachment. False negatives (teratogens which did not inhibit attachment) occurred in 8 of 22 cases (36%), and several of these represented compounds which inhibit macromolecular synthesis and might require longer preincubation times to exert a detectable effect. Another reason for the high number of false negatives could be that certain drugs were not metabolized to active forms. In this regard, BRAUN and DAILEY (1980) subsequently showed that thalidomide inhibited attachment only if it was first preincubated for at least 30 min with a mouse liver microsomal system. It would be of interest to determine whether other compounds known to require metabolic activation are active in inhibiting adhesion only after preincubation with the microsomal system. Although the effects of the teratogens were dose dependent (BRAUN et al. 1979), in some cases the concentrations required to inhibit cell attach-

**Table 3.** Inhibition of tumor cell attachment to plastic disks coated with concanavalin A[a]

| | Inhibit attachment | | | Inhibit attachment | |
|---|---|---|---|---|---|
| *Teratogens* | | | | | |
| Aspirin | + | (14 m*M*) | Chloramphenicol | + | (2.8 m*M*) |
| Phenylbutazone | + | (0.12 m*M*) | Nalidixic acid | + | (0.5 m*M*) |
| Procaine | + | (11 m*M*) | Triton x-100 | + | (0.015 m*M*) |
| Warfarin | + | (0.8 m*M*) | Ethanol | + | (0.54 *M*) |
| Caffeine | + | (35 m*M*) | Busulfan | + | (1.3 m*M*) |
| Diphenylhydantoin | + | (0.84 m*M*) | Carmustine | + | (2.3 m*M*) |
| Diazepam | + | (0.88 m*M*) | Griseofulvin | + | (0.14 m*M*) |
| Chlordiazepoxide | + | (0.17 m*M*) | Diethystilbestrol | + | (0.11 m*M*) |
| Trifluoroperazine | + | (0.1 m*M*) | Estradiol | + | (0.11 m*M*) |
| Chlorpromazine | + | (0.1 m*M*) | Adrenaline-HCl | + | (0.46 m*M*) |
| Pentobarbital | + | (1.4 m*M*) | Noradrenaline | + | (0.24 m*M*) |
| Dexamethasone | + | (0.2 m*M*) | Colchicine | – | (5 m*M*) |
| Prednisolone-21- | | | Thalidomide | – | (1 m*M*) |
| sodium succinate | + | (12 m*M*) | +liver microsomes | + | (0.2 mg/ml)[b] |
| Phenylalanine | | (90 m*M*) | Cortisone acetate | – | (0.3 m*M*) |
| Retinoic acid | + | (0.4 m*M*) | Trypan blue | – | (0.83 m*M*) |
| Cytochalasin B | + | (0.69 m*M*) | Actinomycin D | – | (0.2 m*M*) |
| Dinitrophenol | + | (0.1 m*M*) | Methotrexate | – | (2.2 m*M*) |
| Dimethylsulfoxide | + | (0.9 *M*) | 5-Fluorouracil | – | (1.9 m*M*) |
| Penicillin G | + | (17 m*M*) | Vinblastine | – | (1.1 m*M*) |
| *Nonteratogens* | | | | | |
| Tween | + | (0.38 mg/ml) | Ascorbic acid | – | (75 m*M*) |
| Linoleic acid | + | (0.053 m*M*) | Ouabain | – | (4.5 m*M*) |
| Chloroform | – | (33.5 m*M*) | Ammonium chloride | – | (75 m*M*) |
| Heparin | – | (5 µg/ml) | Ethylenediaminetetrat- | | |
| Hydrocortisone-21- | | | acetic acid | – | (10 m*M*) |
| hemisuccinate | – | (1 m*M*) | Monosodium glutamate | – | (150 m*M*) |
| Lysine | – | (45 m*M*) | Propylene glycol | – | (0.1%) |
| Cysteine | – | (75 m*M*) | Carboxymethylcellulose | – | (9 mg/ml) |
| Thiamine | – | (2.5 m*M*) | Streptomycin | – | (16 m*M*) |

[a] Mean inhibitory concentration for compounds which inhibited attachment (+) or maximum concentration tested for compounds which did not inhibit attachment (–). (Adapted from BRAUN et al. 1979)
[b] A.G. BRAUN (personal communication 1980)

ment were considerably higher than the blood levels associated with malformations in embryos. Nevertheless, the correlation between teratogenicity and inhibition of cell attachment was strong, suggesting that this system may be useful for detecting teratogens, particularly those which might act by disrupting intercellular interactions.

Synapse formation between neurons or between neurons and their target organs represents a highly specific cellular interaction that occurs during development. Cells from spinal cords of 13-day mouse fetuses (PEACOCK et al. 1973) or of 7-day chick embryos (FISCHBACH 1972) can be dissociated and plated as single cells, either alone on in coculture with myoblasts. Such cultures can be examined by electron microscopy and electrophysiologic methods to analyze the synaptic interactions that occur. NELSON (1978) has suggested the use of such cultures to study acute and chronic effects of neuropharmacologic agents. Similar systems might be useful also for detecting teratogens, particularly those which exert their effects late in development and those which may affect behavior.

The extracellular matrix influences migration and differentiation of cells in the embryo (reviewed in LASH and BURGER 1977). Recent studies have shown that certain types of cultured cells attach to collagen substrates by means of the glycoprotein fibronectin (for a review, see YAMADA and OLDEN 1978), and it is likely that fibronectin and other attachment proteins, such as chondronectin (HEWITT et al. 1980) may play a similar role in vivo. The binding of fibronectin to collagen (JILEK and HÖRMANN 1979; JOHANSSON and HÖÖK 1980) and to cells (CULP et al. 1979) can be modulated by proteoglycans which are also present in the matrix. Attachment of cells to fibronectin (KLEINMAN et al. 1978) or to chondronectin (HEWITT et al. 1980) is specific for certain cell types and is mediated by membrane-associated glycoconjugates (KLEINMAN et al. 1979). Attachment is energy dependent (KLEBE 1975) and requires divalent cations (KLEBE et al. 1977) and cytoskeletal changes (JULIANO and GAGALANG 1977).

Fibronectin has been detected in basement membranes and associated with certain cell types in early embryos (WARTIOVAARA et al. 1978, 1979), and it has been suggested that fibronectin is involved in morphogenetic movements during early development (CRITCHLEY et al. 1979). Agents which change the normal interactions of cells with fibronectin and other matrix components might disrupt morphogenesis and tissue-specific inductions. For example, vitamin A (ADAMO et al. 1979) and dexamethasone (RENNARD et al. 1979) which are teratogenic, enhance adhesion of cells to collagen. Since attachment assays are easily performed on numerous replicates, it would be of interest to screen other teratogenic and nonteratogenic compounds for their effects on attachment of certain embryonic cells to collagen substrates in culture, since such a system might provide a rapid and sensitive method for detecting teratogens which affect cell–matrix interactions.

## D. Migration of Cells in Culture

Certain cells, such as primordial germ cells, primary mesenchyme cells, neural crest cells, and corneal fibroblasts, migrate in highly specific pathways in the embryo. Migratory cells require a functioning motility apparatus and must be able to respond to stimuli and form and break associations with other cells or matrix macromolecules. Teratogens could prevent migration by interfering with any of these functions. Movement of cells in culture can be assessed by the phagokinetic track assay (ALBRECHT-BUEHLER 1977). In this assay, coverslips are coated with gold particles, and the rate of movement of cells plated on the gold substrate is reflected by the size of the tracks left by cells as they ingest the gold.

Alternatively, directed cell movement, or chemotaxis, can be measured using a modified Boyden chamber assay (CATES et al. 1978). The Boyden chamber is composed of an upper and lower compartment, separated by a filter. Cells placed in the upper compartment migrate through the filter is response to a gradient which is established by placing an attractant in the lower compartment. The number of cells which migrate to the lower surface of the filter is a measure of the chemotactic response of the cells. It has recently been shown that fibroblasts (POSTLETHWAITE et al. 1976, 1978; GAUSS-MÜLLER et al. 1980; SEPPÄ et al. 1980) and smooth muscle cells (GROTENDORST et al. 1981) migrate in response to chemoattractants in vitro.

It would be of interest to test teratogens for their effects both on motility with the phagokinetic track assay and on chemotaxis with the Boyden chamber assay. Although these systems would not be expected to detect teratogenic activity of as wide a variety of compounds as do differentiating cells (WILK et al. 1980) or cells interacting with lectins (BRAUN et al. 1979), they might be highly specific for detecting teratogens which disrupt cell migration.

## E. Conclusions

In vitro tests are now recognized as useful procedures for first-line screening of carcinogens (Interagency Regulatory Liaison Group 1977). In vitro teratogen testing, however, is much more complex than carcinogen testing because of the greater variety of mechanisms by which teratogens can act, and it is important to devise tests to account for these mechanisms. Embryonic cells which differentiate in culture (WILK et al. 1980) and tumor cells which attach to lectin-coated surfaces (BRAUN et al. 1979) discriminate between known teratogenic and nonteratogenic compounds. A larger group of reference compounds needs to be tested, and other possible tests based on cell–cell and cell–substrate interactions and on cellular migration in vitro should be developed.

Systems which use cells in vitro, however, fail to account for maternal–fetal interactions which might antagonize or enhance the effect of a teratogen. Neither do they directly assess the effect of a substance on tissue interactions or measure the accessibility of the substance to various parts of the developing fetus. Furthermore, in vitro tests are complicated by insolubility of certain test compounds and possible toxicity of solvents.

Despite these difficulties, these systems may provide useful prescreening methods for teratogens, and may help in selecting compounds for subsequent animal testing. In addition, a major advantage in developing in vitro systems may be their usefulness for studying the mechanisms by which teratogens act, the relationship between structure and function of a teratogen, and the metabolism of a compound which results in the proximate teratogen.

*Acknowledgment.* I am grateful to Dr. ANN L. WILK for her valuable comments during the preparation of this manuscript.

## References

Adamo S, DeLuca LM, Akalovsky I, Bhat PV (1979) Retinoid-induced adhesion in cultured, transformed mouse fibroblasts. J Natl Cancer Inst 62:1473–1477

Albrecht-Buehler G (1977) The phagokinetic tracks of 3T3 cells. Cell 11:395–404

Ames BN (1979) Identifying environmental chemicals causing mutations and cancer. Science 204:587–593

Ames BN, Durston WE, Yamasaki E, Lee RD (1973) Carcinogens are mutagens: a simple test system combining liver homogenates for activation and bacteria for detection. Proc Natl Acad Sci USA 70:2281–2285

Bandman E, Walker CR, Strohman RC (1978) Diazepam inhibits myoblast fusion and expression of muscle specific protein synthesis. Science 200:559–560

Bischoff R, Holtzer H (1970) Inhibition of myoblast fusion after one round of DNA synthesis in 5-bromodeoxyuridine. J Cell Biol 44:134–150

Blau HM, Epstein CJ (1979) Manipulation of myogenesis in vitro: reversible inhibition by DMSO. Cell 17:95–108

Braun AG, Dailey JP (1980) Thalidomide metabolite inhibits tumor cell attachment to lectin coated surfaces. Teratology 21:29A

Braun AG, Emerson DJ, Nichinson BB (1979) Teratogenic drugs inhibit tumor cell attachment to lectin-coated surfaces. Nature 282:507–509

Cates KL, Ray CE, Quie PG (1978) Modified Boyden chamber method of measuring polymorphonuclear leukocyte chemotaxis. In: Gallin JI, Quie PG (eds) Leukocyte chemotaxis. Raven Press, New York, pp 67–71

Collins TFX (1978) Reproduction and teratology guidelines: review of deliberations by the national toxicology advisory committee's reproduction panel. J Environ Pathol Toxicol 2:141–147

Critchley DR, England MA, Wakeley J, Hynes RO (1979) Distribution of fibronectin in the ectoderm of gastrulating chick embryos. Nature 280:498–500

Culp L, Murray BA, Rollins BJ (1979) Fibronectin and proteoglycans as determinants of cell-substratum adhesion. J Supramol Struct 11:401–427

Dawson M (1972) Cellular pharmacology. The effects of drugs on living vertebrate cells in vitro. CC Thomas, Springfield IL

Filler R (1980) An in vitro/in vivo coupled prescreen to identify teratogens requiring metabolic activation. Teratology 21:37A–38A

Fischbach GD (1972) Synapse formation between dissociated nerve and muscle cells in low density cell cultures. Dev Biol 28:407–429

Garcia RI, Werner I, Szabo G (1979) Effect of 5-bromo-2′-deoxyuridine on growth and differentiation of cultured embryonic retinal pigment cells. In Vitro 15:779–788

Gauss-Müller V, Kleinman HK, Martin GR, Schiffman E (1980) Role of attachment and attractants in fibroblast chemotaxis. J Lab Clin Med 96:1071–1080

Goetinck PF, Pennypacker JP, Royal PD (1974) Proteochondroitin sulfate synthesis and chondrogenic expression. Exp Cell Res 87:241–248

Greenberg JH, Oliver C (1980) Dimethylsulfoxide reversibly inhibits the pigmentation of cultured neural crest cells. Arch Biochem Biophys 204:1–9

Greenberg JH, Schrier BK (1977) Development of choline acetyltransferase activity in chick cranial neural crest cells in culture. Dev Biol 61:86–93

Greenberg JH, Wilk AL, Horigan EA (1980) Detection of teratogens in vitro using differentiating neural crest cells. Gryder R, Frankos V (eds) In: Fifth Food and Drug Administration science symposium on the effects of foods and drugs on the development and function of the nervous system. HHS Publ (FDA) 80-1076. Government Printing Office, Washington DC

Grotendorst GR, Sëppa HEJ, Kleinman HK, Martin GR (1981) Attachment of smooth muscle cells to collagen and their migration toward platelet-derived growth factor. Proc Natl Acad Sci USA 78:3669–3672

Hamburger V, Hamilton HL (1951)A series of normal stages in the development of the chick embryo. J Morphol 88:49–92

Hassell JR, Pennypacker JP, Lewis CA (1978) Chondrogenesis and cell proliferation in limb bud cell cultures treated with cytosine arabinoside and vitamin A. Exp Cell Res 112:409–417

Hausman RE, Moscona AA (1975) Purification and characterization of the retina-specific cell-aggregating factor. Proc Natl Acad Sci USA 72:916–920

Hewitt AT, Kleinman HK, Pennypacker JP, Martin GR (1980) Identification of an adhesion factor for chondrocytes. Proc Natl Acad Sci USA 77:385–388

Interagency Regulatory Liaison Group (1979) Identification of potential carcinogens and risk estimation. J Natl Cancer Inst 63:241–268
Jilek F, Hörmann H (1979) Fibronectin (cold-insoluble globulin). VI. Influence of heparin and hyaluronic acid on the binding of native collagen. Hoppe Seylers Z Physiol Chem 360:597–603
Juliano RL, Gagalang E (1977) The adhesion of Chinese hamster cells I. Effects of temperature, metabolic inhibitors and proteolytic dissection of cell surface macromolecules. J Cell Physiol 92:209–220
Johansson S, Höök M (1980) Heparin enhances the rate of binding of fibronectin to collagen. Biochem J 187:521–524
Klebe RJ (1975) Cell attachment to collagen: the requirement for energy. J Cell Physiol 86:231–236
Klebe RJ, Hall JR, Rosenberger P, Dickey WD (1977) Cell attachment to collagen: the ionic requirements. Exp Cell Res 110:419–425
Kleinman HK, Murray JC, McGoodwin EB, Martin GR (1978) Connective tissue structure: cell binding to collagen. J Invest Dermatol 71:9–11
Kleinman HK, Martin GR, Fishman PH (1979) Ganglioside inhibition of fibronectin-mediated cell adhesion to collagen. Proc Natl Acad Sci USA 76:3367–3371
Lash JW, Burger MM (eds) (1977) Cell and tissue interactions. Raven Press, New York
Levitt D, Dorfman A (1972) The irreversible inhibition of differentiation of limb-bud mesenchyme by bromodeoxyuridine. Proc Natl Acad Sci USA 69:1253–1257
Lilien JE (1968) Specific enhancement of cell aggregation in vitro. Dev Biol 17:657–678
Madle S, Obe G (1977) In vitro testing of an indirect mutagen (cyclophosphamide) with human leukocyte cultures: activation with liver microsomes and use of a dialysis bag. Mutat Res 56:101–104
Miranda AF, Nette EG, Khan S, Brockbank K, Schonberg M (1978) Alteration of myoblast phenotype by dimethylsulfoxide. Proc Natl Acad Sci USA 75:3826–3830
Moscona AA, Hausman RE (1977) Biological and biochemical studies on embryonic cell-cell recognition. In: Lash JW, Burger MM (eds) Cell and tissue interactions. Raven Press, New York, pp 173–185
Nelson PG (1978) Neuronal cell cultures as toxicologic test systems. Environ Health Perspect 26:125–133
Peacock JH, Nelson PG, Goldstone NW (1973) Electrophysiologic study of cultured neurons dissociated from spinal cords and dorsal root ganglia of fetal mice. Dev Biol 30:137–152
Postlethwaite AE, Snyderman R, Kang AH (1976) The chemotactic attraction of human fibroblasts to a lymphocyte-derived factor. J Exp Med 144:1118–1203
Postlethwaite AE, Seyer JM, Kang AH (1978) Chemotactic attraction of human fibroblasts to type I, II and III collagens and collagen-derived peptides. Proc Natl Acad Sci USA 75:871–875
Rennard SI, Wind ML, Furcht LT (1979) Dexamethasone enhanced matrix formation in transformed human fibroblasts. J Cell Biol 83:466a
Seppä H, Seppä S, Yamada KM, Grotendorst GR (1980) The cell binding fragment of fibronectin and platelet derived growth factor are chemoattractants for fibroblasts. J Cell Biol 87:323a
Umansky R (1966) The effect of cell population density on the developmental fate of reaggregating limb bud mesenchyme. Dev Biol 13:31–56
Wartiovaara J, Leivo I, Virtanen I, Vaheri A, Graham CF (1978) Cell surface and extracellular matrix glycoprotein fibronectin: expression in embryogenesis and in teratocarcinoma differentiation. Ann NY Acad Sci 312:132–141
Wartiovaara J, Leivo I, Vaheri A (1979) Expression of the cell-surface associated glycoprotein, fibronectin, in the early mouse embryo. Dev Biol 69:247–257
Wilk AL, Greenberg JH, Horigan EA, Pratt RM, Martin GR (1980) Detection of teratogenic compounds using differentiating embryonic cells in culture. In Vitro 16:269–276
Yamada KM, Olden K (1978) Fibronectins – adhesive glycoproteins of cell surface and blood. Nature 275:179–184
Yuspa SH, Harris CC (1974) Altered differentiation of mouse epidermal cells treated with retinyl acetate in vitro. Exp Cell Res 86:95–105

CHAPTER 15

# Embryonic Organs in Culture

D. M. KOCHHAR

## A. Introduction

It is not my purpose to review the field of experimental embryology that deals with tissue culture of mammalian embryonic organs (WESSELLS 1967). A number of embryonic organs and tissues are known to undergo morphogenesis and attain functional maturation upon explanation in vitro, and their capabilities have been exploited to a variable degree in investigations on developmental mechanisms and the processes of cell differentiation (SAXÉN and KOHONEN 1969). Some examples are: kidney (GROBSTEIN 1956; SAXÉN et al. 1968), sex organs (ODOR and BLANDAU 1971; HAFFEN 1976), pancreas (SARRAS et al. 1981; MAYLIE-PFENNINGER and JAMIESON 1981; GROBSTEIN 1953), skin (SUGIMOTO and ENDO 1969), tooth (THESLEFF 1976; THESLEFF et al. 1981), palate (MORIARTY et al. 1963; LAHTI et al. 1972; NEWALL and EDWARDS 1976, 1981; GREENE and PRATT 1977), other craniofacial tissues (JOHNSTON and LISTGARTEN 1972; JOHNSTON et al. 1977; GREENBERG and SCHRIER 1977), and limbs (AGNISH and KOCHHAR 1977; KOCHHAR et al. 1976). Any of these or other developing organs are suitable subjects for the development of a teratologic screening system. This chapter, however, is limited to just one example, i.e., limb bud, that may suffice to bring out feasibility, advantages, and shortcomings of organ culture system in general for short-term teratologic screening purposes.

## B. Advantageous Features of In Vitro Systems

As far as studies on teratogenesis are concerned, the following advantages are shared by all types of tissue culture systems:

1. The target organ or tissue is made accessible to direct observation and manipulation. This helps in establishing the stage-specific sensitivity, if any, of the organogenetic process.
2. Better control over dosage and duration of exposure to the agent is exercised than that available in vivo. This helps in establishing precise dose–response relationships and gives more confidence in identification of the selected endpoint or endpoints.
3. Maternal/placental metabolism of the agent is circumvented, permitting assessment of the active form of the agent.
4. The ease of obtaining replicate samples from the same litter, or even from the same embryos, allows more reproducible results than available in vivo.

With an in vitro system, it should be possible to circumvent species differences in teratogenicity which may be due to differences in metabolism, transport and maternal–fetal membrane relationship. In such a system the effect of an agent could be observed on a particular organ, or even on the embryo itself rather than on the maternal–fetal complex as a whole. By culturing whole embryos or a specific developing organ at an early stage of organogenesis, and exposing these to the teratogen directly, it should be possible to remove the complicating influences due to the maternal metabolism and embryonic and placental membranes. It should also be possible to exploit such a culture system in obtaining accurate information about the effects of a chemical on the embryonic metabolism, growth, and many development processes, such as inductive influences, sorting out and aggregation of cells, or cellular interactions, all of which would be of great value in understanding the mechanisms of teratogenesis.

The use of organ cultures adds dimension to the screening procedure not usually attainable in systems that are based on cell culture methology (see Chap. 14). The explanted organ primordium, usually consisting of heterogeneous tissue components, progresses through its organogenetic stages, simulating closely what it would do in vivo. This provides an opportunity to include several developmental phenomena in the repertoire of assayable endpoints, such as localized cell death, differential growth through regional cell proliferation, tissue interactions, and morphogenetic cell movements.

Studies on teratogenesis have identified that an embryo may respond in one of three ways once it is exposed to a hazardous agent during the organogenetic period. It may be killed outright, it may suffer only growth retardation, or it may become malformed with or without growth retardation. Experience shows that organ culture methodology has much more versatility in differentiating among these teratologic outcomes than other types of systems based on cell cultures (KOCHHAR 1975). Our aim in pursuing the limb bud as an organ of choice in the screening system is based on several characteristics it displays which make it more suitable than the culture of other embryonic organs. Foremost among these is its developmental history which is briefly summarized in Sect. C.

## C. Developmental Features of the Limb Bud

The vertebrate limb arises in early embryos as a mass of mesodermal cells, covered by ectoderm of the embryonic flank. The mesodermal mass goes through a complex series of sequential changes (Table 1) on its way to attaining its differentiated structure (HINCHLIFFE and JOHNSON 1980 for review). Initial changes involve cell proliferation and inductive interactions followed by regional changes in proliferation and cell differentiation (STARK and SEARLS 1973, 1974; KOCHHAR 1977). A critical event in the development of the limb bud is the initiation and gradual formation of cartilaginous models of the long bones along the proximodistal axis of the limb (SAUNDERS 1948; KOCHHAR 1973). The morphological differentation of cartilage is associated with biosynthesis of primarily two tissue-specific macromolecules which serve as molecular markers of this differentiation process: type II col-

**Table 1.** Important events in early limb morphogenesis

1. A mass of highly proliferative mesodermal cells
2. Formation of apical ectodermal ridge
3. Reciprocal interactions between apical ectodermal ridge and mesodermal cells
4. Growth in length of the limb bud
5. Blood vessels and nerves enter the limb bud
6. Regional differences in cell proliferation arise in the elongating limb bud
7. Formation of cartilage in the central mesodermal core and muscle in the areas around the core
8. Skeletal primordia first established proximally (e.g., humerus), then elaborated more distally at subsequent stages
9. Morphogenetic cell death occurs in localized areas during several of these phases; it shapes the limb contours and separates the digits

**Table 2.** Development steps involved in differentiation of cartilage

1. Mesodermal cell proliferation slows down
2. Cell aggregation begins
3. Steps 1 and 2 closely associated with elevated levels of intracellular cyclic AMP
4. Change in cell-cell contacts
5. Enhanced biosynthetic activity related to production of extracellular matrix materials
6. Biosynthesis of type I collagen is superseded by that of type II collagen
7. Enhanced synthesis of specific sulfated proteoglycan macromolecules begins

lagen and sulfated proteoglycans (MILLER and MATUKAS 1969; HASCALL et al. 1976; LINSENMAYER and KOCHHAR 1979).

Since the formation of cartilage and deviations in the sequence of cartilaginous limb segments are some of the important characteristics on which the limb bud organ culture screening system is based, a few points about the process of chondrogenic differentiation itself should be noted. It is a complex process and involves many steps (CAPLAN 1981; VON DER MARK and CONRAD 1979). Although many steps of the process are still speculative, a list of sequential events leading to cartilage differentiation is given in Table 2 (SOLURSH et al. 1978). It can be surmised from the list that a great number of possible endpoints are available if a study of chondrogenesis is incorporated in the screening system. It should be pointed out that some of the biochemical and physiologic parameters included in the list are shared by a number of other developing tissues and organs (SUBTELNY and ABBOTT 1981).

In summary, the choice of limb bud as the subject of a screening system is based on the premise that, during its developmental history, it encompasses many of the important phases known to be critical in normal embryogenesis. Hence, its response or responses to different chemicals of known or unknown hazard potential could in theory be interpreted broadly, even when the site of attack in the embryo is other than limb (KOCHHAR 1975; EBERT and MAROIS 1976; HINCHLIFFE and JOHNSON 1980).

# D. Limb Bud Organ Culture

## I. General

Techniques of organ culture in general are easily available in the literature, and many review articles are now available (KOCHHAR and AYDELOTTE 1974; NEUBERT and BARRACH 1977; EBERT and MARIOS 1976; TROWELL 1961; SAXÉN et al. 1976). After initial success with organ cultures of various segments of chick embryo limb cartilages (FELL and LANDAUER 1935), other authors made efforts to grow mammalian limb buds in vitro (SHEPARD and BASS 1970; KOCHHAR 1970). These latter studies utilized the method popularized by TROWELL (1954). The basic methodology is described in Sect. D.II. In short, the system involves removal of limb buds from mouse embryos of known ages. Under sterile conditions, these buds are placed on top of thin filters and incubated for several days in a nutrient medium in the presence or absence of test chemicals. Finally, the cultured limbs are scored in two ways: qualitatively, for the presence or absence of malformations affecting any segment of the limb; and quantitatively, for the amount of cartilage skeleton formed in the whole limb.

## II. Details of the Culture Method

Most commonly, we have employed mouse embryos on the 12th day of gestation. The embryos at this stage are 5–6 mm in length, possess about 40 somite pairs, and their limbs show no distinct histodifferentiation in mesodermal cells (KOCHHAR 1977). The embryo, after removal from the uterine horns, is stripped of its membranes and the somite number is counted under a dissecting microscope. All procedures are carried out in sterile Tyrode's saline solution (KOCHHAR and AYDELOTTE 1974). With sharpened cataract knives the forelimb and hindlimb buds are cut off from the body along a line immediately lateral to the row of somites (Fig. 1). All four limbs from each embryo in the litter are used in the study, thus yielding an average of 40 limbs from each litter. Between one and four explants are pipetted onto a small piece of ultrathin Millipore or Nucleopore filter which, in turn, is inserted into the culture chamber assembly (KOCHHAR and Aydelotte 1974).

The culture medium most commonly employed is $BGJ_b$ (GIBCO), supplemented with ascorbic acid and 25% fetal bovine serum (dialyzed, GIBCO). Recently, we have used homologous adult mouse serum with excellent results; in the latter case, as little as 10% serum supports adequate growth and development (KOCHHAR and PENNER, unpublished work). Other investigators have made efforts to eliminate the need for serum entirely so that the medium could be completely defined chemically (NEUBERT et al. 1976; KWASIGROCH et al. 1981).

The cultures are incubated in a humidified atmosphere of 5% $CO_2$ in air and maintained at 38 °C. The medium is changed only once at the midpoint of the 6-day culture period. At the end of the culture period, the filters, to which the limbs have now become attached, are withdrawn from the culture chamber and rinsed briefly in saline, immersed in Bouin's fixative and immediately stained, either with alcian blue or with toluidine blue, to visualize the cartilage skeleton (KOCHHAR and AYDELOTTE 1974).

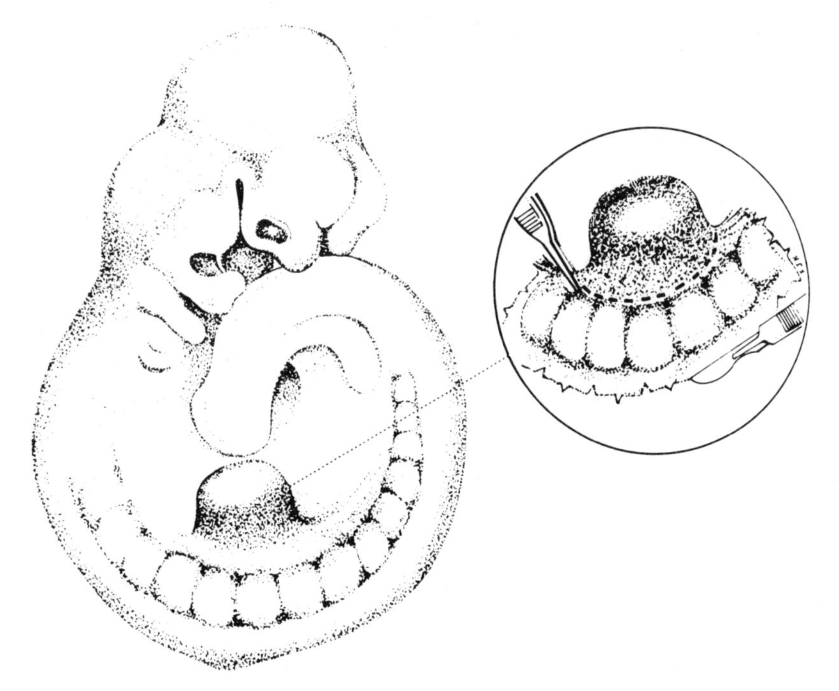

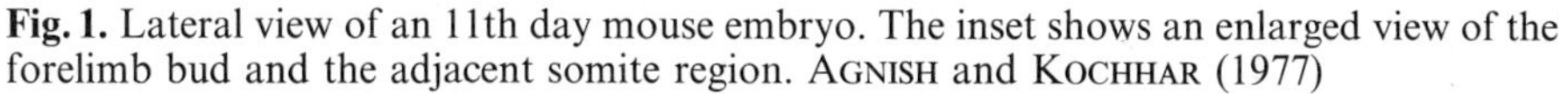

**Fig. 1.** Lateral view of an 11th day mouse embryo. The inset shows an enlarged view of the forelimb bud and the adjacent somite region. AGNISH and KOCHHAR (1977)

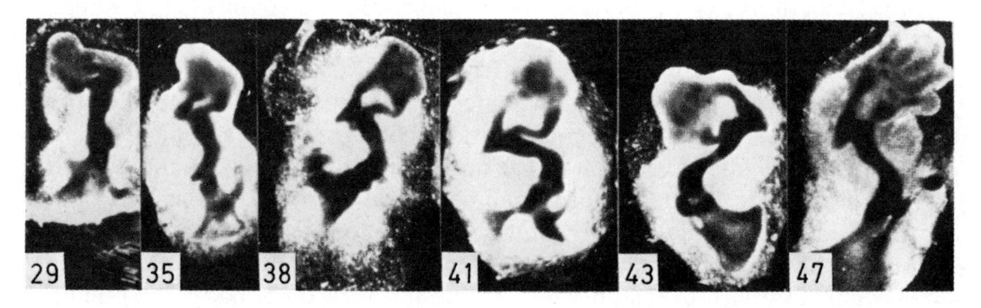


**Fig. 2.** Limb buds cultured for 6 days in control medium and stained with alcian blue. Donor embryos were obtained from mice on the 11th or 12th day of gestation, ranging in somite number from 29 to 47 as shown. Increased amount of cartilage formed as the donor embryos advanced in age (see text). KOCHHAR and AYDELOTTE (1974) × 12.5

## III. Characteristics of the Cultured Limb Buds

Since qualitative comparisons between control and drug-exposed specimens are based on stained limb bud cultures, a few remarks about this aspect are in order. Each of the cartilage segments typical of the vertebrate limb is represented in the limb cultured for 6 days (Fig. 2). The extent of development and growth (size and shape) attained by limbs in culture depends on the initial developmental stage of the donor embryos. In Fig. 2, a series of forelimbs taken from embryos of different chronological ages is shown; the age is represented by the number of somites in the donor embryo – the range in this case is 29–47 somites, i.e., 11th and 12th day embryos.

The scapula develops as a triangular cartilage with a prominent acromion process in all cultured limb buds. At the 29-somite stage, the humerus is most prominent as a straight bar of cartilage. At 35-somite and older stages, ulna and radius also become prominent. Adequate development of the digits is obtained only in 45-somite and older stages; in younger embryos the cartilages of individual digits are not always separately recognized. One flexure is observed in all cultured forelimbs which represents the future elbow joint. The shaft of the humerus shows an additional curvature only in limbs derived from embryos older than 35-somite stage (Fig. 2).

## IV. Quantification of Cartilage in Cultures

It is apparent from Fig. 2 that the amount of cartilage formed in cultures is dependent on the age of the donor embryos. A method is needed to provide actual quantification of the amount of cartilage if the system is to be utilized as a screening device. NEUBERT et al. (1978 a) have published a method of giving numerical ratings to each segment of the limb, e.g., scapula, long bones, and digits, and ending up with a cumulative score for each limb. This method has merit as far as rough estimation is concerned, but may fail to detect minor effects of the test chemicals owing to its semiquantitative approach. AGNISH and KOCHHAR (1976 a, b) have published another method which eliminates to some extent the problems of subjective aspects of quantification: Toluidine-blue-stained and cleared limbs are photographed under low magnification on a Kodachrome color film. After processing, the photographic slides are projected in a Tri-Simplex Micro Projector (Bausch and Lomb, Rochester, New York) onto squared graph paper. The outline of the cartilage is drawn on the graph paper and various cartilage zones (scapula, humerus, radioulna, and digits) are delimited. The number of graph paper squares occupied by each cartilage is counted and this number is referred to as cartilage area units for that particular cartilage. Alternatively, area can be measured by a planimeter and expressed as $mm^2$.

Such an approach to quantifying the amount of cartilage has certain built-in errors. In organ culture, the various cartilages of the limb grow in a three-dimensional aspect, rather than two, as a photograph would record it. Also, sometimes two cartilages overlap, or some parts (especially scapula and humerus) bend downwards in the growing cultures. In most cases, these errors can be easily rectified by comparing the enlarged outline against the original stained limb. The data obtained are very reproducible and the amount of cartilage area units in the limb explants of similarly staged and treated embryos is found to be quite similar and variations in most cases are rather small. In a few cases, where variation is large (for example when the standard eror is more than 10%–15% of the mean value), the experiment is repeated one or more times to collect a larger sample so as to obtain a statistically valid mean value. All measurements are made on toluidine-blue-stained preparations. When no metachromasia is detected, a complete suppression of chondrogenesis is assumed to have occurred (AYDELOTTE and KOCHHAR 1975).

**Table 3.** The extent of cartilage development in the cultured limb[a] explants, as related to the "age" of the donor embryos

| Embryo | Extent of cartilage development (area units) | | | | | |
|---|---|---|---|---|---|---|
| | Somites | Scapula | Humerus | Radioulna | Digits | Total ± SD[b] |
| Mid 11th day | 32–34 | 127 | 63 | 37 | 0 | 227 ± 10 |
| Late 11th day | 35–38 | 245 | 146 | 50 | 0 | 441 ± 42 |
| 12th day | 40–46 | 290 | 184 | 86 | 53 | 613 ± 63 |
| Early 13th day | 52–56 | 523 | 128 | 130 | 148 | 929 ± 52 |
| Mid 13th day | 58–62 | 679 | 187 | 183 | 166 | 1,215 ± 126 |

[a] Forelimbs were organ cultured for 6 Days (9 days for the limbs from the 11th day embryos), fixed and stained in toluidine blue. The amount of cartilage development is expressed as "cartilage area units"

[b] SD = standard deviation

Using this method, we can now interpret quantitatively the morphological data shown in Fig. 2 (Table 3). There is an excellent correlation between embryonic age (somite number) and total amount of cartilage (expressed in area units) formed in the cultured limb. Not only can we compare the area units of different limbs, but the method permits an analysis of growth (and differentiation) of each of the limb segments separately; hence, regional effects, if any, of the test chemicals can be caried out (Table 3).

While our quantification method is simple in design and easy to perform, it suffers from the fact that several steps are involved, such as photography, draftsmanship, and actual counting of cartilage area. Hence, it is not as quick as one would like to have in a rapid screening system. Also, the numerical values are not absolute. Our future efforts would be to use an approach whereby the cultured limbs are evaluated directly by an automatic image analyzer (KWASIGROCH et al. 1981). The image analyzer will have the capability to score and make a file record of several parameters of the cultured limb. Not only the perimeter and area occupied by the cartilage skeleton would be recorded, but volume as well as density of each cartilage (or noncartilaginous soft tissue) segment may also be evaluated. Such equipment is now commercially available, e.g., Quantimet 800 by Cambridge Instruments, Royston, Herts, United Kingdom or Artek 800 Image Analyzer by the Artek Company, Farmington, New York. Successful adaptation of these instruments to our purposes should significantly reduce the time and effort required to complete the screening process. Rapid retrieval of historical control data achieved in this manner would enhance the ability of the screening system to detect even mildly hazardous agents having subtle effects on developmental parameters.

## V. The Use and Efficacy of the Screening System

In 1975, we reported a list of 12 chemicals that were tested for their activity in the organ culture system (KOCHHAR 1975). Included were many potent teratogenic agents, such as vitamin A analogs, aminopterin, 6-aminonicotinamide, and several

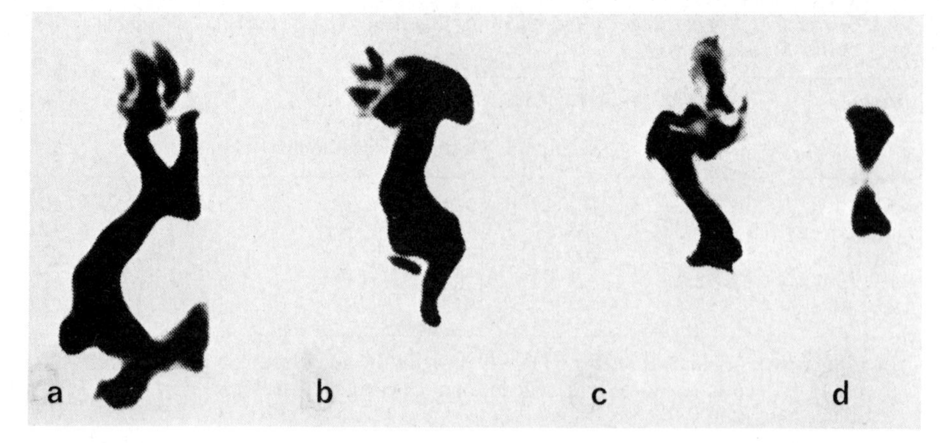


**Fig. 3 a–d.** Toluidine-blue-stained limb bud cultures initiated from embryos on the 12th day of gestation and grown for 6 days in control medium (**a**) or in medium containing ribavirin 10 μg/ml (**b**); 25 μg/ml (**c**); or 50 μg/ml (**d**). Note a dose-dependent inhibition of growth as well as deformation and lack of development of certain segments of the limb cartilages. KOCHHAR et al. (1980) × 6.5

drugs active as anticancer agents: chlorambucil, Diazooxonorleucine (DON), hydroxyurea, and cytosine arabinoside. All of these chemicals altered the appearance of limb buds in a manner which could be termed "malformation", and some agents produced malformations in vitro which were equivalent to reduction deformities actually encountered in fetuses in conventional teratologic studies (KOCHHAR and AYDELOTTE 1974). In assessing the teratologic outsome in vitro, we could isolate the effects which were due to growth retardation versus those produced through interference in certain steps in the process of differentiation, e.g., biosynthesis of collagen or proteoglycans (AYDELOTTE and KOCHHAR 1972, 1975). Mild teratogenic agents such as the lathyrogenic agent $\beta$APN ($\beta$-aminopropionitrile) produced no effect on growth or differentiation, but altered the bending pattern of the cartilage segments. While cytosine arabinoside was a potent teratogenic agent in vitro, its inactive analog, uracil arabinoside was not. The effects of cytosine arabinoside (ara-C) could be counteracted by the presence of 2′-deoxycytidine in the medium. All-*trans* retinoic acid was found to be 4–5-fold more effective in producing deformities than its less toxic analog 13-*cis*-retinoic acid.

Further confidence in the organ culture system as a screening device is engendered by the efficiency and ease with which we can obtain rather precise dose–response relationships. In a recent experiment, we used ribavirin, a new antiviral drug, to asses qualitative aspects of its developmental effects on the limb bud (Fig. 3). The dose was varied between 1 and 100 μg/ml in the culture medium. No detrimental effects on the growth or chondrogenic differentiation were noticed at concentrations of 5 μg/ml or less. Raising the concentration to 10 μg/ml, one could discern a slight inhibition of overall growth (Fig. 3 b) while further increase to 25 or 50 μg/ml resulted in overt deformities (Fig. 3 c, d) of the limb skeleton, such as those encountered in our teratologic studies with the same drug (KOCHHAR et al. 1980).

**Table 4.** Effect of low concentrations of BUDR on the differentiation of cartilage in the limb[a] cultures of 12th day mouse embryos

| [BUDR] | Extent of cartilage development (area units) | | | | |
|---|---|---|---|---|---|
| (μg/ml) | Scapula | Humerus | Radioulna | Digits | Total ± SD[b] |
| 0 | 290 | 184 | 86 | 53 | 613 ± 63 |
| 1 | 250 | 243 | 109 | 55 | 657 ± 47 |
| 2 | 179 | 229 | 81 | 56 | 545 ± 51 |
| 4 | 62 | 194 | 77 | 49 | 382 ± 34 |
| 8 | 15 | 154 | 71 | 34 | 274 ± 36 |
| 16 | 8 | 102 | 58 | 26 | 194 ± 21 |
| 32 | 6 | 53 | 51 | 15 | 125 ± 11 |

[a] Forelimbs were cultured for 6 days and exposed to various concentrations of BUDR for the entire culture period
[b] SD = standard deviation

**Table 5.** Effect of low concentrations of ara-C on the differentiation of cartilage in the limb[a] cultures of 12th day mouse embryos

| [ara-C] | Extent of cartilage development (area units) | | | | |
|---|---|---|---|---|---|
| (μg/ml) | Scapula | Humerus | Radioulna | Digits | Total ± SD[b] |
| 0 | 290 | 184 | 86 | 53 | 613 ± 63 |
| 0.14 | 88 | 118 | 113 | 62 | 381 ± 39 |
| 1.4 | 0 | 21 | 103 | 21 | 145 ± 24 |
| 14.0 | 0 | 0 | 0 | 0 | 0 ± 0 |

[a] Forelimbs were cultured for 6 days and exposed to various concentrations of cytosine arabinoside (ara-C) for the entire culture period
[b] SD = standard deviation

More quantitative aspects of dose–response data from studied on other drugs, i.e., BUDR and ara-C, are given in Tables 4 and 5. These examples clearly illustrate the sensitivity of this system, as well as the type of dose-related studies that can be carried out. Here we were interested in studying the effects of relatively low concentrations of BUDR and ara-C on the differentiation of various cartilage segments in the limbs of 12th day mouse embryos.

## VI. Summary

Studies such as those summarized in Sect. D.V suggest that the in vitro testing of drugs is a reliable means of screening for teratologic effects. The major characteristics of the organ culture technique are summarized here:

a) Cultures can be initiated from the limbs of 11th, 12th, or 13th day embryos, and maintained for an extended period of time, usually 6–9 days.
b) The test compound can be introduced into the culture medium at any time and, once introduced, the duration of treatment can be easily regulated by simply transferring the culture to a control medium.

c) The detrimental effects on growth and differentiation of the organ can be monitored quickly in a preliminary screening, after which more precise qualitative and quantitative studies can be designed.

The major advantages of this technique stem from the flexibility and ease with which it can be combined with other in vivo and in vitro methods, reproducibility of results, and the fact that only small quantities of the test chemicals are needed for initial screening. The last point is important in circumstances where a number of unknown metabolites or pollutants are to be monitored during drug development and industrial processing, respectively.

## E. Current Limitations and Future Improvements

One major shortcoming of in vitro systems is that they usually lack the drug-metabolizing enzymes of the intact animal. Hence, the teratogenic activity of a test chemical may not be apparent, unless such enzyme preparations are added to the culture systems (NEUBERT et al. 1978 b). The major activation (or detoxification) of drugs is carried out by a multicomponent, membrane-bound complex of enzymes called mixed function oxygenases (MFO). Metabolism occurs when the drug, in the presence of molecular oxygen and NADPH, is oxidized by MFO enzymes.

In most experimental animals, typical cytochrome P-450 enzymes are believed not to develop until the late prenatal or even the neonatal stage (FOUTS 1973; FOUTS and ADAMSON 1959; RANE et al. 1973; see also Chap. 4). In contrast, P-450 enzymes are present in liver microsomes of human fetuses as early as 8–15 weeks of gestation (PELKONEN et al. 1973; YAFFEE et al. 1970). This would mean that activation of compounds may not occur in fetuses of laboratory animals, while human fetuses are perfectly capable of such activation. Therefore, development of an efficient and reproducible in vitro activation system would by a very useful advance for in vitro teratologic testing.

Microsomal fractions obtained from livers of phenobarbital-injected animals are commonly used for drug activation in other in vitro systems such as the Ames *Salmonella*/S 9 test for mutagenesis (AMES et al. 1973). In limb bud culture systems, however, MANSON and SIMONS (1979) found that the liver microsomal preparation as such was toxic to the limb bud. These authors have developed another approach which has been successful with at least one tested drug, cyclophosphamide. Cyclophosphamide is teratogenic in a number of mammalian species, including humans (ASHBY et al. 1976; GIBSON and BECKER 1968; TOLEDO et al. 1971). Cyclophosphamide added directly to the culture medium produced no deformities in the explanted limb bud (BARRACH et al. 1978; MANSON and SIMONS 1979). The addition of certain metabolites of cyclophosphamide did result in deformation and lack of normal differentiation in limb bud cartilage. To generate the metabolism of cyclophosphamide in the limb bud culture system, MANSON and SIMONS (1979) used monolayers of hamster embryo cells (HEC) as the source of MFO enzymes. HEC cells were grown for 6 days at the bottom of tissue culture dishes and treated with phenobarbital. Limb buds were set up in the same plates and cyclophosphamide introduced into the medium. Limb bud development was abnormal in this instance, indicating that teratogenically active metabolites were generated by this method. These are preliminary findings and there is some question regarding the authenticity of the metabolites formed in vitro. Yet this has indicated that the organ culture system is reliable enough to respond to in vitro activation of at least conventional drugs.

## F. Conclusions

The need for efficient methods to screen new chemicals, drugs, and environmental pollutants for their teratogenic activity is obvious. The method currently available, i.e., pregnant animal testing, is of considerable value, but there are certain drawbacks which prevent reliance on this method alone as the predictive device. Nutritional state of the mother, variability in the developmental age of embryos from mother to mother and even within the same litter, metabolic differences between species, placental function, and a host of other factors must be taken into account before data obtained from animal testing can be logically extrapolated to humans.

Many of the variables are either eliminated altogether, or at least can be controlled by the use of organ culture techniques. Among other advantages, these procedures allow one to exercise control over the effective concentration of the suspected teratogen to which an embryo is exposed, and also the duration of this exposure. Maternal metabolism or modification of the drug is routinely eliminated as the entire experiment is conducted in a "mother-free" system.

The choice of limb bud in the screeing system may turn out to be ideal since during its development, the limb progresses through a succession of important embryonic processes in achieving its final form. Hence, such a screening system may not only predict teratogenicity, but also provide insight into the mechanisms by which a test chemical is teratogenic. In addition, techniques of limb bud organ cultures are well established and conveniently, limbs are paired organs so that from the same embryo, one limb can be grown in control medium, while the other can be grown in a drug-supplement medium, making direct comparisons a routine matter.

*Acknowledgments.* I am indebted to my colleague Dr. N. D. Agnish who assisted me greatly in completing parts of this manuscript. Original work from my laboratory was supported by National Institutes of Health grant HD-10935-04. Invaluable technical assistance of Mr. John D. Penner and Miss Barbara Kuczynski is gratefully acknowledged. The manuscript was prepared by Mrs. Debra Lundgren.

## References

Agnish ND, Kochhar DM (1976a) Direct exposure of post-implantation mouse embryos to 5-bromodeoxyuridine in vitro and its effects on subsequent chondrogenesis in the limbs. J Embryol Exp Morphol 36:623–638

Agnish ND, Kochhar DM (1976b) Direct exposure of mouse embryonic limb-buds to 5-bromodeoxyuridine in vitro and its effect on chondrogenesis: increasing resistance to the analog at successive stages of development. J Embryol Exp Morphol 36:639–652

Agnish ND, Kochhar (1977) The role of somites in the growth and early development of mouse limb buds. Dev Biol 56:174–183

Ames BN, Lee FD, Durston WE (1973) An improved bacterial test system for the detection and classification of mutagens and carcinogens. Proc Natl Acad Sci USA 70:782–786
Ashby R, Davis L, Dewhurst BB, Espinal R, Penn RN, Upshall DG (1976) Aspects of teratology of cyclophosphamide. Cancer Treat Rep 60:477–482
Aydelotte MB, Kochhar DM (1972) Development of mouse limb buds in organ culture; chondrogenesis in the presence of proline analog, L-azetidine-2-carboxylic acid. Dev Biol 28:191–201
Aydelotte MB, Kochhar DM (1975) Influence of 6-diazo-5-oxo-L-norleucine (DON), a glutamine analogue, on cartilaginous differentiation in mouse limb buds in vitro. Differentiation 4:73–80
Barrach HJ, Bauman I, Neubert D (1978) The applicability of in vitro systems for the evaluation of the significance of pharmacokinetic parameters for the induction of an embryonic effect. In: Neubert D, Merker HJ, Nau H, Langman J (eds) Role of pharmacokinetics in prenatal and perinatal toxicology. G Thieme, Stuttgart, pp 323–336
Caplan AI (1981) The molecular control of muscle and cartilage development. In: Subtelny S, Abbott UK (eds) Levels of genetic control in development. AR Liss, New York, pp 37–68
Ebert JD, Marois M (1976) Tests of teratogenicity in vitro. North-Holland, Amsterdam
Fell HB, Landauer W (1935) Experiments on skeletal growth and development in vitro in relation to the problem of avian phokomelia. Proc R Soc Lond [Biol] 118:133–154
Fouts JR (1973) Microsomal mixed-function oxidases in the fetal and newborn rabbit. In: Boreus L (ed) Fetal pharmacology. Raven Press, New York, pp 305–320
Fouts JR, Adamson RH (1959) Drug metabolism in the newborn rabbit. Science 129:897–898
Gibson JE, Becker BA (1968) The teratogenicity of cyclophosphamide in mice. Cancer Res 28:475–480
Greenberg JH, Schrier BK (1977) Development of choline acetyltransferase activity in chick cranial neural crest cells in culture. Dev Biol 61:86–93
Greene RM, Pratt RM (1977) Inhibition by DON of rat palatal glycoprotein synthesis and epithelial cell adhesion in vitro. Exp Cell Res 105:27–37
Grobstein C (1953) Morphogenetic interaction between embryonic mouse tissues separated by a membrane filter. Nature 172:869–871
Grobstein C (1956) Transfilter induction of tubules in mouse metanephric mesenchyme. Exp Cell Res 10:424–440
Johnston MC, Listgarten MA (1972) The migrations, interactions, and early differentiation of oro-facial tissues. In: Slavkin HC, Bavetta LA (eds) Developmental aspects of oral biology. Academic Press, New York, pp 53–80
Johnston MC, Morriss GM, Kuchner DC, Bingle GJ (1977) Abnormal organogenesis of facial structures. In: Wilson JG, Fraser FC (eds) Handbook of teratology, vol 2. Plenum Press, New York, pp 421–451
Haffen K (1976) Organ culture and determination of sex organs. In: Ebert JD, Marois M (eds) Tests of teratogenicity in vitro. North-Holland, Amsterdam, pp 285–301
Hascall VC, Oegema TR, Brown M, Caplan AI (1976) Isolation and characterization of proteoglycans from chick limb bud chondrocytes grown in vitro. J Biol Chem 251:3511–3519
Hinchliffe JR, Johnson DR (1980) The development of the vertebrate limb. Clarendon Press, Oxford
Kochhar DM (1970) Effects of azetidine-2-carboxylic acid, a proline analog, on chondrogenesis in cultured limb buds. In: Bass R, Beck F, Merker HJ, Neubert D, Randham B (eds) Metabolic pathways in mammalian embryos during organogenesis and its modification by drugs. Freie Universität Press, Berlin, pp 475–482
Kochhar DM (1973) Limb development in mouse embryos. I. Analysis of teratogenic effects of retinoic acid. Teratology 7:289–298
Kochhar DM (1975) The use of in vitro procedures in teratology. Teratology 11:273–288
Kochhar DM (1977) Cellular basis of congenital limb deformity induced in mice by vitamin A. In: Bergsma D, Lenz W (eds) Morphogenesis and malformation of the limb. AR Liss, New York, pp 111–154

Kochhar DM, Agnish ND (to be published) Teratogenesis testing in vitro. In: Nardone RM (ed) Toxicity testing in vitro. Academic Press, New York
Kochhar DM, Aydelotte MB (1974) Susceptible stages and abnormal morphogenesis in the developing mouse limb, analyzed in organ culture after transplacental exposure to vitamin A (retinoic acid). J Embryol Exp Morphol 31:721–734
Kochhar DM, Aydelotte MB, Vest TK (1976) Altered collagen fibrillogenesis in embryonic mouse limb cartilage deficient in matrix granules. Exp Cell Res 102:213–222
Kochhar DM, Penner JD, Knudsen TB (1980) Embryotoxic, teratogenic and metabolic effects of ribavirin in mice. Toxicol Appl Pharmacol 52:99–112
Kwasigroch TE, Skalko RG, Church JK (1981) Development of limb buds in organ culture: examination of hydroxyurea enhancement of bromodeoxyuridine toxicity using image analysis. In: Neubert D, Merker H-J (eds) 5th symposium on prenatal development: applicability of culture techniques for studies on prenatal differentiation and toxicity. W de Gruyter, Berlin, pp 237–253
Lahti A, Antila E, Saxén L (1972) The effect of hydrocortisone on the closure of the palatal shelves in two inbred strains of mice in vivo and in vitro. Teratology 6:37–42
Linsenmayer TF, Kochhar DM (1979) In vitro cartilage formation: effects of 6-diazo-5-oxo-L-norleucine (DON) on glycosaminoglycan and collagen synthesis. Dev Biol 69:517–528
Manson JM, Simons R (1979) In vitro metabolism of cyclophosphamide in limb bud culture. Teratology 19:149–158
Maylie-Pfenninger M-F, Jamieson JD (1981) Effect of 5-bromodeoxyuridine on appearance of cell-surface saccharides in organ cultures of embryonic pancreas. Dev Biol 87:16–23
Miller EJ, Matukas VJ (1969) Chick cartilage collagen: a new type of $\alpha 1$ chain not present in bone or skin of the species. Proc Natl Acad Sci USA 64:1264–1268
Moriarty TM, Weinstein S, Gibson RD (1963) The development *in vitro* and *in vivo* of fusion of the palatal processes of rat embryos. J Embryl Exp Morphol 11:605–619
Neubert D, Barrach HJ (1977) Significance of in vitro techniques for the evaluation of embryotoxic effects. In: Neubert D, Merker HJ, Kwasigroch TE (eds) Methods in prenatal toxicology: evaluation of embryotoxic effects in experimental animals. G Thieme, Stuttgart, pp 202–209
Neubert D, Merker H-J, Barrach H-J, Lessmollmann U (1976) Biochemical and teratological aspects of mammalian limb bud development in vitro. In: Ebert JD, Marois M (eds) Tests of teratogenicity in vitro. North-Holland, Amsterdam, pp 335–365
Neubert D, Hinz N, Baumann I, Barrach HJ, Schmidt K (1978a) Attempt upon a quantitative evaluation of the degree of differentiation of or the degree of interference with development in organ culture. In: Neubert D, Merker HJ, Nau H, Langman J (eds) Role of pharmacokinetics in prenatal and perinatal toxicology. G Thieme, Stuttgart, pp 337–349
Neubert D, Merker HJ, Nau H, Langman J (eds) (1978b) Role of pharmacokinetics in prenatal and perinatal toxicology. G Thieme, Stuttgart
Newall DR, Edward JRG (1976) In vitro fusion of the human secondary palate. Cleft Palate J 13:54–56
Newall DR, Edwards JRG (1981) The effect of vitamin A on fusion of mouse palates. II. Retinyl palmitate, retinol, and retinoic acid in vitro. Teratology 23:125–130
Odor DL, Blandau RJ (1971) Organ cultures of fetal mouse ovaries. I. Light microscopic structure. Am J Anat 131:387–414
Pelkonen O, Jouppila P, Karki NT (1973) Attemps to induce drug metabolism in human fetal liver and placenta by administration of phenobarbital to mothers. Arch Int Pharmacodyn 202:288–297
Rane A, Berggren M, Yaffee S, Ericsson JLE (1973) Oxidative drug metabolism in the perinatal rabbit liver and placenta. Xenobiotica 3:37–48
Sarras MP Jr, Maylie-Pfenninger M-F, Manzi RM, Jamieson JD (1981) The effects of tunicamycin on development of the mammalian embryonic pancreas. Dev Biol 87:1–15
Saunders JW Jr (1948) The proximo-distal sequence of the origin of the parts of the chick wing and the role of ectoderm. J Exp Zool 108:363–404

Saxén L, Kohonen J (1969) Inductive tissue interactions in vertebrate morphogenesis. Int Rev Exp Pathol 8:57–128
Saxén L, Koskimies O, Lahti A, Miettinen H, Rapola J, Wartiovaara J (1968) Differentiation of kidney mesenchyme in an experimental model system. Adv Morphog 7:251–293
Saxén L, Karkinen-Jääsklainen M, Saxen I (1976) Organ culture in teratology. In: Gropp A, Benirschke K (eds) Current topics in pathology. Springer, Berlin Heidelberg New York, pp 123–143
Shepard TH, Bass GL (1970) Organ culture of limb buds from riboflavin-deficient and normal rat embryos in normal and riboflavin-deficient media. Teratology 3:163–168
Solursh M, Ahrens PB, Reiter RS (1978) A tissue culture analysis of the steps in limb chondrogenesis. In Vitro 14:51–61
Stark RJ, Searls RL (1973) A description of chick wing bud development and a model of limb morphogenesis. Dev Biol 33:138–153
Stark RJ, Searls RL (1974) The establishment of the cartilage pattern in the embryonic chick wing and evidence for a role of the dorsal and ventral ectoderm in normal wing development. Dev Biol 38:51–63
Subtelny S, Abbott UK (1981) Levels of genetic control in development. AR Liss, New York
Sugimoto M, Endo H (1969) Effects of hydrocortisone on the keratinization of chick embryonic skin growing in a chemically defined medium. Nature 222:1270–1272
Thesleff I (1976) Differentiation of odontogenic tissues in organ culture. Scand J Dent Res 84:353–356
Thesleff I, Barrach H-J, Foidart JM, Vaheri A, Pratt RM, Martin GR (1981) Changes in distribution of type IV collagen, laminin, proteoglycan and fibronectin during mouse tooth development. Dev Biol 81:182–192
Toledo TM, Harper RC, Moser RH (1971) Fetal effects during cyclophosphamide and irradiation therapy. Ann Intern Med 74:87–91
Trowell OA (1954) A modified technique for organ culture in vitro. Exp Cell Res 6:246–248
Trowell OA (1961) Problems in the maintenance of mature organs in vitro. In: La culture organotypique. Editions du Centre National de la Recherche Scientifique, Paris, pp 237–249
von der Mark K, Conrad G (1979) Cartilage cell differentiation. Clin Orthop 139:185–205
Wessells NK (1967) Avian and mammalian organ culture. In: Wilt FH, Wessells NK (eds) Methods in developmental biology. TY Crowell, New York, pp 445–456
Yaffee SJ, Rane A, Sjogvist F, Boreus LO, Orrenius S, (1970) The presence of a monoxygenase system in human fetal liver microsomes. Life Sci 9:1189–1200

CHAPTER 16

# Whole Embryos in Culture

N. W. Klein and L. J. Pierro

## A. Introduction

The postimplantation rat embryo can be separated rather easily from the decidual tissues of the maternal uterus, and induced to pursue normal development in culture. For example, embryos explanted prior to the appearance of the major organ primordia will, in a 48-h culture period, undergo marked organogenesis of the brain, spinal cord, sense organs, and branchial region. Studies from a number of laboratories have shown that the developmental processes occurring in these organ regions can also be made to proceed abnormally by manipulation of culture conditions. These studies have demonstrated the possibility, therefore, of testing a variety of chemical agents and physical factors for teratogenic effects on organogenesis in whole embryos developing independently of the maternal organism.

The capacity for in vitro development is not restricted to the postimplantation embryo. Nor is it limited to rat embryos. Mouse embryos, for example, can be removed from the uterine environment at the two-cell stage and induced to continue development in vitro. Indeed, fertilization can be accomplished in vitro, and development to the blastocyst stage observed. Reports published during the past 20 years have shown that physical, chemical, and biologic agents can also interfere with developmental processes taking place in preimplantation stage embryos cultured in vitro.

Although it is possible to carry out teratogenic testing with in vitro whole embryo cultures, and a number of laboratories are so engaged, there is some question as to how widely this approach should be adopted. Facilities needed to establish embryo culture programs exceed those needed for the more traditional approaches. Embryo culture is labor intensive and time consuming; not all methodological problems have been solved. Moreover, although in vitro systems offer certain advantages over systems in which the maternal organism serves as a continuing intermediary between the embryo and its environment, the converse is also true. In this chapter, we will review studies involving test systems in which the whole embryo is asked to pursue its development in the absence of the maternal organism for the purpose of testing a response to a potential teratogenic agent. Our objective is to evaluate the contributions which in vitro testing for teratologic assessment can make, in order to suggest situations in which this approach may be more appropriate than the traditional testing methods.

Our discussion will be organized in terms of the developmental stage attained by the embryo at the initiation of in vitro culture, using the rodent (mouse, rat) embryo as a standard since it is the most popular subject for teratologic investigation.

The three developmental phases recognized are: preimplantation (cleavage through blastocyst); peri-implantation (egg cylinder through primitive streak stages); postimplantation (head fold and somite stages).

## B. Preimplantation

### I. General Considerations

In 1973, SPINDLE and PEDERSEN described a culture system which supported development of preimplantation embryos in vitro to an egg cylinder stage in which two germ layers, ectoderm and endoderm, could be readily distinguished in the inner cel mass (ICM). Prior to this time, most studies on in vitro development of the preimplantation embryo terminated at the blastocyst stage. Embryos introduced into culture at the one-cell or two-cell stage developed into blastocysts within a 2–3-day period. An 8-day culture period can sustain the mouse blastocyst through egg cylinder stages equivalent to 7 days gestation (WILEY and PEDERSEN 1977). During this period, not only the ectoderm and endoderm, but also the mesoderm layer, are established, and the embryonic and extraembryonic (amnion, chorion, allantois) regions of the egg cylinder become recognizable. Continued developmental progress in vitro, i.e., into the stages of organogenesis, has been reported less frequently. Early somite stage embryos have been reported by HSU (1979) using a culture system incorporating human placental cord serum into the medium, either at the time that the egg cylinder is reached, or at the initiation of culture (HSU 1971, 1972, 1973). For the most part, however, investigators concerned with determining the capacity of cultured preimplantation embryos to carry out organogenesis have relied on transferring blastocysts into pseudopregnant females whose uteri have reached the equivalent of 3–4 days gestation (BOWMAN and MCLAREN 1970).

Traditional teratologic studies involving treatment of the maternal organism have consistently indicated that challenge during the preimplantation period of gestation may produce relatively high mortality, but surviving embryos appear normal. The availability of in vitro culture systems for preimplantation embryos has made it possible to examine this phenomenon in greater detail. The range of possible approaches can be illustrated with studies on the embryonic response to X-irradiation.

The incidence of embryonic death is greater in pregnant mice irradiated during the preimplantation period of gestation than during organogenesis (RUSSELL 1965 for review). Except for differences in relative radiosensitivity, direct X-irradiation of two-cell stage mouse embryos in vitro and X-irradiation in utero produce comparable results (FISHER and SMITHBERG 1972). X-irradiation in vitro with 121 R or more results in a significant decrease in the number of blastocysts that can implant and develop into fetuses upon transfer from culture to the uteri of pseudopregnant females. No anomalies related to X-irradiation have been reported in living fetuses examined. Analysis of the postirradiation period by prolonged culture in vitro has shown that X-irradiation at cleavage stages interferes with developmental progress at a number of steps leading to the egg cylinder stage, and that some steps are more radiosensitive than others. Hatching of the blastocyst from the zona pellucida is interfered with by smaller doses of X-rays than are needed to prevent blastocyst formation (ALEXANDRE 1974; GOLDSTEIN et al. 1975). Trophoblast outgrowth shows radiosensitivity comparable to that of hatching; growth of the ICM shows the greatest radiosensitivity. Since X-irradiation at precise developmental stages is possible with in vitro systems, GOLDSTEIN et al. (1975) have been able to establish similar patterns of radiosensitivity for two-cell and four-cell embryos and for morulae. Sensitivity of ICM growth, as indicated by the number of trophoblast outgrowths devoid of ICM, or with only a few scattered ICM cells, appears greater if X-irradiation is delivered to blastocysts than to earlier embryonic stages. Thus, depending on dosage and developmental stage at the time of X-irradiation, embryo lethality resulting from exposure during the preimplantation period can be due to interference with ICM growth in embryos that manage to implant, failure of blastocysts to hatch, or even failure of embryo to develop into blastocysts.

## II. The All-or-None Response

The repeated observation that exposure of preimplantation embryos to noxious agents, physical or chemical, may result in high embryo mortality, but survivors appear normal, has led to fairly wide acceptance of the concept of an all-or-none response of preimplantation embryos. Frequently overlooked is the fact that the test of normality is generally a morphological one, often applied at only the gross level. Increased interest in the application of behavioral tests to apparently normal survivors in teratologic experiments may well change this situation. In the meantime, even observations made at the morphological level in teratologic studies involving in vitro culture of preimplantation embryos suggest caution in assessing apparent all-or-none phenomena. The key observation is that when studies are designed to detect it, growth of the ICM (increase in cell number) is more sensitive to experimental treatments than is trophoblast outgrowth, or such preceding steps as blastulation and hatching (GOLBUS and EPSTEIN 1974; ROWINSKI et al. 1975; SHERMAN and ATIENZA 1975; POLLARD et al. 1976; GLASS et al. 1976; SPINDLE 1977; and other papers reviewed in more detail in the preceding and following paragraphs).

Heightened radiosensitivity of the ICM has already been noted in the studies of ALEXANDRE (1974) and GOLDSTEIN et al. (1975). Trophoblast outgrowth devoid of ICM or with only a few scattered ICM cells was implicated as one situation associated with embryonic death around the time of implantation. But what number of ICM cells must the embryo contain in order to survive? What number is required for normal development? Only partial answers to these questions are becoming available.

Interrelationships involving cell number, development of the ICM, and embryo survival during the postimplantation period are fairly well outlined in studies of the effects of cytochalasin B (CB) on preimplantation mouse embryos. Studies of blastocyst formation indicate that culture of cleavage stage embryos in the continuous presence of CB produces dosage-dependent developmental retardation or arrest (GRANHOLM and BRENNER 1976). Developmental arrest is reversible following CB pulses of 6–24 h and subsequent culture in control medium, but even a short pulse of 6 h (4 μg/ml CB) produces latent effects, later manifested in interference with growth of the trophoblast and ICM (GRANHOLM et al. 1979). SNOW (1973) has reported that when two-cell embryos were cultured in CB (10 μg/ml for 12 h) and then transferred to control medium, 40%–75% developed into blastocysts. Two groups of blastocysts could be distinguished on the basis of size. Group I blastocysts were comprised of 54±2 diploid cells; group II blastocysts were comprised of 20±1 tetraploid cells (SNOW 1976). Approximately 98% of the diploid blastocysts hatched and produced outgrowths. After outgrowth, mean cell number was 80±3, with 68±4 trophoblast cells. Approximately 59% of the tetraploid blastocysts hatched and produced outgrowths. Only 40% of the trophoblast outgrowths contained ICM; mean cell number was 30±3, of which 27±3 were trophoblast cells. Trophoblast outgrowths that lacked ICM were made up of only 17±2 cells. After transfer of the tetraploid blastocysts to pseudopregnant mothers, 233 blastocysts implanted, but only 19% of the sites examined at various stages from 8½ days gestation to term showed that embryos had developed in the implants, and only 2% were living at the time of collection (SNOW 1975). Numerous developmental aberrations were detected in 14½- and 16½-day embryos, but even histologic examination did not reveal any apparent abnormalities in embryos collected at 6½–13½ days gestation. Two live births were reported. TARKOWSKI et al. (1977) also reported induction of tetraploidy in the mouse with CB pulses (3–8½ h, 12 μg/ml), followed by culture in control medium to the blastocyst stage. Subsequent transfer of blastocysts to pseudopregnant females produced successful implantations; developmental defects were observed as early as day 8 of pregnancy. No live births were recorded. The studies of SNOW then suggest that the average presence of three ICM cells at the time of trophoblast outgrowth is only marginally successful in supporting embryonic development, even abnormal. This may define the lower limit for ICM number, but it remains to be determined at which level development will become normal, or proceed with aberrations consistent with embryo viability and birth.

The possibility that, at some level, ICM number may not only be reduced, but also sufficiently altered to leave a teratologic residue in surviving embryos needs to be explored. Perhaps extension of the studies reported by EIBE and SPIELMAN (1977) will be productive in this direction. EIBE and SPIELMAN recently examined the embryo lethal effect of cyclophosphamide (CPA), another chemical that appears to exert all-or-none effects on preimplantation embryos. Embryos were challenged by maternal treatment on day 2 of gestation, and subsequent development in vivo and in vitro was compared. When blastocysts were flushed from uteri of CPA-treated mothers on day 3 of gestation, significantly fewer cells were counted in embryos from mothers that had received 40–80 mg/kg body weight than in control embryos. During subsequent culture in vitro (in the absence of CPA), dosage-related effects on trophoblast attachment and outgrowth, and on differentiation of ectoderm and endoderm in the ICM, were observed. At any given dosage, differentiation of the germ layers appeared to be more sensitive than the other parameters measured. The implications of interference with germ layer differentiation need to be assessed, particularly as additional markers for early differentiation stages become available. Observations on mothers permitted to continue with gestation showed the expected resorptions and decrease in living embryos reaching stages of organogenesis. What is interesting is that, although no gross malformations were observed, embryos appeared to lag by about 24 h. It is conceivable that, in the case of complex structures such as the eye, differential developmental lag in the several interacting tissues could result in subtle, but important, aberrations. Tests of normality applied at other levels of organization (cellular/molecular/behavioral) were not reported.

## C. Peri-Implantation

### I. General Considerations

Mouse embryos begin implantation on day 5 of gestation. Implantation is a complex sequence, involving establishment of contact with the antimesometrial surface of the uterine horn, obliteration of the uterine cavity, initiation of a stable implantation on the mesometrial surface of the uterine horn, and reestablishment of a uterine cavity between the antimesometrial uterine wall and the decidua capsularis sorrounding the embryo chamber. While the implantation process is taking place, the embryo develops to the egg cylinder stage, the primitive streak appears and mesoderm formation ensues, and the various extraembryonic structures are formed. It would be expected that in vitro culture systems initiated at the egg cylinder stage would provide an opportunity for detailed examination of the formation of primitive streak, amnion, yolk sac, allantois, and the placenta itself, as well as of the susceptibility of these critical processes to teratologic insult. In practice, however, very little information on these processes has been derived from cultures initiated at the egg cylinder stage. Indeed, much of the information available has been derived from studies of embryos introduced into culture at the blastocyst stage.

### II. Technical Obstacles

In vitro studies of embryos introduced into culture at egg cylinder stages have perhaps not focused on the phenomena associated with formation of the primitive streak and extraembryonic structures, because of the dramatic observations reported in early attempts to culture rat egg cylinders. Embryos explanted at 7½–8½ days gestation into culture medium consisting of rat serum generally showed developmental retardation and characteristically possessed double hearts (New and Daniel 1969). It was subsequently found that double heart formation could be prevented by the simple expedient of separating serum from whole blood by immediate centrifugation, rather than allowing clot formation (Steele 1972; Steele and New 1974). Presumably, some significant serum component, probably a protein (Klein et al. 1978), is removed when blood is allowed to clot. Although the use of immediately centrifuged serum abolished the heart defects, it did not appreciably correct for the retardation of embryonic development. Somites were still poorly formed and only about one-quarter of the embryos showed signs of axial rotation in a 48-h culture period.

Early studies using rat egg cylinders explanted at the primitive streak stage were also hampered by the use of excessively high oxygen levels and static watch glass cultures. For example, Steele et al. (1974) cultured embryos in static watch glass cultures under an atmosphere of 40% oxygen. Only 11 of 36 embryos cultured on the control medium developed a heartbeat. Subsequent studies have shown that organogenesis and growth rates (protein accumulation) similar to those observed in vivo can be obtained if rat embryos are cultured in rotating bottles under an atmosphere of 5% oxygen, and using heat-inactivated, immediately centrifuged serum (BUCKLEY et al. 1978). More recently, TAM and SNOW (1980) have described an in vitro culture system for primitive streak stage mouse embryos which permits growth for 24 h, comparable to that observed in vivo. Approximately 90% of late streak embryos continue to grow and develop for an additional 24 h, but only 60% of early streak embryos do so. Presumably, continued technical refinements will help to focus renewed attention on this critical development period.

### III. Blastocyst Cultures

Embryos introduced into culture at the blastocyst stage hatch out of the zona pellucida and begin to adhere to the coverslip substratum by day 2 of culture (WILEY and PEDERSEN 1977). At this time, the ICM consists of two distinct layers, endoderm and ectoderm, capped by polar trophoblast and enclosed by a continuous layer of endoderm cells resting on a sheet of mural trophoblast cells. One region of the elongate structure, referred to as distal, contains a solid mass of cells derived from the ICM; another region, referred to as proximal, includes the polar trophoblast. A small cavity appears in the distal segment late on day 4, and expands during the next 4 days of culture. During the same period, a hollow middle segment is formed between the proximal and distal segments. During days 6–7 of culture, mesoderm cells appear in association with a thickened portion of embryonic ectoderm (primitive streak) near the junction of the distal and middle segments. Mesoderm comes to occupy the space between the ectoderm and visceral endoderm as a mass of loosely arranged small cells.

On day 8, each of the three segments contains a cavity. The proximal segment has a crescent-shaped cavity bounded on one end by the mass of ectoplacental core cells and on the other by the extraembryonic ectoderm (chorion), both derived from the polar trophoblast, according to GARDNER et al. (1973) and GARDNER and JOHNSON (1975). The cavity of the middle segment (exocoelom) is lined by mesoderm, and often contains a sac-like structure which appears to consist of endodermal cells and is attached to the wall of the exocoelom by a narrow stalk. The double-layered wall of the middle segment corresponds to the visceral yolk sac. The cavity of the distal segment (proamniotic cavity) is lined with the ectoderm of the amnion and of the embryo proper. The embryo thus has reached the late egg cylinder stage characteristic of approximately 7 days gestation in the mouse.

## D. Postimplantation

For teratologic studies with embryo culture, postimplantation stages of rodent embryos have been used more extensively than other stages. To some extent this may be attributed to the work D. A. T. NEW and his associates, whose efforts established the technique of culturing whole embryos at this particular stage (for reviews see NEW 1970, 1976, 1978). However, other factors have contributed to the extensive use of this stage. For example, postimplantation stages are convenient for isolation and manipulation, morphological organogenesis is dramatic and rapid at this time, and embryo nutritional and gaseous requirements can be satisfied by the yolk sac without the need for a functional placenta. Although the use of embryo culture during this limited developmental period continues to be of value to teratology, attempts to extend the culture period to include both earlier (BUCKLEY et al. 1978; TAM and SNOW 1980) and later periods (COCKROFT 1973) have been reported. Hopefully, these efforts will serve to increase the application of embryo culture to teratology by providing access to additional developmental events, such as limb or palate formation (KOCHHAR 1975 a; AGNISH and KOCHHAR 1976 a, b).

In spite of the technical progress that has been made in mammalian embryo culture, procedures have not been standardized between laboratories engaged in this work. For this chapter, variations were noted in composition of the gaseous and nutritional environments, the number of embryos cultured per unit volume of medium as well as per culture vessel, fluid: air space ratio within the culture vessel, and the duration of the in vitro culture period. Although these variables could influence the outcome of a teratologic study, the absence of comparative data precludes considerations of the possible problems. The important variable of the embryo stage at which the study began has received some consideration. Thus, in studies of directly added cadmium (KLEIN et al. 1980), as well as directly added glucose (SADLER 1980 b), earlier stages were clearly more sensitive than later developmental stages. Therefore, the researcher is left with the dilemma of either using a sharply defined narrow stage or allowing stage-related responses to become part of the study.

The analyses of cultured embryo responses have usually involved morphology at the gross, histologic, or even electron microscopic levels and quantitative estimates of embryo size based on accumulated amounts of protein, DNA, or RNA. An interesting attempt to provide a quantitative morphological scoring system for cultured rat embryos was recently published (BROWN and FABRO 1981). In addition, radioactive compounds have been used with cultured embryos and recently tissues from cultured embryos have been analyzed for sister chromatid exchange frequencies. The question of embryo survival in relation to teratogenicity remains an important consideration with cultured embryos as with in vivo studies. Thus, while some investigators consider only morphological abnormalities in live embryos as relevant to teratogenicity, others consider embryo lethality during the course of culture as the most extreme teratogenic response. The objective of this section has been to evaluate the many possible applications of postimplantation rodent embryo cultures to teratology. The headings were selected to encompass as much of the relevant literature as possible.

## I. Direct Additions

The responses of cultured embryos to a potential teratogen by simply adding it to the culture medium have served as a starting point for many studies. For this purpose the approach has appeared reasonable, but as a study in itself, adding substances to the culture medium may have little merit. For example, the proximal or actual teratogen may not be identified if the parent compound has some limited teratogenicity prior to metabolic activation. Similarly, the often stated value of "demonstrating a direct effect in the absence of maternal influence" seems of little merit, as a substance may be capable of acting directly on an embryo in culture, but in the reality of in vivo existence may require maternal activation.

### 1. Chemical Inhibitors

In one of the first teratologic studies with cultured mammalian embryos, the niacin inhibitor, 6-aminonicotinamide was added to the medium with 10-day rat embryos for periods of up to 32 h (TURBOW and CHAMBERLAIN 1968). The development of somites was particularly sensitive to this drug which the authors suggested was related to the skeletal abnormalities produced in vivo. The addition of nicotinamide to the medium reversed the inhibitory effects of this compound, as had been previously demonstrated by LANDAUER (1957) using injections into chicken eggs.

This approach was combined with the use of radioactive compounds to study the direct action of several DNA inhibitors (KOCHHAR 1975b; AGNISH and KOCHHAR 1976a; SADLER and KOCHHAR 1976; KOCHHAR et al. 1980). In one of the first studies, chlorambucil was used with 11-day mouse embryos cultured for 4 or 8 h (SADLER and KOCHHAR 1976). Cuts were made in the tissue of the yolk sac in order to permit direct access of the inhibitor and radioactive precursor molecules to the embryo. Chlorambucil caused reduced incorporation of thymidine into DNA, but did not reduce either incorporation of uridine into RNA or leucine into protein. The second study was directly concerned with an abnormality, gastroschisis, caused by hydroxyurea (MILLER and RUNNER 1978). Mouse embryos of 8.5 days were given the drug for periods of only 15 min prior to a 30-min exposure to radioactive thymidine. Autoradiography showed that drug treatment caused reduced labeling in all tissues. The tissue most directly involved with gastroschisis, the samotopleure, showed labeling differences between right and left sides in control but not drug-treated groups. MILLER and RUNNER speculated that this loss of somatopleure side differences in cellular proliferation could ultimately lead to abnormal morphogenesis.

### 2. Environmental Factors

Temperatures between 37° and 40 °C did not appear to influence the growth and development of 9½-day rat embryos appreciably during 48 h of culture (COCKROFT and NEW 1975, 1978). However, at 40.5 °C or as little as a 12-h exposure to 41 °C, embryo protein accumulation was severely inhibited and embryos developed with a variety of abnormalities, including microcephaly, edema of the pericardium, and abnormal posterior body rotation. A careful analysis, involving comparisons between brain and whole body protein content, showed that microcephaly occurred even at 40 °C, although this was not apparent by gross observations.

Considerable attention has been given to oxygen effects in the development of the embryo culture technique. Thus, the benefit of a low oxygen level during the first 24 h of culture with 9½-day embryos has been reported (NEW et al. 1976) and the use of 2–3 atmospheres oxygen pressure appeared to have some advantage for rat embryo cultures started at 11½ days gestation (NEW and COPPOLA 1970). However, in a later report (COCKROFT 1976) with 12½- and 13½-day embryos, hyperbaric oxygen was not employed. The teratogenicity of oxygen has also been considered. In an interesting early study, SHEPARD et al. (1969) found that rat embryos of 10.3 days could survive hypoxia for 30 min without adverse effects while embryos of 11 and 12 days could not survive pure nitrogen for as little as 10 min. In a most elegant study, MORRISS and NEW (1979) studied the exencephaly resulting from culturing 9½-day rat embryos at elevated (20% or 40%) levels of oxygen. Using scanning as well as transmission electron microscopy, these authors implicated failure of the lateral edges of the neural folds to curve properly as the cause of failure of the neural tube to close. Furthermore, they suggested that this in turn may have resulted from failures of the neural crest cells to migrate, normal cell death to occur, and the persistence of microfilament bundles on the apical surface of the neural epithelium.

## 3. Substances Implicated in Human Exposure

The possible need for surgery during pregnancy and the reproductive problems associated with operating room workers has led to "direct effect" studies using anesthetics. Using an anesthetic, Avertin, KAUFMAN and STEELE (1976) found that a teratogenic response in cultured rat embryos could only be produced by using an airtight culture vessel and by severely limiting the air space in the vessel. Under these conditions, adverse effects on somites, hearts, and embryo protein accumulation were observed. In another study (O'SHEA and KAUFMAN 1980) the local anesthetic, Xylocaine, was added to cultures of mouse embryos and resulted in failure of the neural tube to close. Examination by electron microscopy indicated that, in Xylocaine-treated embryos, the neuroepithelial cells failed to elevate, and this was associated with a lack of microfilament bundles and microtubules in these cells.

Although it was not surprising to learn that cultures of 9½-day rat embryos were sensitive to alcohol when added to the medium, it was of interest that the level of sensitivity (1.5 mg and 3.0 mg/ml medium) was within the range of blood levels found in human subjects who consume large amounts of alcohol (BROWN et al. 1979). During 48 h of culture the embryo growth parameters of protein, DNA, and crown to rump length were reduced by alcohol. The authors state that alcohol retarded development, but did not cause gross structural defects. This distinction between delayed development and an abnormality was difficult to reconcile with the observation made in this same study that alcohol caused microcephaly. It appears essential to determine if microcephaly represented delayed development or a lasting defect. In this regard, SNOW and TAM (1979) have reported that the injection of mitomycin C into pregnant mice led to growth inhibition of embryos during early gestation which was overcome by the time of birth. However, these animals subsequently showed high mortality rates and motor defects.

In view of the concern that hypervitaminosis may represent a reproductive risk to humans, vitamin A was shown to be teratogenic in vivo (KOCHHAR 1967, 1977) and in cultures of 8-day of 9-day rat embryos (MORRISS and STEELE 1976). On the basis of weight (5 μg/ml medium), retinoic acid appeared more detrimental than retinol in this latter study. Although both forms of the vitamin caused reduced embryo protein accumulation and various abnormalities in common, the acid form caused a unique abnormality, involving the extension of the posterior embryo trunk through the yolk sac tissue, while the alcohol form caused large lipid droplet accumulations in the endoderm of the yolk sac.

## II. Beyond Direct Additions

In the next series of studies, further attempts were made to evaluate the responses of embryos to direct additions. Three general approaches have been used. First, teratogens were injected into the contents of the yolk sac or amnion. In this approach, achieving sufficient internal concentrations should be of concern. Second, direct addition responses have been compared with those observed in vivo. For this type of study to be of value, embryos should be examined after comparable periods of exposure and hopefully, a teratogen-specific abnormality would be observed. Finally, direct effects have been compared with those observed with embryos cultured on the serum from teratogen-treated animals. An important consideration in this latter approach has been the time between teratogen administration and bleeding. Clearly, a variety of exposure times and dosage levels should be used when considering this approach.

### 1. Chemical Inhibitors

In what appears to have been the first application of whole rat embryo culture to problems of teratology, TURBOW (1966) demonstrated two possible uses of embryo culture with the teratogen, trypan blue. First, he compared sites of administration. Since addition of the dye to the medium produced the same embryo responses as direct injection into the cavity of the yolk sac, the embryo was implicated as the site of action. Second, he was able to demonstrate the importance of the intact trypan blue molecules because "half trypan blue", a modification of the parent molecule, failed to harm embryos. More recently, trypan blue has been studied in embryo culture with an interesting variation in experimental design. In these studies, embryos were exposed to the dye in vivo by injecting pregnant rats either 4 or 24 h prior to embryo removal for in vitro culture. Such an approach would be particularly useful in establishing teratogen exposure times and possible recovery capacity, as shown by recent work with several teratogenic agents (KOCHHAR et al. 1978, 1980). Indeed, in the case of trypan blue, as little as 4 h appeared to be sufficient in vivo exposure time to inhibit embryo accumulation of protein, RNA, and DNA in vitro (FISHER 1981). In the second paper (BEAUDOIN and FISHER 1981), a variety of teratogens were studied, including trypan blue, using the same in vivo/in vitro procedure as the previous paper. All compounds were inhibitory to cultured embryos, and the nature of the abnormalities produced in vitro were more severe than would be expected from previous observations in vivo. BEAUDOIN and FISHER suggested that this difference could have resulted from either embryo recoveries or the death of severely affected embryos in vivo.

An attempt to compare rat embryo responses to three different routes of teratogen administration has been reported (MCGARRITY et al., to be published). In general, they appeared to suggest that in vivo embryo responses to sodium salicylate were comparable to responses to directly added compound in vitro. Similar responses were observed when embryos were cultured on serum from injected rats. However, available data were insufficient to provide a critical evaluation of this study and the authors noted that in vivo sodium salicylate caused embryo death and resorptions, while embryos survived treatment in vitro.

## 2. Heavy Metals

In a study mainly concerned with the demonstration that rat embryo cultures could be used to monitor serum teratogenicity, serum samples taken from rats injected with cadmium chloride were used as culture media (KLEIN et al. 1980). In 9½-day rat embryos, serum samples taken 1 and 4 h after dosing were embryo lethal. Serum taken 8 h after dosing allowed 48-h survival but caused exencephaly and reduced embryo protein and DNA content, while 16- and 24-h posttreatment serum samples caused only reduced protein and DNA content relative to controls. Distinct differences were observed between these results and those obtained from embryos cultured on serum to which cadmium chloride was directly added. For example, with directly added teratogen, extensive brain hemorrhages were observed, but neural tubes were closed. Unfortunately, in vivo comparisons were not provided in this study, making it impossible to determine which of these two procedures more closely approached the in vivo condition. It should be noted that embryo responses to the same concentration of directly added cadmium ranged from embryo death to no effect embryos with small differences in developmental stage (early to late head fold) at the start of culture.

Injections of copper sulfate into pregnant mice led to failure of the neural tube to close and caused heart enlargement during the narrow period of 8–9 days of gestation (O'SHEA and KAUFMAN 1979). Similar defects were produced by adding precise concentrations of copper sulfate to the culture medium with 9-day mouse embryos. These authors note that, although early somite stage embryos in culture were sensitive to copper, this stage in vivo did not appear to be adversely affected. Although this may represent a maternal interaction with copper, it could have simply resulted from exposures in vitro to greater concentrations of the teratogen than those in vivo.

## 3. Nutrition

Pregnant rats given a diet deficient in vitamin E resorb their litters on approximately day 13 of gestation. In one of the first studies using serum from treated animals as a culture medium, STEELE et al. (1974) cultured 8½-day rat embryos on serum from rats fed a diet deficient in vitamin E for 3 months. Embryos were cultured for as long as heart pulsations were observed. Those provided with serum which was deficient in vitamin E accumulated an average of 12 μg protein, while those given the same serum supplemented with vitamin E accumulated an average of 68 μg protein. One antioxidant tested could in part replace the vitamin requirement. These studies suggested that the lack of vitamin E in serum from animals receiving a deficient diet was the direct cause of reduced embryo growth.

Starvation for periods of up to 36 h prior to 10½ days of pregnancy, caused reductions in embryo protein content and somite number, but gross abnormalities were not apparent (ELLINGTON 1980). When 9½-day rat embryos were cultured on serum from rats starved for 36 h, small reductions in embryo protein content and somite number were again observed. This could be overcome by the addition of glucose to this same serum. The importance of glucose as a constituent of embryo culture medium was previously noted in studies of glucose utilization (COCKROFT and COPPOLA 1977), as well as in studies of embryo culture on human serum (CHATOT et al. 1980).

## III. Metabolic Activation

One of the most important applications of whole embryo culture to teratology has come in the area of metabolic activation of potential teratogenic substances. One approach that has been used follows directly from the work of AMES on bacterial mutagenesis and carcinogenesis in that rat liver extracts are combined in a single culture vessel with embryos and drugs. In another approach, embryos are simply cultured on a medium of serum taken from an animal previously exposed to the drug. Both types of study have provided important insights into the nature of teratogenesis, including identification of proximal teratogenic substances and the establishment of a basis for species and individual differences in drug sensitivities.

CPA has served as a model compound for metabolic activation because of the striking contrast between inactivity of the parent compound and activity of the metabolites. In the presence of CPA, a liver supernatant was also required in order to demonstrate an adverse effect on cultured rat embryos (FANTEL et al. 1979). In this study, 10-day rat embryos were cultured for only 24 h, but a rather unusual abnormality was observed, involving protrusions from the prosencephalon. This specific abnormality referred to as "hammer head" was subsequently used in a most elegant manner to identify the active or proximal teratogen (MIRKES et al. 1981). Three metabolites of CPM were compared. Acrolein at equimolar concentrations to that used with activated cyclophosphamide had no effect on cultured embryos; 4-keto-cyclophosphamide caused abnormalities, but they were distinct from those caused by the activated parent compound; and finally only phosphoramide mustard caused the unique "hammer head" embryos found previously with the activated parent compound. The requirement that cyclophosphamide be activated for teratogenicity with cultured embryos was confirmed and the involvement of the cytochrome P-450 enzyme system was clearly implicated by demonstrating a requirement for NADPH in conjunction with the activating microsome fraction (KITCHIN et al. 1981 a). In subsequent papers, optimum concentrations of metabolic activation ingredients were determined (KITCHIN et al. 1981 b) and two alkylating agents (TEM and nitrogen mustard) were found to be teratogenic to cultured rat embryos without the need for metabolic activation (SANYAL et al. 1981). Although technical concern has arisen from using teratogenic substances to induce cytochrome P-450 enzyme systems for use in in vitro teratologic assays, of greater concern has been the possibility that in vitro activation produces metabolites distinct from those produced in vivo (BIGGER et al. 1980).

In this regard, KLEIN et al. (1980) demonstrated that serum samples from animals injected with CPA were teratogenic to cultured rat embryos. The possibility that metabolites of CPA produced in vivo and in vitro were different might be implied by the presence of exencephaly in cultured embryos in the one study (KLEIN et al. 1980) and "hammer heads" in the other study (FANTEL et al. 1979). However, this difference might simply reflect differences between the two groups due to the embryo stages selected for the start of culture.

Cultures of 7½–8½-day mouse embryos were recently found to be sensitive to the polycyclic hydrocarbon, benzo[*a*]pyrene without the need for an exogenous metabolic activating system (GALLOWAY et al. 1980). This finding in itself is important in view of the apparent inability of rat embryos to metabolize CPA. In addition, this study provided other important findings of considerable relevance to teratology. First, the sensitivity to directly added benzo[*a*]pyrene was shown to be genetically related to the *Ah* locus. Second, sister chromatid exchange frequencies in the cells of the cultured embryos, rather than embryo growth or abnormalities, were used to evaluate the response. Clearly these findings provide a basis for studying individual differences in drug sensitivity, but of greater importance, they challenge the classical methods of evaluating teratogenicity. Does sister chromatid exchange provide a sensitive measure of teratogenicity? With regard to this question, the ability of cultured rat embryos to metabolize CPA directly was reconsidered with this technique (ALLEN et al. 1981). Considering only the cells from the yolk sac, CPA failed to increase the frequency of sister chromatid exchanges, but an increase was found when the metabolite phosphoramide mustard was added to the culture medium.

Following the observation that rat embryos could be cultured on human serum (CHATOT et al. 1980), one of the first studies has involved anticonvulsants (CHATOT et al. 1981). A comparative study using rat embryos cultured on serum from human epileptics receiving single anticonvulsant drugs (diphenylhydantoin, carbamazepine, Valproic acid, and Phenobarbital) has recently been completed. Teratogenic activity has been demonstrated in the serum from each of these drug groups. However, it was not possible to demonstrate a direct relationship between serum parent drug levels and teratogenic activity and this directed attention to individual drug metabolism. With diphenylhydantoin direct addition of up to 100 μg/ml had no effect on 9½-day rat embryos cultured for 48 h. However, serum samples taken from monkeys following diphenylhydantoin administration produced severe embryo abnormalities at serum drug levels of only 30 μg/ml. To further implicate the genetics of drug metabolism: (1) responses to human serum samples at the same level of serum diphenylhydantoin ranged from embryo lethal, through various abnormalities, to no affect; (2) the teratogenicity of monkey serum depended on time after administration of drug, and not diphenylhydantoin blood levels; and (3) it has been impossible to produce teratogenic serum from rats, regardless of dosage or time of bleeding following drug administration. It should be clearly noted that many factors other than those related to drugs could lead to human serum teratogenicity. For example, nutritional factors as well as an epileptic "background" have also been implicated as possible factors in the high incidence of birth defects among epileptics. Hopefully, embryo cultures on human serum will help to identify the potential teratogenic factors in individuals.

## IV. Teratogen Identification

The following studies represent recent departures from the characteristic teratologic approach. Rather than studying the effects of known or potential teratogens, a search for undefined substances which produce abnormalities in cultured embryos was attempted.

### 1. Diabetes

The first studies with cultured embryos and diabetes were started by the late ELIZABETH M. DEUCHAR. Using pregnant rats, she found that streptozotocin or alloxan induced diabetes and caused a preponderance of open neural tubes, heart defects, and resorptions (DEUCHAR 1977). Although injections of streptozotocin 5 days before mating resulted in resorptions, she was still concerned that the drug itself, rather than the diabetic state, interfered with embryonic development. Thus, prior to the start of her proposed in vitro studies, she showed that the addition of streptozotocin directly to the culture medium of 10-day rat embryos caused reduced embryo size and yolk sac circulatory problems, but not the neural tube or heart defects observed in vivo (DEUCHAR 1978). Subsequently, it was observed (SADLER 1980a) that serum from streptozotocin-treated rats caused open neural tubes and reduced embryo protein content in cultures of mouse embryos. These responses were related to the age of the embryo at the start of culture (2–3-somite stages were more sensitive than 4–6-somite stages) as well as to the severity of the induced diabetes. Although the addition of excess glucose to the culture medium caused open neural tubes in both rat (COCKROFT and COPPOLA 1977) and mouse embryos (SADLER 1980b), this did not appear to be responsible for the teratogenicity of the diabetic serum. The most severe diabetic serum had a blood glucose level of 6.11 mg/ml while 12–15 mg/ml added glucose was required to produce an adverse effect in the rat study (COCKROFT and COPOLLA 1977) and 9.2 mg/ml in the mouse study (SADLER 1980b). The possibility that reduced insulin levels could have contributed to the serum teratogenicity could not be excluded, but mildly diabetic serum was teratogenic with insulin levels comparable to controls. Hopefully, the analysis of serum will continue using both the rat model and human diabetic subjects.

### 2. Immunologic Responses

In an early study (BERRY 1971), it was reported that rabbit IgG and IgM fractions prepared against rat heart actin-myosin complexes were lethal to 11-day cultured rat embryos. By showing that the pulsations of isolated hearts were sensitive to the antisera, and that ferritin from labeled immunoglobulin could be detected by electron-micrographs of the heart, BERRY suggested that these proteins pass from the medium to the embryo. In another early study, NEW and BRENT (1972) tested the effect of goat anti-rat yolk sac immunoglobulins on cultured rat embryos. At high levels, the immunoglobulin fraction was embryo lethal and, at lower levels, developmental retardations were observed. Injection of the immunoglobulins into the yolk sac or amniotic cavities failed to cause an adverse response. This suggested that only the visceral yolk sac endoderm was sensitive to the antibody. In studies of human serum, a female human subject was identified with serum that was embryo lethal (CAREY et al. 1980). Through a sequence of analytic steps it was found that her IgG was the cause of this toxicity, and that it could be absorbed by yolk sac tissue, but not embryo tissue. It was interesting to note that the embryos described by NEW and BRENT appeared quite similar to those observed with the embryo lethal human serum. The studies with human serum were primarily designed to show that rat embryo responses could be used in a systematic manner to analyze serum. The relevance of an IgG toxic to cultured rat embryos to the reproductive function of the donor remains to be elucidated.

### 3. Fetal Wastage

The most striking indication that cultured rat embryo responses to serum are relevant to the reproductive risk of the serum donor has come from studies of monkeys with histories of fetal wastage (KLEIN et al. 1982). As part of the development of a teratologic screening procedure incorporating primate metabolism, rat embryos were cultured for 48 h on serum from 18 different female rhesus monkeys. Regardless of the relationship to menstrual cycle, serum from only 2 monkeys caused distinct abnormalities with cultured embryos. Subsequently, it was learned that these 2 monkeys, unlike the other 16, had failed to become pregnant in over 2 years of regular breeding. In order to extend this study, serum samples were obtained from a group of pig-tailed monkeys, including 12 with excellent reproductive histories and 14 with histories of spontaneous abortions, stillbirths, or neonatal deaths. In blind studies, cultured embryo abnormalities coincided with reproductive histories for 8 of the 12 good breeders and 12 of the 14 poor breeders. These results were generally reproducible with additional blood samples from the same animal. On gross morphological examination, only four cultured embryo abnormality types were identified, and the abnormality frequencies were found to be more closely related to donor reproductive histories than either embryo protein content or somite number. The actual relevance of these findings to teratology must await serum analysis.

*Acknowledgments*. This chapter is dedicated to the memory of ELIZABETH M. DEUCHAR.
This work forms Scientific Contribution 926, Storrs Agricultural Experiment Station, University of Connecticut and was supported in part by U.S. Department of Energy Contract EVO 3139 (Office of Health and Environmental Research). We wish to thank S. CAREY, C. CHATOT, M. CLAPPER, H. FISH, and J. PLENEFISCH for their help in the preparation of this chapter.

## References

Agnish ND, Kochhar DM (1976a) Direct exposure of post-implantation mouse embryos to 5-bromodeoxyuridine in vitro and its effects on subsequent chondrogenesis in the limbs. J Embryol Exp Morphol 36:623–638
Agnish ND, Kochhar DM (1976b) Direct exposure of mouse embryonic limb-buds to 5-bromodeoxyuridine in vitro and its effect on chondrogenesis: increasing resistance to the analog at successive stages of development. J Embryol Exp Morphol 36:639–652
Alexandre HL (1974) Effects of x-irradiation on preimplantation mouse embryos cultured in vitro. J Reprod Fertil 36:417–420

Allen JW, El-Nahass E, Sanyal MK, Dunn RL, Gladen B, Dixon RL (1981) Sister-chromatid exchange analyses in rodent material, embryonic and extra-embryonic tissues. Mutat Res 80:297–311
Beaudoin AR, Fisher DL (1981) An in vivo/in vitro evaluation of teratogenic action. Teratology 23:57–61
Berry CL (1971) The effects of an antiserum to the contractile proteins of the heart on the developing rat embryo. J Embryol Exp Morphol 25:203–212
Bigger CAH, Tomaszewski JE, Dipple A (1980) Limitations of metabolic activation systems used with in vitro tests for carcinogens. Science 209:503–505
Bowman P, McLaren A (1970) Viability and growth of mouse embryos after in vitro culture and fusion. J Embryol Exp Morphol 23:693–704
Brown NA, Fabro S (1981) Quantitation of rat embryonic development in vitro: A morphological scoring system. Teratology 24:65–78
Brown NA, Goulding EH, Fabro S (1979) Ethanol embryotoxicity: Direct effects on mammalian embryos in vitro. Science 206:573–575
Buckley SKL, Steele CE, New DAT (1978) In vitro development of early postimplantation rat embryos. Dev Biol 65:396–403
Carey SW, Chatot CL, Klein NW (1980) In vitro cultures of rat embryos on human serum: A case study of embryo lethality. Teratology 21:33A
Chatot CL, Klein NW (1981) Teratogenic activity of serum from human epileptic subjects studied by rat embryo cultures. Teratology 23:30A
Chatot CL, Klein NW, Piatek J, Pierro LJ (1980) Successful culture of rat embryos on human serum: Use in the detection of teratogens. Science 207:1471–1473
Cockroft DL (1973) Development in culture of rat foetuses explanted at 12.5 and 13.5 days of gestation. J Embryol Exp Morphol 29:473–483
Cockroft DL (1976) Comparison of in vitro and in vivo development of rat foetuses. Dev Biol 48:163–172
Cockroft DL, Coppola PT (1977) Teratogenic effects of excess glucose on head-fold rat embryos in culture. Teratology 16:141–146
Cockroft DL, New DAT (1975) Effects of hyperthermia on rat embryos in culture. Nature 258:604–606
Cockroft DL, New DAT (1978) Abnormalities induced in cultured rat embryos by hyperthermia. Teratology 17:277–284
Deuchar EM (1977) Embryonic malformations in rats, resulting from maternal diabetes: preliminary observations. J Embryol Exp Morphol 41:93–99
Deuchar EM (1978) Effects of streptozotocin on early rat embryos grown in culture. Experientia 34:84–85
Eibe HG, Spielmann H (1977) Inhibition of post-implantation development of mouse blastocysts in vitro after cyclophosphamide treatment in vivo. Nature 270:54–56
Ellington SKL (1980) In vivo and in vitro studies on the effects of maternal fasting during embryonic organogenesis in the rat. J Reprod Fertil 60:383–388
Fantel AG, Greenaway JC, Juchau MR, Shepard TH (1979) Teratogenic bioactivation of cyclophosphamide in vitro. Life Sci 25:67–72
Fisher DL (1981) Accumulation of DNA, RNA, and protein by cultured rat embryos following maternal administration of a teratogenic dose of trypan blue. J Exp Zool 216:415–422
Fisher DL, Smithberg M (1972) In vitro and in vivo x-irradiation of preimplantation mouse embryos. Teratology 7:57–64
Galloway SM, Perry PE, Meneses J, Nebert DW, Pedersen RA (1980) Cultured mouse embryos metabolize benzo[a]pyrene during early gestation: genetic differences detectable by sister chromatid exchange. Proc Natl Acad Sci USA 77:3524–3528
Gardner RL, Johnson MH (1975) Investigation of cellular interaction and deployment in the early mammalian embryo using interspecific chimaeras between the rat and mouse. In: Cell patterning, 29. CIBA foundation symposium. Associated Scientific, New York, pp 183–200
Gardner RL, Papaioannou VE, Barton SC (1973) Origin of the ectoplacental cone and secondary giant cells in mouse blastocysts reconstituted from isolated trophoblast and inner cell mass. J Embryol Exp Morphol 30:561–572

Glass RH, Spindle AI, Pedersen RA (1976) Differential inhibition of trophoblast outgrowth and inner cell mass growth by actinomycin D in cultured mouse embryos. J Reprod Fertil 48:443–445
Golbus MS, Epstein CJ (1974) Effect of 5-bromodeoxyuridine on pre-implantation mouse embryo development. Differentiation 2:143–149
Goldstein LS, Spindle AI, Pedersen RA (1975) X-ray sensitivity of the preimplantation mouse embryo in vitro. Radiat Res 62:276–287
Granholm NH, Brenner GM (1976) Effects of cytochalasin B (CB) on the morula-to-blastocyst transformation and trophoblast outgrowth in the early mouse embryo. Exp Cell Res 101:143–153
Granholm NH, Brenner GM, Rector JT (1979) Latent effects on in vitro development following cytochalasin B treatment of 8-cell mouse embryos. J Embryol Exp Morphol 51:97–108
Hsu Y (1971) Post-blastocyst differentiation in vitro. Nature 231:100–102
Hsu Y (1972) Differentiation in vitro of mouse embryos beyond the implantation stage. Nature 239:200–202
Hsu Y (1973) Differentiation in vitro of mouse embryos to the stage of early somite. Dev Biol 33:403–411
Hsu Y (1979) In vitro development of individually cultured whole mouse embryos from blastocyst to early somite stage. Dev Biol 68:453–461
Kaufmann MH, Steele CE (1976) Deleterious effect of an anaesthetic on cultured mammalian embryos. Nature 260:782–783
Kitchin KT, Schmid BP, Sanyal MK (1981 a) Teratogenicity of cyclophosphamide in a coupled microsomal activating/embryo culture system. Biochem Pharmacol 30:59–64
Kitchin KT, Sanyal MK, Schmid BP (1981 b) A coupled microsomal-activating/embryo culture system: toxicity of reduced B-nicotinamide adenine dinucleotide phosphate (NADPH). Biochem Pharmacol 30:985–992
Klein NW, Minghetti PP, Jackson SK, Vogler MA (1978) Serum protein depletion by cultured rat embryos. J Exp Zool 203:313–318
Klein NW, Vogler MA, Chatot CL, Pierro LJ (1980) The use of cultured rat embryos to evaluate the teratogenic activity of serum: cadmium and cyclophosphamide. Teratology 21:199–208
Klein NW, Plenefisch JD, Carey SW, Fredrickson WT, Sackett GP, Burbacher TM, Parker RM (1982) Serum from monkeys with histories of fetal wastage causes abnormalities in cultured rat embryos. Science 215:66–69
Kochhar DM (1967) Teratogenic activity of retinoic acid. Acta Pathol Microbiol Scand 70:398–404
Kochhar DM (1975 a) The use of in vitro procedures in teratology. Teratology 11:273–288
Kochhar DM (1975 b) Assessment of teratogenic response in cultured postimplantation mouse embryos: effects of hydroxyurea. In: Neubert D, Merker H-J (eds) New approaches to the evaluation of abnormal embryonic development. G Thieme, Stuttgart, pp 250–277
Kochhar DM (1977) Cellular basis of congenital limb deformity induced in mice by vitamin A. In: Bergsma D, Lenz W (eds) Morphogenesis and malformation of the limbs. AR Liss, New York, pp 111–154
Kochhar DM, Penner JD, McDay JA (1978) Limb development in mouse embryos: II. Reduction defects, cytotoxicity and inhibition of DNA synthesis produced by cytosine arabinoside. Teratology 18:71–92
Kochhar DM, Penner JD, Knudsen TB (1980) Embryotoxic, teratogenic and metabolic effects of ribavirin in mice. Toxicol Appl Pharmacol 52:99–112
Landauer W (1957) Niacin antagonists and chick development. J Exp Zool 136:509–530
McGarrity C, Samani N, Beck F, Gulamhusein A (to be published) The effect of sodium salicylate on the rat embryo in culture: an in vitro model for the morphological assessment of teratogenicity. J Anat
Miller SA, Runner MN (1978) Tissue specificity for incorporation of [$^3$H]thymidine by the 10- to 12-somite mouse embryo: alteration by acute exposure to hydroxyurea. J Embryol Exp Morphol 44:181–189

Mirkes PE, Fantel AG, Greenaway JC, Shepard TH (1981) Teratogenicity of cyclophosphamide metabolites: phosphoramide mustard, acrolein, and 4-ketocyclophosphamide in rat embryos cultured in vitro. Toxicol Appl Pharmacol 58:322–330
Morriss GM, New DAT (1979) Effect of oxygen concentration on morphogenesis of cranial neural folds and neural crest in cultured rat embryos. J Embryol Exp Morphol 54:17–35
Morriss GM, Steele CE (1976) Comparison of the effects of retinol and retinoic acid on postimplantation rat embryos in vitro. Teratology 15:109–120
New DAT (1970) Culture of fetuses in vitro. Adv Biosci 6:367–380
New DAT (1976) Techniques for assessment of teratologic effects: embryo culture. Environ Health Perspect 18:105–110
New DAT (1978) Whole-embryo culture and the study of mammalian embryos during organogenesis. Biol Rev 53:81–122
New DAT, Brent RL (1972) Effect of yolk-sac antibody on rat embryos grown in culture. J Embryol Exp Morphol 27:543–553
New DAT, Coppola PT (1970) Development of explanted rat fetuses in hyperbaric oxygen. Teratology 3:153–162
New DAT, Daniel JC (1969) Cultivation of rat embryos explanted at 7.5 and 8.5 days of gestation. Nature 223:515–516
New DAT, Coppola PT, Cockroft DL (1976) Improved development of head-fold rat embryos in culture resulting from low oxygen and modifications of the culture serum. J Reprod Fertil 48:219–222
O'Shea KS, Kaufman MH (1979) Influence of copper on the early post-implantation mouse embryo: an in vivo and in vitro study. Rouxs Arch Dev Biol 186:297–308
O'Shea KS, Kaufman MH (1980) Neural tube closure defects following in vitro exposure of mouse embryos to xylocaine. J Exp Zool 214:235–238
Pollard DR, Baran MM, Bachvarova R (1976) The effect of 5-bromodeoxyuridine on cell division and differentiation of preimplantation mouse embryos. J Embryol Exp Morphol 35:169–178
Rowinski J, Solter D, Kiprowski H (1975) Mouse embryo development in vitro: Effects of inhibitors of RNA and protein synthesis on blastocyst and post-blastocyst embryos. J Exp Zool 192:133–142
Russell LB (1965) Death and chromosome damage from irradiation of pre-implantation stages. In: O'Connor M, Wolstenholme GEW (eds) CIBA Foundation Symposium on preimplantation stages of pregnancy. Little, Brown, Boston, pp 217–241
Sadler TW (1980a) Effects of maternal diabetes on early embryogenesis: I. The teratogenic potential of diabetic serum. Teratology 21:339–347
Sadler TW (1980b) Effects of maternal diabetes on early embryogenesis: II. Hyperglycemia-induced exencephaly. Teratology 21:349–356
Sadler TW, Kochhar DM (1976) Biosynthesis of DNA, RNA and proteins by mouse embryos cultured in the presence of a teratogenic dose of chlorambucil. J Embryol Exp Morphol 36:273–281
Sanyal MK, Kitchin KT, Dixon RL (1981) Rat conceptus development in vitro: Comparative effects of alkylating agents. Toxicol Appl Pharmacol 57:14–19
Shepard TH, Tanimura T, Robkin M (1969) In vitro study of rat embryos: I. Effects of decreased oxygen on embryonic heart rate. Teratology 2:107–110
Sherman MI, Atienza SB (1975) Effects of bromodeoxyuridine, cytosine arabinoside and colcemid upon in vitro development of mouse blastocysts. J Embryol Exp Morphol 34:467–484
Snow MHL (1973) Tetraploid mouse embryos produced by cytochalasin B during cleavage. Nature 244:513–515
Snow MHL (1975) Embryonic development of tetraploid mice during the second half of gestation. J Embryol Exp Morphol 34:707–721
Snow MHL (1976) The immediate postimplantation development of tetraploid mouse blastocysts. J Embryol Exp Morphol 35:81–86
Snow MHL, Tam PPL (1979) Is compensatory growth a complicating factor in mouse teratology? Nature 279:555–557

Spindle AI (1977) Inhibition of early postimplantation development of cultured mouse embryos by bromodeoxyuridine. J Exp Zool 202:17–26
Spindle AI, Pedersen RA (1973) Hatching, attachment, and outgrowth of mouse blastocysts in vitro: fixed nitrogen requirements. J Exp Zool 186:305–318
Steele CE (1972) Improved development of rat egg-cylinders in vitro as a result of fusion of the heart primordia. Nature New Biol 237:150–151
Steele CE, Jeffery EH, Diplock AT (1974) The effect of vitamin E and synthetic antioxidants on the growth in vitro of explanted rat embryos. J Reprod Fertil 38:115–123
Steele CE, New DAT (1974) Serum variants causing the formation of double hearts and other abnormalities in explanted rat embryos. J Embryol Exp Morphol 31:707–719
Tam PPL, Snow MHL (1980) The in vitro culture of primitive-streak-stage mouse embryos. J Embryol Exp Morphol 59:131–143
Tarkowski AK, Witkowska A, Opas J (1977) Development of cytochalasin B-induced tetraploid and diploid/tetraploid mosaic mouse embryos. J Embryol Exp Morphol 41:47–64
Turbow MM (1966) Trypan blue induced teratogenesis of rat embryos cultivated in vitro. J Embryol Exp Morphol 15:387–395
Turbow MM, Chamberlain JG (1968) Direct effects of 6-aminonicotinamide on the developing rat embryo in vitro and in vivo. Teratology 1:103–108
Wiley LM, Pedersen RA (1977) Morphology of mouse egg cylinder development in vitro: A light and electron microscopic study. J Exp Zool 200:389–402

CHAPTER 17

# The Role of an Artificial Embryo in Detecting Potential Teratogenic Hazards

E. M. JOHNSON and B. E. G. GABEL

## A. Introduction

The teratogenic potential of drugs, chemicals, food additives, etc., is routinely tested in experiments patterned after the (U.S. Food and Drugs Administration Segment II protocol which calls for administration of a test substance to pregnant rodents and/or rabbits during the period of major organogenesis characteristic of the species. This is considered an acceptable and state-of-the-art means for detecting substances hazardous to normal development of the conceptus. Careful examination of data from such experiments establishes the fact that the overwhelming majority of substances so tested are determined to be capable of disrupting development only at doses approaching or exceeding those also toxic to the adult. It can be further determined that the ratio between the teratogenic and adult toxic doses of a chemical not requiring species-specific metabolism remains relatively consistent from species to species, provided the dose levels compared are those produced by similar routes of administration. One can even rank substances according to their ability to manifest toxicity to the conceptus in relationship to the adult toxic dose. For example, in the mouse, the teratogenic dose of sodium chloride is 1,900 mg/kg and the adult toxic dose is 2,500 mg/kg (NISHIMURA and MIYAMOTO 1969). Dividing the adult toxic dose level $A$ by the developmentally toxic dose level $D$ gives a value of approximately 1. The $A/D$ value for aspirin is 2; for actinomycin $D$, 5; and nonacetylated isoniazid, 50. One cannot determine with exactitude, but the ratio for the active component of thalidomide may be as large as 60.

It follows then that the question: is table salt teratogenic? is answered in the affirmative, as is the same question for isoniazid. From the viewpoint of "safety in the workplace", however, the qestion is trivial and the answer superfluous (JOHNSON 1980). From the broad view of developmental toxicology, every substance has the potential to disrupt or kill a conceptus at some dose, and those doing so in the absence of adult toxicity are considered as potential developmental hazards. Assume for a moment that table salt and isoniazid were environmental chemicals A and B, respectively and that neither has been evaluated for teratogenicity. The workplace exposure levels (optimistically) will be kept below the adult toxic level according to the U.S. National Institute of Occupational Safety and Health standards, coupled with a modest safety factor. This is the real-life situation throughout the developed world and chemicals such as A are coeffective teratogens (JOHNSON 1981) and pose no unique threat to the conceptus. They are capable of disrupting development of the conceptus only at dose levels near those toxic to adults. Those rare substances represented by B are the developmental hazards –

placing the conceptus at risk because safety factors based on adult toxicity do not allow for unique vulnerabilities of developmental events to that particular substance. We clearly recognize and classically acknowledge two populations in the workplace: adult males and adult females, and we know that each has substances to which it is uniquely vulnerable. Lacking has been our full recognition that there are actually three populations in that workplace and the third – the conceptus, also has its own unique vulnerabilities (JOHNSON et al. to be published).

One could hold that, with an understanding of this concept, substances can be evaluated in pregnant rats and/or rabbits and the conceptus protected as adequately as adults. Unfortunately, this will not occur because such tests are too expensive and time consuming to permit evaluation of teratogenic potential in the 70,000 chemicals already in commerce, or even the several hundred new formulations appearing each year. An inexpensive method is needed to sift through large numbers of chemicals and identify those needing further evaluation because of their ability to disrupt development at levels markedly below those toxic to the adult. Lacking such a method, the degree and breadth of protection we offer to the conceptus is going to lag increasingly behind the extent of protection we provide for ourselves, the adults.

An assay developed with adults of the freshwater cnidarian, *Hydra attenuata*, and its artificial "embryo" shows remarkable ability to detect substances uniquely toxic to the conceptus. With development, validation, and application of such a rapid testing procedure, we procure the means to identify and isolate substances and mixtures injurious to the unborn. Total ability to do this would not prevent all congenital defects, but rapid identification of the most flagrant of the bad actors could, for the first time in human history, perhaps reduce their incidence.

## B. Basic Aspects of Hydra Biology

The system to be described may be unknown to some. An understanding of its characteristics and of the ontogenic structure into which it can be manipulated, however, is essential as a basis for understanding the system's abilities.

### I. Nurture of Adult Hydra

The freshwater cnidarian, *Hydra attenuata*, is readily grown in the laboratory by a semiautomated means (Fig. 1), capable of maintaining the large animal census required. The genus is a favorite of developmental biologists and hundreds of papers employing the genus have been published since 1744. There are many species of *Hydra*, but *H. attenuata* seems most amenable to the studies proposed as it is not complicated by associated organisms (i.e., algae). The usual method (LOOMIS and LENHOFF 1956) is adequate for their growth, though we have modified the method somewhat to fit our goal. The organisms reproduce asexually by budding and it is possible for a population of over 100,000 to be housed in an area 1.5 $m^2$. Once or twice each day they are fed freshly hatched brine shrimp *Artemia salina*. Either the brine shrimp themselves or their "eggs" are treated with 20 parts/$10^6$ io-

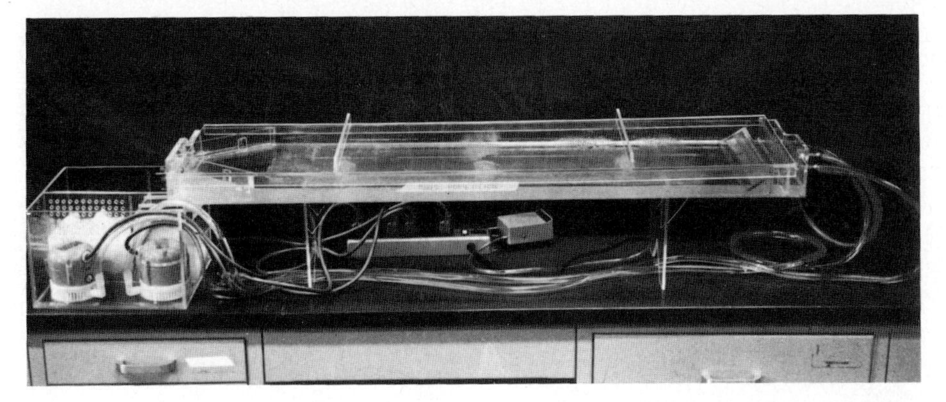

**Fig. 1.** The aquatic environmental apparatus for the care and feeding of large *Hydra* populations

dine to kill their associated bacteria and fungi. This precaution, along with adequate oxygenization and constant temperature regulation between 10° and 20 °C, keeps the organisms essentially free of the gram-negative rods and the more rapidly growing water molds which otherwise would flourish and preclude use of the system.

## II. The Nature of Artificial Hydra "Embryos"

Adult *H. attenuata* are rather easily dissociated into their component cells. Several methods are available for this. Some date back over 100 years, but we use that developed by GIERER et al. (1972). Approximately 300 adult organisms (Fig. 2) are incubated for 30 min at room temperature in a 70 mosmol cell culture medium containing: 3.9 m*M* KCl, 6.6 m*M* $CaCl_2$, 1.3 m*M* $MgSO_4$, 6.6 m*M* Na-citrate, 6.6 m*M* Na-pyruvate, 13.1 m*M* TES buffer, 100 mg/l phenol red, 150 mg/l amikacin, pH 6.9. The animals are then sheared into small pieces of tissue and individual cells through a narrow orificed pipette (Fig. 3). The suspension is allowed to sediment for 7 min and the supernatant transferred to another tube and centrifuged for 3 min at 200 *g*. The cells are resuspended and drawn up into 0.5-mm diameter polyethylene tubing (Fig. 4) which is placed in to small, conical Eppendorf tubes. The tubing is clamped at one end, and centrifuged for 3 min at 100 *g*. The resulting cell pellets are ejected (Figs. 5–7) into wells containing 4 ml 70 mosmol cell culture medium. The osmolarity of the medium is gradually reduced over 26 h, so that at the end of this time the aggregates are back in the original medium of optimal osmolarity for adults. The normal sequence of development of the preparation is evident in Figs. 8–14. It takes somewhat longer than 1 week for a pellet "embryo" to develop into multiple free-standing adults, but the actual test need not exceed 42–90 h, because during this period the "embryo" achieves its basic development.

Studies of regeneration have shown that in order for new adults to be formed the cells must achieve; survival, changes in cell size and shape (GIERER 1977; WEBSTER and HAMILTON 1972), selective cell death (GIERER et al. 1972), cells must be-

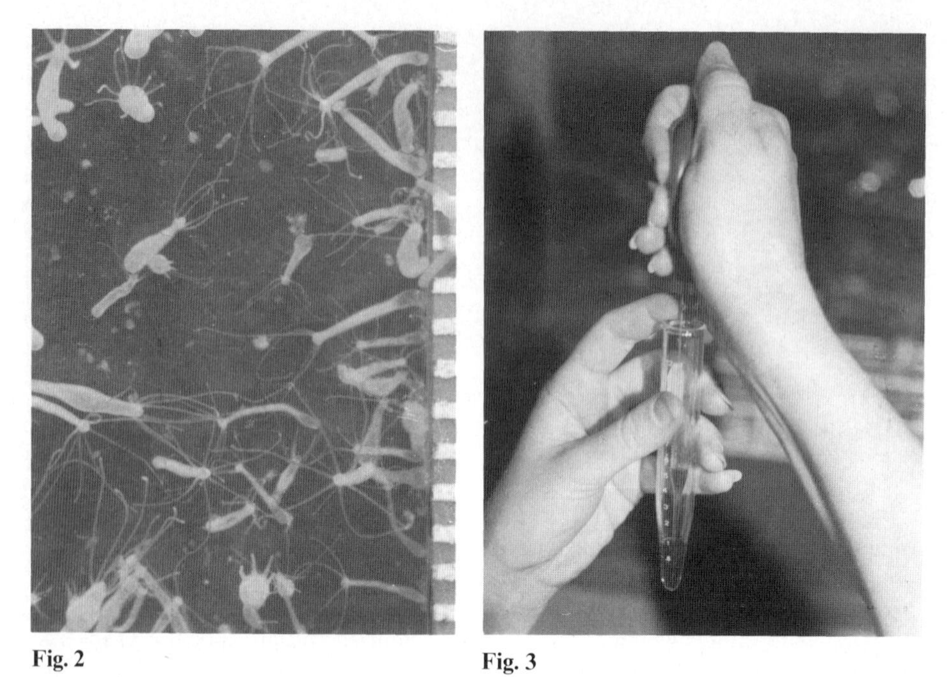

Fig. 2 Fig. 3

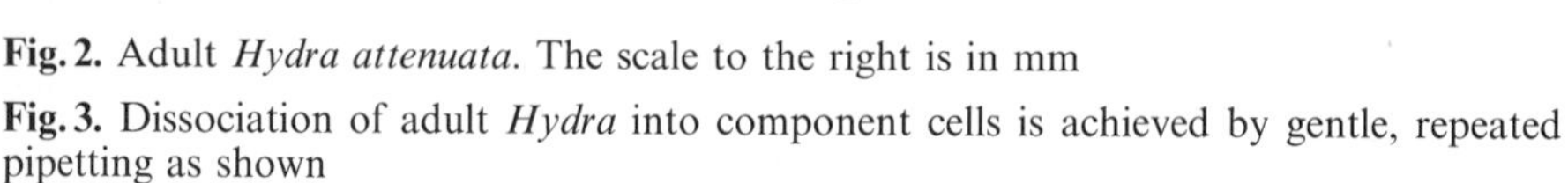

**Fig. 2.** Adult *Hydra attenuata.* The scale to the right is in mm

**Fig. 3.** Dissociation of adult *Hydra* into component cells is achieved by gentle, repeated pipetting as shown

come spatially oriented, must recognize neighbors and form specialized junctions (FILSKIE and FLOWER 1977; WAKEFORD 1979), form selective adhesive associations and migrate (WEBSTER and HAMILTON 1972), induce differentiation of other cells less differentiated than themselves (BROWNE 1909; LEE and CAMPBELL 1979; SUGIYAMA and FUJISAWA 1979), form intercellular matrix (EPP et al. 1979), be responsive to inductive stimuli and differentiate (BERKING 1979; BERKING and GIERER 1977; BODE et al. 1976; BROWNE 1909; SCHALLER 1976a; SCHALLER 1976b), form cell-specific organelles and products (LENTZ 1965), undergo mitotic division and then differentiate (BURNETT et al. 1973; DAVID and CAMPBELL 1972), form organ fields (BROWNE 1909; GIERER 1977; OTTO and CAMPBELL 1977), regulate organ field size (BODE et al. 1973; WEBSTER and HAMILTON 1972), and become associated into tissues (DAVIS 1975) capable of functioning as parts of an integrated, coordinated adult. This is essentially the same list of phenomena required of a zygote in becoming an embryo and then a fetus. It also encompasses all of the phenomena considered vulnerable to abnormality during the pathogenesis of a developmental abnormality (WILSON 1973; JOHNSON et al. to be published). It is not being implied that these phenomena are all the same as in higher forms. Perhaps the molecular mechanisms to achieve them, however, are more similar than different. A basis for this rather speculative thought is that an agent held to disrupt microtubules (vinblastine) interferes with a reaggregated pellet's activities during the time of most active cell migration and shape changing, while an agent perturbing DNA synthe-

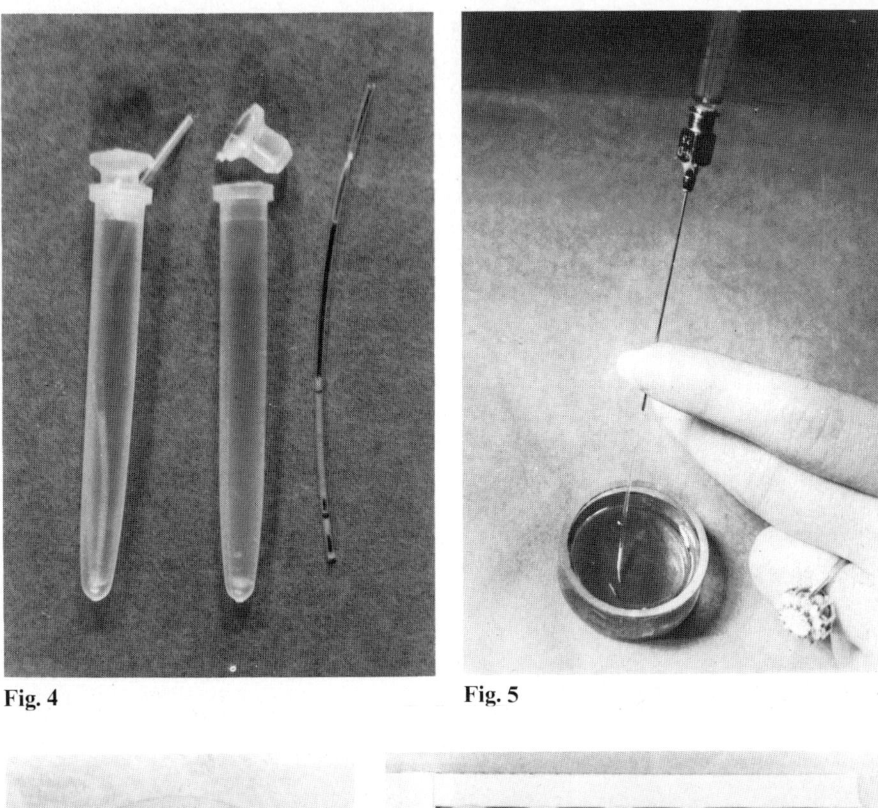

Fig. 4

Fig. 5

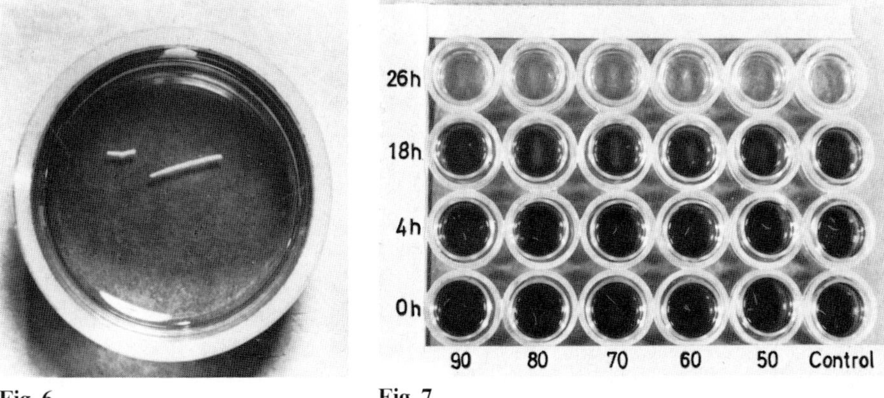


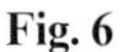

Fig. 6

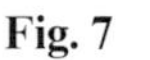

Fig. 7

**Fig. 4.** Polyethylene tubing after second centrifugation, showing the pellet in the bottom one-third of the tubing

**Fig. 5.** Ejecting the pellet into a test well

**Fig. 6.** Ejected pellets

**Fig. 7.** Tray of test wells, showing the concentration of test substance

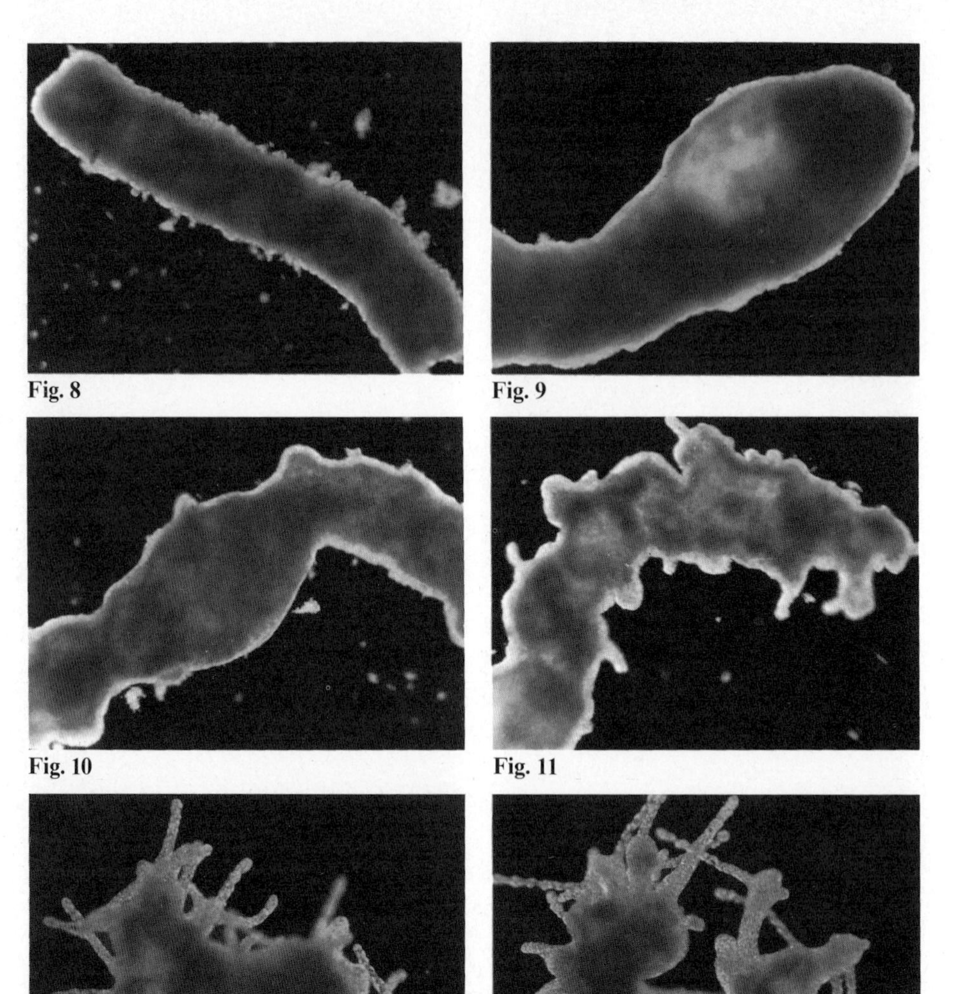

Fig. 8 Fig. 9

Fig. 10 Fig. 11

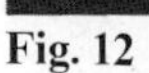

Fig. 12 Fig. 13

**Fig. 8.** Pellet at 4 h, showing smoothed surface

**Fig. 9.** Pellet at 18 h, showing hollowing into a trilaminar vesicle

**Fig. 10.** Pellet at 26 h, showing tentacle bud formation

**Fig. 11.** Pellet at 42 h. The tentacle buds have elongated

**Fig. 12.** Pellet at 66 h. The tentacles have formed and hypostomes are developing

**Fig. 13.** Pellet at 90 h, showing elongated tentacles around the developed hypostomes and body columns

| Silhouette of "embryo" | Designation | Developmental elapsed time (h) |
|---|---|---|
| | Solid pellet | 4 |
| | Hollowed and laminar | 18 |
| | Tentacle buds | 26 |
| | Tentacle buds elongated | 42 |
| | Hypostomes | 66 |
| | Polyps | 90 |

**Fig. 14.** Drawings representing the normal development of the artificial embryo

sis (methotrexate) disrupts regeneration at the time of greatest cell proliferation (JOHNSON 1982 unpublished work). Methotrexate did not affect the "embryo" until after 90 h of regeneration, when there is normally a marked increase in mitotic activity of the preparation, and even markedly increased dosage did not speed up the time to effect. The point of this discussion is to indicate that the system may, in some respects, be considered an artificial "embryo" of sorts.

### 1. The Testing Procedure

#### a) "Embryos"

Freshly made pellets are ejected into each of several glass dishes containing 4 ml 70 mosmol cell culture medium and the substance being tested at logarithmic interval concentrations. Fresh test compound is added to the wells with each medium change until the end of the experiment. At 4 h after pellet formation the 70 mosmol culture medium is diluted to 35 mosmol. At this time the irregular cell clump has developed into a solid, smooth sphere; 14 h later the medium is further diluted to

17 mosmol and the sphere shows signs of becoming hollow. By 26 h, when the cell culture medium is replaced with 5 mosmol medium, the process of hollowing is complete. The aggregates are placed into fresh medium and test substance once each day and the observations are made at this time. From 24 to 48 h, tentacle buds emerge on the surface of the hollow sphere. The tentacles then elongate, hypostomes form by 4 days, and body columns elongate and become sculpted by day 5. Within about 1 week the aggregates have begun separating into individual and free-standing normal adult *H. attenuata*, themselves capable of budding.

Observations are made under ×35 magnification each time the medium is changed which is also coincident with the developmental stages. Their development in treated medium is compared with the normal course of development of concurrent untreated preparations. The lowest concentration producing an effect is subdivided at lower concentrations (1/10 logarithmic intervals) and the experiment repeated to give the "embryo" effective dose and time to effect. Disruption of the "embryo's" development is followed quickly by death and dissolution of the pellet and the concentration of test substance needed to produce this endpoint is considered the developmental minimal effective dose.

b) Adult Hydra

Adult *H. attenuata* are placed in a series of dishes containing 4 ml medium containing logarithmic interval concentrations of the substance being tested. They are observed, as are the "embryos". The animals being treated are compared with normal animals for body column and tentacle size and shape, and for body column and tentacle movements. The lowest (logarithmic interval) dose affecting an adult is divided into tenths and the experiment repeated to give the lowest dose (1/10 logarithmic interval) adversely affecting adults. This is considered the adult minimal effective dose.

In Figs. 15–18 and 19, the progressive response of adult *Hydra* to a test compound are depicted. This sequence is encountered, at some concentration and duration of exposure, with each substance evaluated. The endpoint determination of the adult minimal effective dose is the tulip stage, because animals at this stage tend not to recover, even when removed to a normal medium, and also because animals dissociate after only a few hours at the tulip stage.

## C. Evaluation of Results

As can be seen in Fig. 20, the assay must be made for both adult *H. attenuata* and for the artificial embryos. The assay is repeated in a similar manner at four levels (I, II, III, and IV) for each. Level I represents a range-finding experiment to establish the lowest whole-log concentration (mg/l) of *p*-phenylenediamine (PPD), pro-

**Fig. 15.** Norman adult *Hydra*

**Fig. 16.** Adult *Hydra*, showing clubbing of the tentacle

**Fig. 17.** Adult *Hydra*, showing shortened tentacles

**Fig. 18.** Adult *Hydra* which has reached the tulip stage

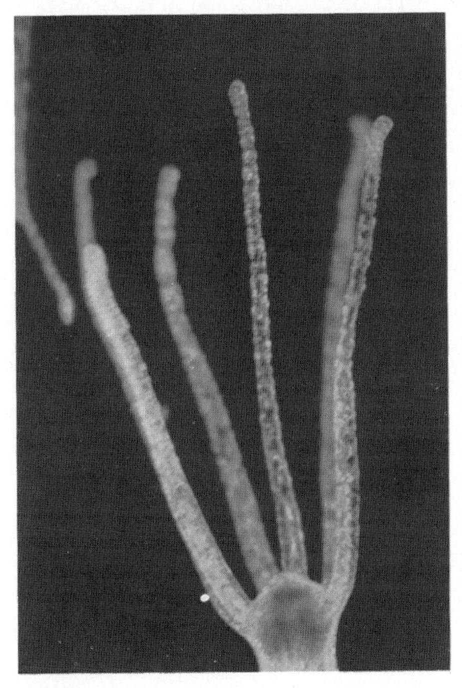

Fig. 15

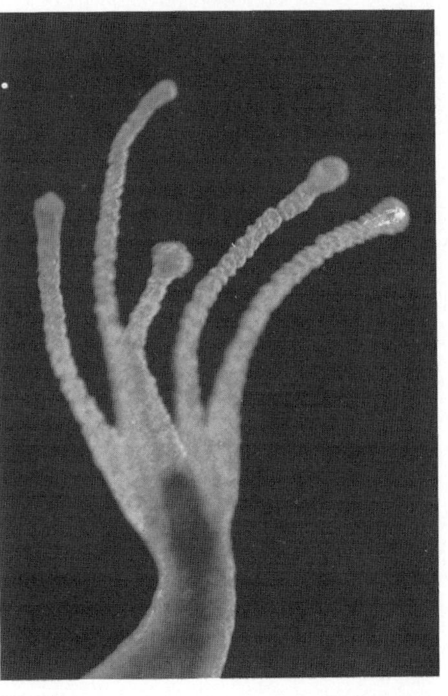

Fig. 16

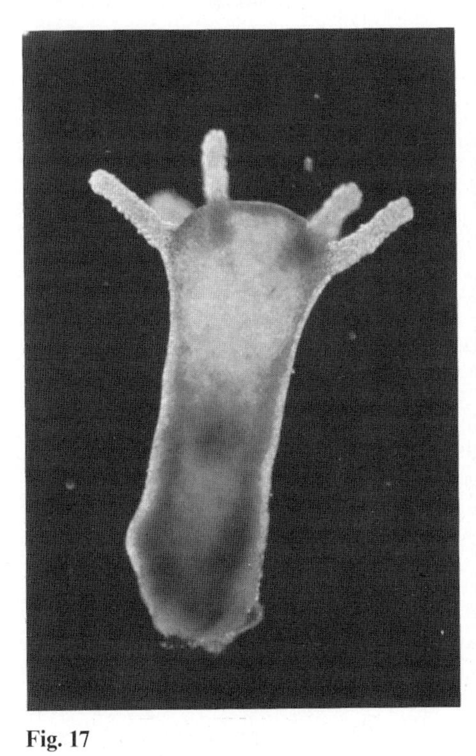

Fig. 17

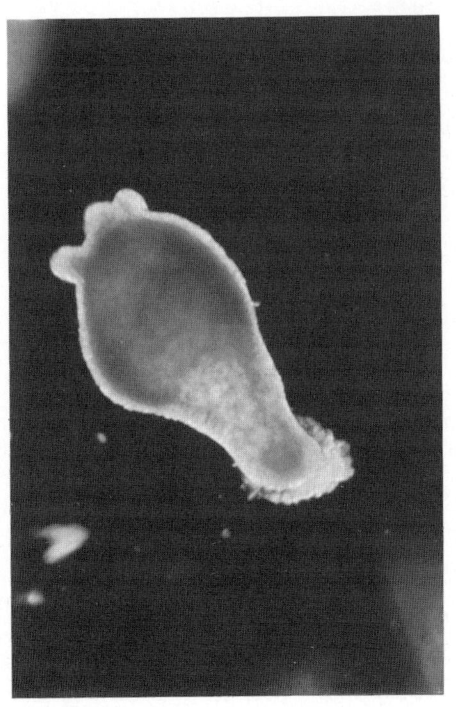

Fig. 18

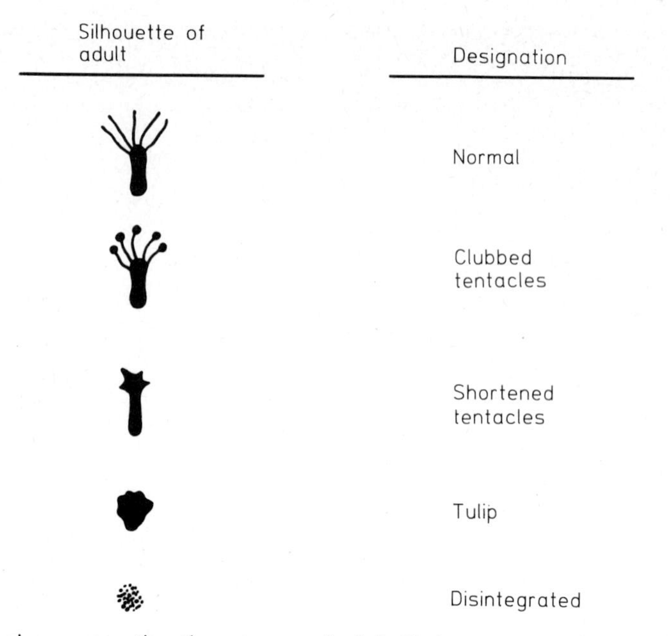


**Fig. 19.** Drawing representing the response of adult *Hydra* to a test substance

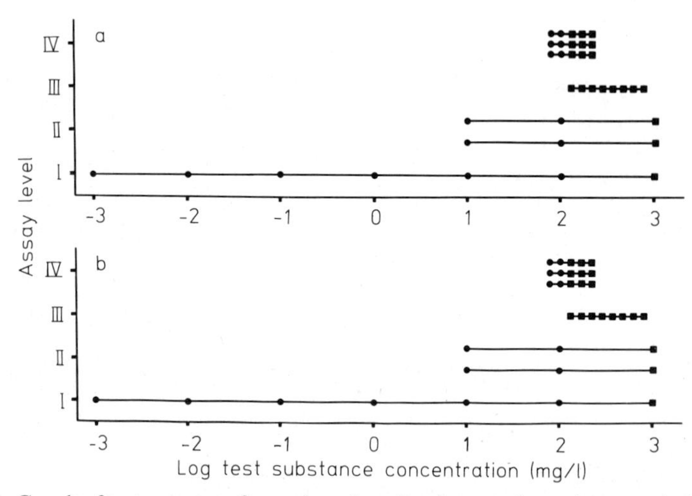


**Fig. 20 a, b.** Graph of test sequence for *p*-phenylenediamine, *circles* and *squares* indicate concentrations tested, (*squares* indicate endpoints). Minimal effective dose 200 mg. **a** adult *Hydra attenuata;* **b** "embryo" *H. attenuata*

cuding an adverse effect. These endpoints are indicated by squares in Fig. 20. As few as one adult or one embryo is used at each logarithmic interval dose level. In level II the whole-log effective dose is confirmed by making the assay in (usually) two or more specimens. At the end of this level of testing, one is confident that the lowest effective logarithmic concentration (3 in this case) has been established.

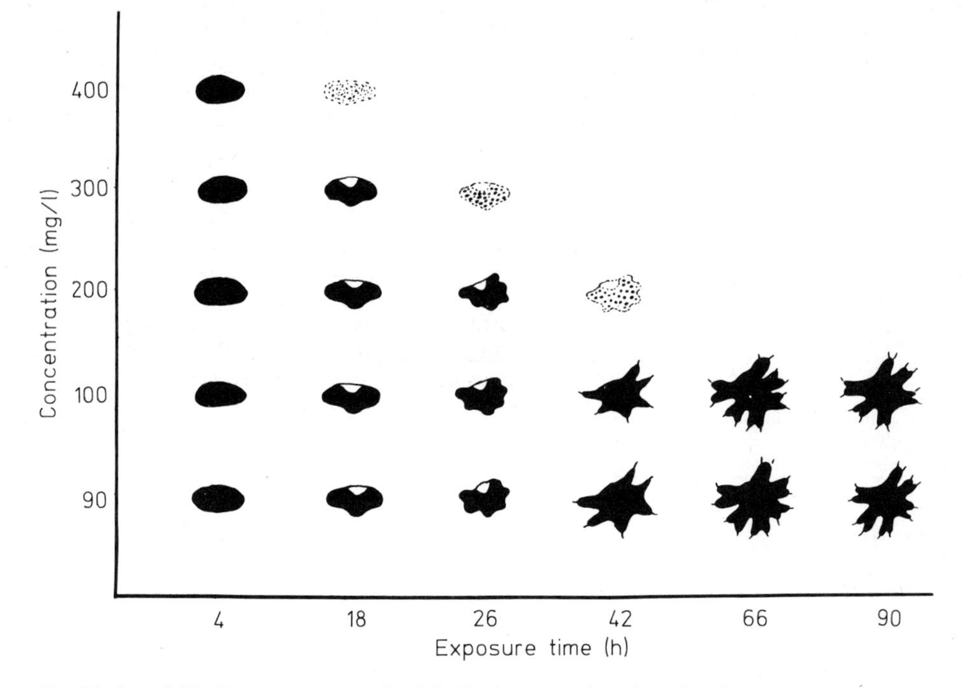


**Fig. 21.** Level IV. Dose–response of adult *Hydra* to *p*-phenylenediamine

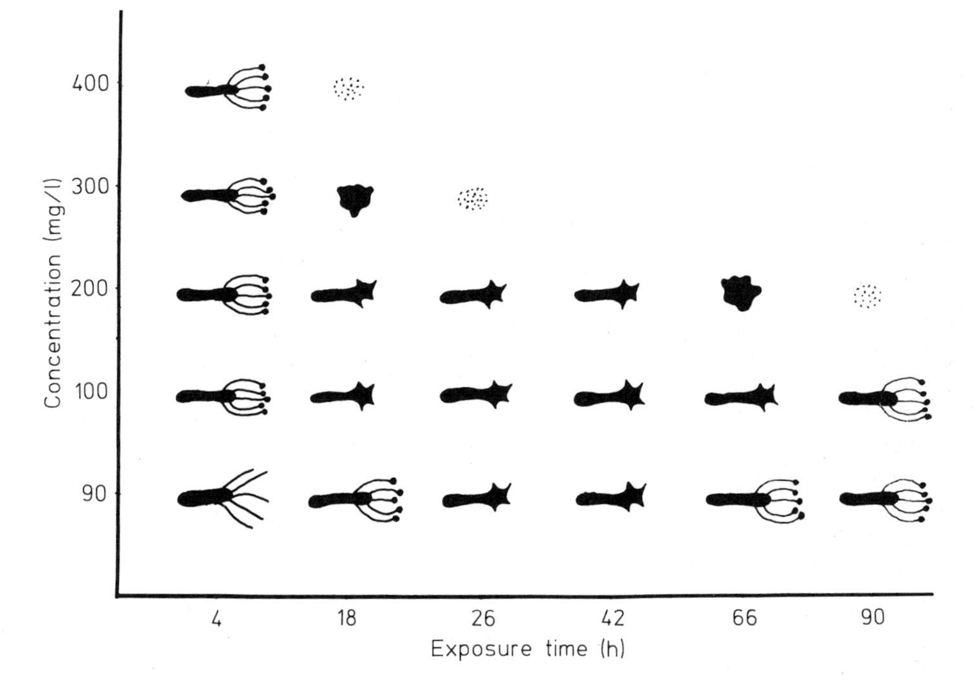


**Fig. 22.** Level IV. Dose–response of the "artificial embryo" to *p*-phenylenediamine

(Level II assay may be done in the same week as level I or in the following week, depending on the time to effect for the test chemical.) Level III assay is similar to level I, except the goal is to determine the lowest effective logarithmic concentration to within one-tenth. Once found, the concentration is confirmed by level IV assay. The uniform endpoint assays or determinations are death and its attendent dissolution for the embryo and tulip stage reaction (or its immediately ensuing death) for the adult. Note that level IV experiments routinely are repeated to assure that the minimal effective doses for both the adult and the embryo are accurate.

Figures 21 and 22 are sketches of the data derived from the level IV tests of PPD. The adult minimal effective dose (Fig. 21) determined by this test in *H. Attenuata* was 200 mg/l; the embryo or developmental toxic minimal effective dose (Fig. 22) was 200 mg/l. This *A/D* value of 1 directly predicts data of a more complex evaluation.

## D. Discussion

The test substances employed in this explanation was PPD, which is a constituent of some hair dye preparations. The *H. attenuata* system predicted that PPD is not a teratogenic hazard, as the low *A/D* value is indicative of a coeffective teratogen. That is, *H. attenuata* predicted that PPD was a substance capable of disrupting development only at or near the concentration or dose toxic to the adult. If the prescreen were valid, than a similar *A/D* value should be calculable from the data of a standard Segment II safety evaluations.

THOMAS et al. (to be published) administered PPD to Sprague-Dawley rats by gavage on days 6–15 of gestation in a standard Segment II safety evaluation. The single daily doses were 5, 10, 15, 20, or 30 mg/KG. A pair-fed control group was restricted to the food intake of the 30 mg kg/day test group. Dams given either 30 or 20 mg/kg PPD did not gain weight at the same rate as controls. This decrement was dose related, but the group treated with 15 mg/kg gained the same amount of weight as did normal controls. Therefore, the demonstrated adult minimal effective dose in these rats is 20 mg/kg. None of the dose levels increased the incidence of frank gross anatomic malformations, but the incidence of supernumerary ribs and skeletal variations was increased in a dose-related manner with treatment a low as 15 mg/kg/day. THOMAS et al. concluded appropriately that the test compound is not a teratogenic hazard. This is borne out by the demonstrated *A/D* value near unity (1.33). The *H. attenuata* assay gave the value as 1, and it follows that the results of a complex and expensive Segment II study would have been accurately predicted, i.e., at that dose producing minimal adult toxicity, there would be produced a minimal perturbation of development. The prescreen, if it had been the only test made, would have accurately predicted that PPD was not a developmental hazard as it had no unique capability of disrupting development at a small fraction of the adult toxic dose. In other words, this prescreen would provide a basis, as accurate as the Segment II evaluation in rodent, for concluding PPD not to be a high priority substance for evaluation of developmental toxicology. As far as the conceptus is concerned, the exposure level only needs regulation on the basis of the more easily determined adult toxic level. Application of a modest safety factor to this would also be considered adequate to protect the conceptus from adverse effects.

*Acknowledgments*. This work was supported by funds from Hoffman LaRoche Inc. and Mobil Oil Corp. The Hydra Farms were purchased from Rockhill Enterprises Inc. P.O. Box 2324, Philadelphia, PA 19103.

## References

Berking S, Gierer A (1977) Analysis of early stages of budding in hydra by means of an endogenous inhibitor. Wilhelm Rouxs Arch Dev Biol 182:117–129

Berking S, (1979) Control of nerve cell formation from multipotent stem cells in hydra. J Cell Sci 40:192–205

Bode HR, Berking S, David CN, Gierer A, Schaller H, Trenkner E (1973) Quantitative analysis of cell types during growth and morphogenesis in hydra. Wilhelm Rouxs Arch Dev Biol 171:269–285

Bode HR, Flick K, Smith G (1976) Regulation of interstitial cell differentiation in *Hydra attenuata*. J Cell Sci 20:29–46

Browne EM (1909) The production of new hydranths in *Hydra* by the insertion of small grafts. J Exp Zool 7:1–24

Burnett AL, Lowell R, Cyslin MN (1973) Regeneration of a complete *Hydra* from a single, differentiated somatic cell type. In: Burnett AL (ed) Biology of hydra. Academic Press, New York

David CN, Campbell RD (1972) Cell cycle kinetics and development of *Hydra attenuata*. J Cell Sci 11:557–568

Davis LE (1975) Histological and ultrastructural studies of the basal disk of *Hydra*. III. The gastrodermis and the mesoglea. Cell Tissue Res 162:107–118

Epp LG, Tardent P, Banninger R (1979) Isolation and observation of tissue layers in *Hydra attenuata* pall (cnidaria, hydrozoa). Trans Am Micros Soc 98:392–400

Filskie BK, Flower NE (1977) Junctional structures in *Hydra*. J Cell Sci 23:151–172

Gierer A (1977) Physical aspects of tissue evagination and biological form. Q Rev Biophys 10:529–593

Gierer A, Berking S, Bode H et al. (1972) Regeneration of hydra from reaggregated cells. Nature New Biol 239:98–105

Johnson EM (1980) Screening for teratogenic potential: are we asking the proper question? Teratology 21:259

Johnson EM (1981) Screening for teratogenic hazards: nature of the problems. Annu Rev Pharmacol Toxicol 21:417–429

Johnson EM, Gorman RM, Gabel BEG, George ME (to be published) The *Hydra attenuata* system for detection of teratogenic hazards. Teratog Mutag Carcinog

Lee H, Campbell R (1979) Development and behavior of an intergeneric chimera of Hydra (Pelmatohydra oligactis interstitial cells: *Hydra attenuata* epithelial cells). Biol Bull 157:288–296

Lentz TL (1965) Fine structural changes in the nervous system of the regenerating *Hydra*. J Exp Zool 159:181–194

Loomis WF, Lenhoff HM (1956) Growth and asexual differentiation of *Hydra* in culture. J Exp Zool 132:555–573

Nishimura H, Miyamoto S (1969) Teratogenic effects of sodium chloride in mice. Acta Anat Nippon 74:121–124

Otto J, Campbell R (1977) Budding in *Hydra attenuata:* bud stages and fate map. J Exp Zool 200:417–427

Schaller HC /1976 a) Action of the head activator as a growth hormone in *Hydra*. Cell Differ 5:1–11

Schaller HC (1976b) Action of the head activator on the determination of interstitial cells in *Hydra*. Cell Differ 5:13–20
Sugiyama T, Fujisawa T (1979) Genetic analysis and developmental mechanisms in *Hydra*. VII. Statistical analysis of developmental-morphological characters and cellular compositions. Dev Growth Differ 21:361–375
Thomas AR, Loehr RF, Rodwell DE, D'Aleo CJ, Burnett CM (to be published) The nonteratogenicity of p-phenylenediamine in Sprague-Dawley rats. Fund Appl Toxicol
Wakeford RJ (1979) Cell contact and positional communication in hydra. J Embryol Exp Morphol 54:171–183
Webster GW, Hamilton S (1972) Budding in hydra: the role of cell multiplication and cell movement in bud initiation. J Embryol Exp Morphol 27:301–316
Wilson JG (1973) Environment and birth defects. Academic Press, New York

# Subject Index

Page numbers in *italics* refer to illustrations, diagrams, graphs or tables.

# Chemical Index

# Handbook of Experimental Pharmacology

Continuation of "Handbuch der experimentellen Pharmakologie"



Volume 19
**5-Hydroxytryptamie and Related Indolealkylamines**

Volume 20: Part 1
**Pharmacology of Fluorides I**

Part 2
**Pharmacology of Fluorides II**

Volume 21
**Beryllium**

Volume 22: Part 1
**Die Gestagene I**

Part 2
**Die Gestagene II**

Volume 23
**Neurohypophysial Hormones and Similar Polypeptides**

Volume 24
**Diuretica**

Volume 25
**Bradykinin, Kallidin and Kallikrein**

Volume 26
**Vergleichende Pharmakologie von Überträgersubstanzen in tiersystematischer Darstellung**

Volume 27
**Anticoagulantien**

Volume 28: Part 1
**Concepts in Biochemical Pharmacology I**

Part 3
**Concepts in Biochemical Pharmacology III**

Volume 29
**Oral wirksame Antidiabetika**

Volume 30
**Modern Inhalation Anesthetics**

Volume 32: Part 2
**Insulin II**

Volume 34
**Secretin, Cholecystokinin, Pancreozymin and Gastrin**

Volume 35: Part 1
**Androgene I**

Part 2
**Androgens II and Antiandrogens/Androgene II und Antiandrogene**

Volume 36
**Uranium - Plutonium - Transplutonic Elements**

Volume 37
**Angiotensin**

Volume 38: Part 1
**Antineoplastic and Immunosuppressive Agents I**

Part 2
**Antineoplastic and Immunosuppressive Agents II**

Volume 39
**Antihypertensive Agents**

Volume 40
**Organic Nitrates**

Volume 41
**Hypolipidemic Agents**

Volume 42
**Neuromuscular Junction**

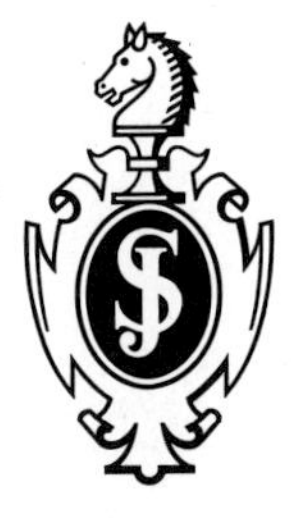

Springer-Verlag
Berlin
Heidelberg
New York

# Handbook of Experimental Pharmacology

Continuation of "Handbuch der experimentellen Pharmakologie"



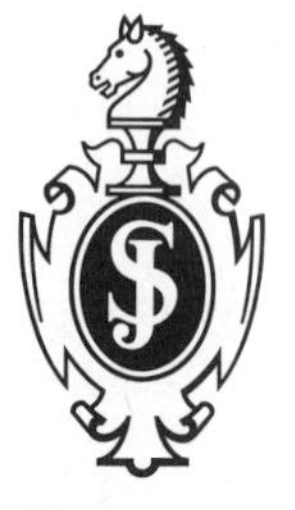

Springer-Verlag
Berlin
Heidelberg
New York

Volume 43
**Anabolic-Androgenic Steroids**

Volume 44
**Heme and Hemoproteins**

Volume 45: Part 1
**Drug Addiction I**

Part 2
**Drug Addiction II**

Volume 46
**Fibrinolytics and Antifibrinolytics**

Volume 47
**Kinetics of Drug Action**

Volume 48
**Arthropod Venoms**

Volume 49
**Ergot Alkaloids and Related Compounds**

Volume 50: Part 1
**Inflammation**

Part 2
**Anti-Inflammatory Drugs**

Volume 51
**Uric Acid**

Volume 52
**Snake Venoms**

Volume 53
**Pharmacology of Ganglionic Transmission**

Volume 54: Part 1
**Adrenergic Activators and Inhibitors I**

Part 2
**Adrenergic Activators and Inhibitors II**

Volume 55
**Psychotropic Agents**

Part 1
**Antipsychotics and Antidepressants I**

Part 2
**Anxiolytis, Gerontopsychopharmacological Agents and Psychomotor Stimulants**

Part 3
**Alcohol and Psychotomimetics, Psychotropic Effects of Central Acting Drugs**

Volume 56, Part 1 + 2
**Cardiac Glycosides**

Volume 57
**Tissue Growth Factors**

Volume 58
**Cyclic Nucleotides**
Part 1: **Biochemistry**
Part 2: **Physiology and Pharmacology**

Volume 59
**Mediators and Drugs in Gastrointestinal Motility**
Part 1: **Morphological Basis and Neurophysiological Control**
Part 2: **Endogenis and Exogenous Agents**

Volume 60
**Pyretics and Antipyretics**

Volume 61
**Chemotherapy of Viral Infections**

Volume 62
**Aminoglycosides**